Medical Management of Neurosurgical Patients

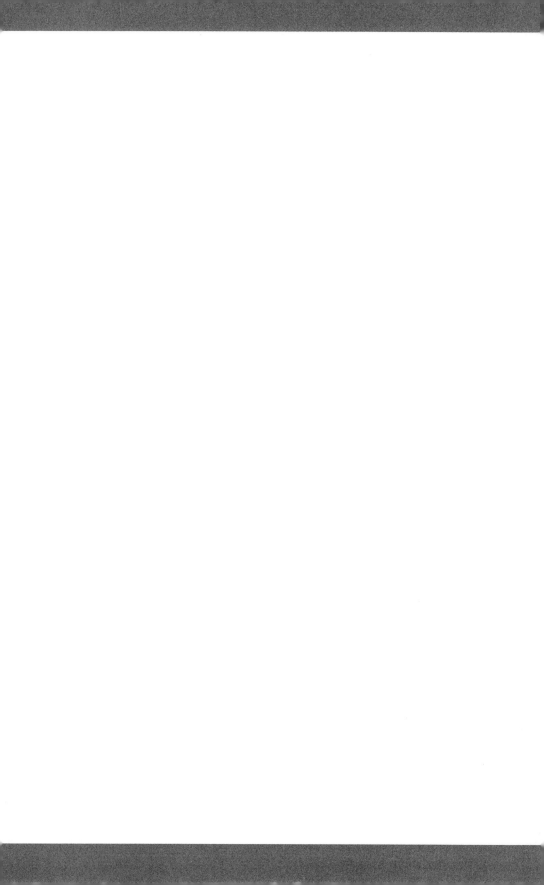

MEDICAL MANAGEMENT OF NEUROSURGICAL PATIENTS

Edited by

Rene Daniel, MD, PhD

Vickie and Jack Farber Institute for Neuroscience at Jefferson

Departments of Medicine and Neurological Surgery

Thomas Jefferson University

Philadelphia, PA

Catriona M. Harrop, MD, FACP, SFHM

Vickie and Jack Farber Institute for Neuroscience at Jefferson

Departments of Medicine and Neurological Surgery

Thomas Jefferson University

Philadelphia, PA

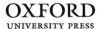

OXFORD
UNIVERSITY PRESS

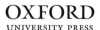

Oxford University Press is a department of the University of Oxford. It furthers
the University's objective of excellence in research, scholarship, and education
by publishing worldwide. Oxford is a registered trade mark of Oxford University
Press in the UK and certain other countries.

Published in the United States of America by Oxford University Press
198 Madison Avenue, New York, NY 10016, United States of America.

Library of Congress Cataloging-in-Publication Data
Names: Daniel, Rene, author. | Harrop, Catriona M., author.
Title: Medical management of neurosurgical patients / Rene Daniel and Catriona M. Harrop.
Description: New York, NY : Oxford University Press, [2020] |
Includes bibliographical references.
Identifiers: LCCN 2019012370| ISBN 9780190913779 (pbk.) |
ISBN 9780190913786 (UPDF) | ISBN 9780190913793 (EPUB) |
Subjects: | MESH: Neurosurgical Procedures | Patient Care Management | Nervous System Diseases
Classification: LCC RD593 | NLM WL 368 | DDC 617.4/8—dc23
LC record available at https://lccn.loc.gov/2019012370

This material is not intended to be, and should not be considered, a substitute for medical or other
professional advice. Treatment for the conditions described in this material is highly dependent on the
individual circumstances. And, while this material is designed to offer accurate information with respect
to the subject matter covered and to be current as of the time it was written, research and knowledge about
medical and health issues is constantly evolving and dose schedules for medications are being revised
continually, with new side effects recognized and accounted for regularly. Readers must therefore always
check the product information and clinical procedures with the most up-to-date published product
information and data sheets provided by the manufacturers and the most recent codes of conduct and
safety regulation. The publisher and the authors make no representations or warranties to readers, express
or implied, as to the accuracy or completeness of this material. Without limiting the foregoing, the
publisher and the authors make no representations or warranties as to the accuracy or efficacy of the drug
dosages mentioned in the material. The authors and the publisher do not accept, and expressly disclaim,
any responsibility for any liability, loss, or risk that may be claimed or incurred as a consequence of the use
and/ or application of any of the contents of this material.

9 8 7 6 5 4 3 2 1

Printed by Sheridan Books, Inc., United States of America

Contents

Foreword

The Farber Hospitalist Service was created by the Department of Neurological Surgery to provide co-management care for neurosurgery patients from their preoperative evaluation through their postoperative care. From this experience the group compiled a book of 14 chapters co-authored by neurosurgery hospitalists and specialists to address the major issues encountered by hospitalists managing this patient population.

The first chapter lays the groundwork by reviewing the most commonly encountered neurosurgical procedures and their associated indications and outcomes. This is followed by the preoperative risk stratification and management of this patient population in preparation for neurologic surgery. Chapters 3, 4, 5, and 6 take into consideration the management of the patient with specific neurologic issues, which include subarachnoid hemorrhage, intraparenchymal bleeding, brain tumors, seizure disorders, and acute spinal cord injury. These chapters aim to define the co-management strategies with the neurosurgeon. In Chapters 7–11 the focus is on the most common complications encountered in the postoperative period. Bleeding disorders, fevers, electrolyte disorders, hyperglycemia, and pressure injuries are reviewed with respect to etiology, assessment, and management. The final three chapters focus on the important management issues that face the neurosurgery hospitalist in the co-management of neurosurgical patients. Pain management can be extremely challenging and may often require a team approach along with psychiatry, anesthesia pain management, and neurosurgery. Understanding the role of physical and occupational therapy will allow hospitalists to better plan for the disposition of their patients to home, skilled nursing facilities, or rehabilitation centers. The final chapter focuses on the unfavorable outcomes from neurosurgical procedures. Hospitalist need to understand when and how to engage palliative care in the management of this patient group.

Providers who participate in the medical management of neurosurgery patients, including hospitalists, residents, nurse practitioners, physician assistants, and medical students, will find the information practical and the management strategies easy to implement in the care of the neurosurgical patient.

—R. H. Rosenwasser, MD, MBA, FACS, FAHA, Jewell L. Osterholm
Professor and Chairman
Department of Neurological Surgery Professor of Radiology
Neurovascular Surgery, Interventional Neuroradiology
President/CEO, Farber Institute for Neuroscience
Medical Director, Jefferson Neuroscience Network
Senior Vice President, Jefferson Enterprise Neuroscience
Thomas Jefferson University Jefferson Hospital for Neuroscience

—Geno J. Merli, MD, MACP, FHM, FSVM
Professor of Medicine & Surgery
Sr. Vice President, Associate CMO
Co-Director, Jefferson Vascular Center
Division Director, Vascular Medicine
Thomas Jefferson University

Contributors

Babak Abai, MD, FACS
Department of Surgery
Thomas Jefferson University
Philadelphia, PA

Rakhshanda Akram, MD
Division of Infectious Diseases
Department of Medicine
Thomas Jefferson University
Philadelphia, PA

Timothy Ambrose, MD
Jefferson Comprehensive
Epilepsy Center
Department of Neurology
Thomas Jefferson University
Philadelphia, PA

Katherine A. Belden, MD
Division of Infectious Diseases
Department of Medicine
Thomas Jefferson University
Philadelphia, PA

Crystal Benjamin, MD
Vickie and Jack Farber
Institute for Neuroscience
at Jefferson
Departments of Medicine and
Neurological Surgery
Thomas Jefferson University
Philadelphia, PA

James Bresnehan, MD
Department of Physical Medicine and
Rehabilitation
Thomas Jefferson University
Philadelphia, PA

Rene Daniel, MD, PhD
Vickie and Jack Farber Institute for
Neuroscience at Jefferson
Departments of Medicine and
Neurological Surgery
Thomas Jefferson University
Philadelphia, PA

Jesse Edwards, MD
Vickie and Jack Farber Institute for
Neuroscience at Jefferson
Departments of Medicine and
Neurological Surgery
Thomas Jefferson University
Philadelphia, PA

**Alexandra Emes, Bachelor of Science,
and MD is in progress (class of 2021)**
Department of Neurological Surgery
Vickie and Jack Farber Institute for
Neuroscience at Jefferson
Sidney Kimmel Medical College
Thomas Jefferson University
Philadelphia, PA

James J. Evans, MD, FACS, FAANS
Department of Neurological Surgery
Vickie and Jack Farber Institute for
Neuroscience at Jefferson
Department of Otolaryngology
Thomas Jefferson University
Philadelphia, PA

Kevin Furlong, DO
Division of Endocrinology
Diabetes and Metabolic Diseases
Department of Medicine
Thomas Jefferson University
Philadelphia, PA

Vedavyas Gannamani, MD
Vickie and Jack Farber Institute for
Neuroscience at Jefferson
Departments of Medicine and
Neurological Surgery
Thomas Jefferson University
Philadelphia, PA

Tomas Garzon-Muvdi, MD
Department of Neurological Surgery
Vickie and Jack Farber Institute for
Neuroscience at Jefferson
Thomas Jefferson University
Philadelphia, PA

M. Reid Gooch, MD
Department of Neurological Surgery
Vickie and Jack Farber Institute for
Neuroscience at Jefferson
Thomas Jefferson University
Philadelphia, PA

Rakesh Gulati, MD
Division of Nephrology
Department of Medicine
Thomas Jefferson University
Philadelphia, PA

Kristin Gustafson, DO
Department of Physical Medicine and
Rehabilitation
Thomas Jefferson University
Philadelphia, PA

**Catriona M. Harrop, MD,
FACP, SFHM**
Vickie and Jack Farber Institute for
Neuroscience at Jefferson
Departments of Medicine and
Neurological Surgery
Thomas Jefferson University
Philadelphia, PA

James Harrop, MD, FACS
Department of Neurological Surgery
Vickie and Jack Farber Institute for
Neuroscience at Jefferson
Thomas Jefferson University
Philadelphia, PA

Kevin Hines, MD
Department of Neurological
Surgery
Vickie and Jack Farber Institute for
Neuroscience at Jefferson
Thomas Jefferson University
Philadelphia, PA

Pascal M. Jabbour, MD
Department of Neurological Surgery
Vickie and Jack Farber Institute for
Neuroscience at Jefferson
Thomas Jefferson University
Philadelphia, PA

Omaditya Khanna, MD
Department of Neurological Surgery
Vickie and Jack Farber Institute for
Neuroscience at Jefferson
Thomas Jefferson University
Philadelphia, PA

Philip Koehler, DO
Department of Physical Medicine and
Rehabilitation
Thomas Jefferson University
Philadelphia, PA

John Liantonio, MD
Department of Family and Community
Medicine
Division of Palliative Care
Division of Geriatric Medicine
Thomas Jefferson University
Philadelphia, PA

Michael Liquori, MD
Division of Primary Care and
Population Health
Section of Hospice and Palliative
Medicine
Stanford University School of
Medicine, Hospice, & Palliative
Medicine
Division of Primary Care & Population
Health
Stanford University
Palo Alto, CA

Swathi Maddula, MD
Vickie and Jack Farber Institute for
Neuroscience at Jefferson
Departments of Medicine and
Neurological Surgery
Thomas Jefferson University
Philadelphia, PA

Megan Margiotta, MD
Jefferson Comprehensive
Epilepsy Center
Department of Neurology
Thomas Jefferson University
Philadelphia, PA

Kathleen Mechler, MD
Department of Family and
Community Medicine
Division of Palliative Care
Thomas Jefferson University
Philadelphia, PA

Newton Mei, MD
Vickie and Jack Farber Institute for
Neuroscience at Jefferson
Departments of Medicine and
Neurological Surgery
Thomas Jefferson University
Philadelphia, PA

**Geno Merli, MD, MACP,
FHM, FSVM**
Departments of Medicine and Vascular
Surgery
Thomas Jefferson University
Philadelphia, PA

Aditya Munshi, MD
Vickie and Jack Farber Institute for
Neuroscience at Jefferson
Departments of Medicine and
Neurological Surgery
Thomas Jefferson University
Philadelphia, PA

Linda Mwamuka, MD
Vickie and Jack Farber Institute for
Neuroscience at Jefferson
Departments of Medicine and
Neurological Surgery
Thomas Jefferson University
Philadelphia, PA

Adam Pennarola, MD
Department of Medicine
Thomas Jefferson University
Philadelphia, PA

Sage P. Rahm, BA
Department of Neurological
Surgery
Vickie and Jack Farber Institute for
Neuroscience at Jefferson
Thomas Jefferson University
Philadelphia, PA

Sanaa Rizk, MD, FACP
Cardeza Foundation Hemophilia and
Thrombosis Center
Thomas Jefferson University
Philadelphia, PA

**Robert H. Rosenwasser, MD, MBA,
FACS, FAHA**
Department of Neurological
Surgery
Vickie and Jack Farber Institute for
Neuroscience at Jefferson
Thomas Jefferson University
Philadelphia, PA

Ashwini D. Sharan, MD, FACS
Department of Neurological
Surgery
Vickie and Jack Farber Institute for
Neuroscience at Jefferson
Thomas Jefferson University
Philadelphia, PA

Sharad Sharma, MD
Division of General Internal Medicine
Department of Medicine
University of Pittsburgh Medical
Center Montefiore
Pittsburgh, PA

Geoffrey Stricsek, MD
Department of Neurological Surgery
Vickie and Jack Farber Institute for
Neuroscience at Jefferson
Thomas Jefferson University
Philadelphia, PA

Ahmad Sweid, MD
Department of Neurological Surgery
Vickie and Jack Farber Institute for
Neuroscience at Jefferson
Thomas Jefferson University
Philadelphia, PA

Thana Theofanis, MD
Department of Neurological Surgery
Vickie and Jack Farber Institute for
Neuroscience at Jefferson
Thomas Jefferson University
Philadelphia, PA

Stavropoula Tjoumakaris, MD
Department of Neurological Surgery
Vickie and Jack Farber Institute for
Neuroscience at Jefferson
Thomas Jefferson University
Philadelphia, PA

Satya Villuri, MD
Vickie and Jack Farber Institute for
Neuroscience
Departments of Neurological Surgery
and Medicine
Thomas Jefferson University
Philadelphia, PA

Donald Y. Ye, MD
Department of Neurological Surgery
Vickie and Jack Farber Institute for
Neuroscience at Jefferson
Thomas Jefferson University
Philadelphia, PA

1 Common Neurosurgical Procedures

Kevin Hines, Stavropoula Tjoumakaris, Pascal M. Jabbour, Robert H. Rosenwasser, and M. Reid Gooch

GENERAL PRINCIPLES

In general, when caring for neurosurgical patients perioperatively, hemorrhage at the surgical site can be more injurious than in other specialties. Therefore a strong emphasis is placed on maintaining coagulation and platelet parameters pre- and postoperatively for these patients. As a rule of thumb, surgeons are comfortable with most neurosurgical procedures if the platelet count is greater than 100,000 and the INR is less than 1.5. In addition, patients will often need to hold antiplatelet and anticoagulant agents 1–2 weeks preoperatively. Whether from consumption, nutritional deficiency, alcoholism, or other bleeding disorders, it is important for physicians to keep these parameters in mind to prevent devastating hemorrhages in both cranial and spinal procedures.

VENTRICULOPERITONEAL SHUNTING
Indications

Hydrocephalus is one of the most common and dangerous problems encountered in neurosurgery. In accordance with the Monro-Kellie doctrine, inappropriate accumulation of cerebral spinal fluid directly impacts intracranial blood volume, brain parenchyma, and can cause neuronal dysfunction and/or disruption of cerebral blood flow.

Commonly encountered causes of hydrocephalus include subarachnoid hemorrhage, meningitis, neoplasm, meningeal carcinomatosis, congenital hydrocephalus, idiopathic intracranial hypertension (pseudotumor cerebri), and normal pressure hydrocephalus.

Hydrocephalus is essentially a plumbing problem and is treated with cerebrospinal fluid (CSF) diversion. Temporary diversion is achieved with a lumbar puncture, lumbar drain, or external ventricular drain. Persistent hydrocephalus requires permanent drainage with a shunting procedure or endoscopic third ventriculostomy in cases where an intracranial obstruction can be internally bypassed.

Table 1.1 Perioperative signs associated with procedural complications, followed by immediate next steps in workup/management

Procedure	Signs/symptoms	Associated complication	Immediate diagnosis and intervention
Ventricular peritoneal shunt	Lethargy/headache/ neurological deficit Sudden focal neurological deficit Severe abdominal pain/fever/sepsis/ nausea or vomiting Coughing/shortness of breath/desaturation	Shunt failure Pericatheter hemorrhage Bowel perforation Pneumothorax	Head CT to assess ventricles Head CT to assess size of hemorrhage Upright abdominal x-ray or CT abdomen, general surgery consult Chest x-ray and general surgery consult for chest tube
Craniotomy/ Craniectomy	Decreased consciousness/ focal neurological deficit	Surgical bed hemorrhage, hydrocephalus	STAT head CT
Anterior cervical discectomy and fusion	Difficulty breathing Hoarseness/difficulty swallowing Difficulty swallowing/ fevers/sepsis	Hematoma, soft tissue edema Recurrent laryngeal nerve injury Esophageal injury	Emergent NS evaluation Speech and swallow evaluation, potential laryngoscopy Chest x-ray and swallow study, general surgery evaluation
Posterior cervical fusion	New weakness, pain out of proportion to surgery, altered consciousness	Epidural hematoma	STAT CT vs. MRI C spine, immediate evacuation
Anterior lumbar fusion	Abdominal pain, nausea/vomiting, distension	Bowel perforation vs. ileus	Abdominal x-ray, abdominal CT, general surgery evaluation

Table 1.1 Continued

3

Chapter 1: Common Neurosurgical Procedures

Procedure	Signs/symptoms	Associated complication	Immediate diagnosis and intervention
Posterior lumbar laminectomy/ fusion	Positional headaches worse when sitting up, surgical site leakage Urinary retention, new weakness, abnormal rectal exam	Cerebrospinal fluid leak Epidural hematoma	Flat bedrest, lumbar drain, surgical repair CT vs MRI L spine, immediate evacuation
Cerebral angiogram	Decreased consciousness, focal neurological deficit Severe limb pain, loss of pulses, cold limb, bruising/ hematoma Hypotension, tachycardia, pale skin	Ischemic vs. hemorrhage stroke Hematoma with vascular compromise of limb Retroperitoneal hematoma	STAT head CT, possible decompression vs intervention STAT vascular surgery evaluation, possible cutdown with thrombectomy Check labs, CT abdomen/pelvis, general surgery evaluation, transfuse RBCs if needed

In every scenario, open communication with the surgical team allows for quicker detection and correction of perioperative issues.

Two main options exist for long-term CSF diversion: endoscopic third ventriculostomy and extrathecal drainage (shunting). Endoscopic third ventriculostomy is used primarily for hydrocephalus caused by obstructive pathology blocking flow between the third and fourth ventricle along the cerebral aqueduct. The procedure involves using a neuroendoscope to visualize and fenestrate the floor of the third ventricle, thus connecting the lateral ventricles and third ventricle with the perimesencephalic cistern and the rest of the patient's normal subarachnoid anatomy. Although this technique has enjoyed growing acceptance for applicable pathology, extrathecal drainage remains the gold standard for treatment. The procedures for shunting are named by the cavities they connect: ventriculoperitoneal, ventriculojugular, ventriculopleural, lumboperitoneal. By far the most common of these procedures is the ventriculoperitoneal shunt.[1]

Procedural Highlights

A ventriculoperitoneal shunt has three components. The *proximal catheter* resides in the ventricle and is connected to the *valve*, which is then connected to the *distal catheter*, which courses underneath the skin down the scalp, neck, chest, and abdominal wall before terminating in the peritoneal cavity. The proximal catheter can have several different trajectories, but the most common is a frontal entry point where the catheter traverses the frontal lobe, entering the frontal horn of the lateral ventricle and terminating in the foramen of Monroe or third ventricle.[2] A more posterior entry point can be used where the catheter passes through the parietal-occipital lobe to enter the atrium of the lateral ventricle and end in the anterior frontal horn. Regardless of the trajectory, placement of the proximal catheter is accomplished by drilling a burr hole, incising the dura, and passing the catheter into the ventricular space. This is done with traditional landmarks or navigation depending on the complexity of the shunt and surgeon preference.

The shunt valve regulates the pressure needed to drain CSF and thus the amount of CSF flow through the shunt system while also providing a reservoir where CSF can be sampled or contrast introduced to evaluate shunt flow under fluoroscopy. Programmable valves are commonly used today and can be adjusted at the bedside or in the clinic using a simple magnetic shunt programmer based on the clinical or radiographic picture.

The distal catheter is the final part of the shunt system. This tube connects to the distal end of the valve and courses beneath the scalp, then down subcutaneously across the neck, chest, and abdominal wall before taking a deep turn into the peritoneal cavity. Thus CSF drained from the proximal catheter passes through the valve, through the distal catheter, and into the peritoneal cavity where it is resorbed.

Perioperative Considerations

The most feared complication in postoperative ventriculoperitoneal shunt placement is intracranial hemorrhage. Placement of the proximal catheter requires passing the catheter through normal brain parenchyma with a stylet or without a stylet through an already present tract due to prior external CSF diversion (soft passing). Trauma from the catheter, with or without the stylet, may result in parenchymal hemorrhage around the tract. Asymptomatic hemorrhage is relatively common, with rates reported as high as 18.1–43.1%.[3] These are often diagnosed on a postoperative head CT routinely obtained to confirm placement of the catheter. However, approximately 2.3% of patients without coagulopathy may experience symptomatic intraparenchymal hemorrhage postoperatively.[3,4] Consequences of such bleeding can be life-threatening, requiring emergent neurosurgical intervention for clot evacuation. Therefore physicians caring for patients undergoing ventriculoperitoneal shunt procedures should monitor neurological status as well as coagulation studies perioperatively and check the head CT for intraparenchymal hemorrhage.

Injury can also occur anywhere along the body where the distal catheter is passed from the head to the belly. When pushing the tunneler underneath the scalp in line with the neck aiming for the subcutaneous tissue of the chest, a crucial step for the surgeon is ensuring the shunt passer moves superficial to the clavicle. Unintended movements here can injure vascular structures in the neck or dive into the pleural space, resulting in a pneumothorax. Postoperatively, abdominal injury is also important to consider because approximately 10–30% of ventriculoperitoneal shunt complications arise within the abdominal portion of the procedure.[5] Bowel perforation, if suspected, requires emergent upright abdominal x-rays, CT of the abdomen, and concomitant emergent general surgery consultation. Delayed abdominal complications include cerebrospinal loculation or pseudocyst formation, catheter migration into the subcutaneous tissue, pericapsular hepatic cystic formation, or even remote perforation due to catheter erosion into the bowel wall over time. Suspected pathology can be evaluated with an abdominal ultrasound (can be used to visualize a pseudocyst), upright x-rays, or, most definitively, a CT scan with and without contrast.

Shunt infection and shunt failure are the other two main postoperative problems that require a formulaic approach to both diagnose and properly manage. Shunt failure is defined as failure of the shunt's ability to meet the drainage requirements of the CSF in an individual. This can be due to obstruction (partial or complete), hardware/valve failure, or increased CSF production outstripping drainage capabilities. If either is suspected, the workup starts with the clinical exam and history, lab work, and cultures, and then proceeds to noninvasive imaging. If this does not identify an obvious shunt malfunction (e.g., ventricles are larger than the patient's baseline), more invasive testing can be performed that is aided by the shunt valve itself. All shunt valves include a reservoir that the neurosurgeon can tap to sample CSF for cultures and cell counts. Also, contrast can be injected under fluoroscopy to visualize the patency of the system.

Patients with infected shunts often present with two main symptoms: fever and shunt failure. Routinely a noncontrasted CT scan of the head is needed as well as a shunt series consisting of x-ray films to demonstrate the continuity and location of the system. Ventriculomegaly compared to a previous scan indicates shunt malfunction, and kinks or disconnections can be diagnosed on the shunt series. In the patient with abdominal pain, an ultrasound is a good first step to evaluate for a pseudocyst, although the most helpful image will be a CT of the abdomen and pelvis with and without contrast. Fever, especially within the first 6 months of implantation, should raise suspicion for device infection, yet tapping the shunt is avoided if possible until other sources of fever are ruled out. This is because interrogation of the shunt by percutaneous tap has a small but understandable risk of infecting a previously sterile shunt system.[6] Bacterial etiology of shunt infections are most often skin flora; *Staphylococcus epidermidis*, *Staphylococcus aureus*, *Escherichia coli*, *Pseudomonas* spp., and *Klebsiella* spp. are the bacteria with the highest incidence of shunt infection with *S. epidermidis* being the most common.[3,5] Shunt infections require shunt removal, hospitalization for extracorporeal CSF drainage during an extended course of antibiotic treatment, and then reimplantation of a new shunt once the infection has cleared.

CRANIOTOMY AND CRANIECTOMY
Indications

Craniotomy refers to temporarily removing a portion of the skull. When the bone is left off after the intracranial operation is complete, this is a *craniectomy*. Both craniotomies and craniectomies are very common procedures indicated for a wide variety of reasons. Only several scenarios will be discussed here. The first is craniotomy or craniectomy for tumor resection. Reasons for tumor resection can be divided into diagnostic, neurologic, and oncologic. In order to begin treatment, whether systemic or local, radiation and medical oncologists generally require pathology to plan treatment. If no safer lesion for biopsy is identified with a systemic workup (PET scan, CT C/A/P, lumbar puncture, etc.), then a craniotomy may be performed to obtain tissue for pathology in the form of a stereotactic brain biopsy or open resection. Mass effect causing neurological impairment or even hydrocephalus may also require craniotomy for tumor resection or debulking. Finally, depending on the type and location of the tumor as well as the patient's condition and comorbidities, resection or debulking can help with oncologic control and improve survival.

Craniectomy, or leaving the bone off after a craniotomy, is performed in order to allow for severe brain swelling usually caused by large ischemic strokes (malignant middle cerebral artery [MCA] syndrome), intracranial hemorrhages, or trauma. This is done to prevent or relieve pressure on the uninjured brain. There is a wide body of literature supporting craniectomy for the treatment of such patients.[7–9]

Procedural Highlights

In positioning for many craniotomy/craniectomy procedures, the surgeon may elect to have patients placed in a Mayfield three-prong head holder to keep the head fixed in position during a delicate procedure. This device is used to apply 60–80 pounds of force clamping the skull in rigid fixation. Calvarial exposure is accomplished with incisions designed to respect the scalp's blood supply and avoid tissue ischemia during wound healing. Once the skull is exposed, the craniotomy is planned and carried out with several burr holes that are placed with a high-speed drill and then connected using the same drill with a saw attachment. The bone flap is then removed. Of note, the neurosurgical "workhorse" is the pterional craniotomy, which requires dissection and detachment of the temporalis muscle—an aspect of the procedure that often can cause pain during talking and chewing in the postoperative period. The bone removal exposes the dura, which is then cut open, reflected, and then tacked up to reveal the underlying brain.

At this point, the procedure will vary depending on the goal of surgery: dissection begins, and the tumor is resected, the aneurysm is clipped, the clot is removed. During the final phase of surgery, dural edges are reopposed and sutured shut. The bone is then reimplanted using a metal plating system. For craniectomies, the bone is either discarded or sent to a freezer for storage and the scalp is sewn shut, covering the dura. These patients return months later to undergo a cranioplasty procedure where the bone flap or a synthetic implant is placed. Both craniectomy and craniotomy procedures commonly have a temporary drain with bulb suction, which helps to prevent hematoma accumulation in the surgical site and is often removed on post operative day 1 or 2.

Perioperative Considerations

Depending on the pathology being addressed by the craniotomy or craniectomy, specific medical issues arise perioperatively. Many of these will be discussed in subsequent chapters, but some general issues applicable to craniotomies deserve mention. First, and perhaps most importantly, is close attention to the neurological exam. Any negative changes should be emergently relayed to the neurosurgical team and will usually mandate a head CT. Strict blood pressure control based on either mean arterial pressures or systolics is meant to prevent postoperative hemorrhage in the tumor bed. Antiepileptics are often given perioperatively at the discretion of the surgeon. Tumor patients are commonly on high-dose dexamethasone to combat vasogenic edema preoperatively, and a plan for the steroid taper usually starts after the operation. Mannitol and furosemide (Lasix) are commonly given during the case to combat brain swelling and so renal function and fluid balance should be monitored postoperatively.[10,11] Deep vein thrombosis prophylaxis can usually resume on postoperative day 1, but should be judiciously dosed by weight to avoid increasing the risk of hemorrhagic complications. Complications of the procedure will also dictate perioperative medical concerns. For instance sacrificing a draining vein or sinus during the course of the surgery will predispose a patient to venous infarction, and so this patient will require generous hydration.

Finally, while cranial incisions are planned to respect the scalp's major blood supply, these patients are at high risk of wound breakdown and infection. Factors that may be modified to improve outcomes include glycemic control perioperatively and nutritional status.[12,13] Especially in oncologic patients, nutritional supplementation provides support to wounds that often undergo postoperative radiation. Hyperglycemia in postoperative patients is associated with increased infections and return to the operating room for cranial wound revision. By modifying these factors perioperatively, outcomes may be improved.

CERVICAL DECOMPRESSION AND FUSION
Indications

Cervical decompression and fusion procedures have many indications including myelopathy, radiculopathy, trauma, deformity, and instability. By far the most common are cervical myelopathy and traumatic fractures or nonunions. These tend to require central canal decompression and fusion of multiple levels. Depending on the extent and location of pathology (ventral or dorsal), patients may undergo anterior or posterior approaches, or both. If the primary indication is radiculopathy, patients may only require decompression in the form of foraminotomies or laminectomies. In general, the less bony work necessary to achieve neural decompression, the lower the chance of creating iatrogenic instability requiring fusion.

Procedural Highlights

Surgeons may take either an anterior or posterior approach to the cervical spine. The choice of approach is patient-specific, taking into account location of pathology (ventral vs. dorsal) and the goals of surgery. The anterior approach involves an incision off the midline of the neck, often in a natural fold or crease in the skin. Platysma is divided and an avascular plane medial to the sternocleidomastoid dissected, leading to the carotid sheath. The carotid is then retracted laterally and the esophagus medially, exposing the anterior vertebral body. Discectomy is performed and an interbody fusion device is placed, usually along with a plate and screws in adjacent vertebrae. In this way anterior decompression and fusion is achieved. Bleeding is controlled, a drain can be placed, and the platysma is reapproximated with sutures. Skin may be sutured or closed with a topical skin adhesive (Dermabond) per surgeon preference.

Cervical pathology may also be addressed with a posterior cervical decompression and fusion. For this procedure, the patient normally has the head placed in cranial pins to hold the neck in alignment during the procedure. The paraspinal musculature is dissected down to the spinous processes and off the edge of the lateral masses. Screws are placed in the lateral masses to stabilize the spine for bony fusion. Spinous process and lamina are drilled off to create more room in the spinal canal for the neural elements. Afterward a drain is placed and layers of muscle, fascia, fat, and skin are closed.

Perioperative Considerations

During the anterior cervical approach, critical structures encountered include the esophagus, trachea, carotid artery, internal jugular vein, vagus nerve, recurrent laryngeal nerve, and superior laryngeal nerve. From working around these structures, common perioperative medical issues are centered around breathing and swallowing function. Esophageal perforation is a rare but feared complication occurring with an incidence of 0.02–1.52%.[14] Patients may encounter increased sputum production, cough, pain on swallowing, vomiting, and sepsis. The workup may require a swallowing study or CT imaging, antibiotics, and corrective surgery if these concerning symptoms are observed.

While intubation may cause irritation and trauma, hoarse voice, coughing, or aspiration raises concern for the possibility of recurrent laryngeal or superior laryngeal nerve injury during surgery.[14,15] This is a concerning morbidity as nerve damage here will raise the long-term risk of aspiration for patients. Disruption of swallowing function is especially a concern in elderly patients. If swallowing function is a concern, patients may receive a course of steroids to decrease swelling from intubation and surgery. Often this is enough to alleviate symptoms. Further workup of these symptoms includes speech and swallow evaluation, and subsequent laryngoscopy by an otolaryngologist will be required to investigate vocal cord function. On occasion, the vocal folds may be injected with a collagen-like substance to address glottal insufficiency in postoperative patients with vocal cord paresis.[16]

Lastly, careful attention should be paid to respiratory function in the immediate postoperative care of anterior cervical procedures. If bleeding is uncontrolled, damage to the carotid sheath occurs; or, if the drain left intraoperatively does not function correctly, a hematoma may form and compress the airway. In these instances intubation is can be difficult and the patient may need the surgical wound emergently opened at bedside to relieve pressure on the airway.[14]

Whereas the dissection for the anterior approach takes advantage of natural tissue planes between the neck musculature to reach the ventral spine, the posterior approach cuts and retracts the musculature overlying the dorsal spine. Therefore, while possible injury to the esophagus, jugular vein, recurrent laryngeal nerve, and carotid artery is avoided, this approach invariably results in more postoperative pain compared to the anterior approach. The pain should be managed with judicial use of narcotics and muscle relaxants. Severe pain, especially pain that increases after a period of initial improvement, should raise suspicion for a postoperative hematoma and requires emergent attention. Since the lamina has been removed in most cases, a mass lesion here can directly compress the spinal cord, leading to potentially irreversible sensory changes or weakness.[17] Usually emergent imaging (MRI provides a better image but a CT can also demonstrate a postoperative hematoma more quickly) will be followed by an emergent return to the operating room for evacuation.

Regardless of the approach, patients who undergo cervical decompression or fusion are at risk for a postoperative C5 palsy which manifests as deltoid weakness. This is a phenomenon that is well described but not completely understood. The C5 nerve root is presumed to be at greater risk for injury after a decompressive procedure due to the angle at which it leaves the spinal cord. One of the proposed mechanisms is tethering of the nerve root after the spinal cord is decompressed and moved dorsally. However, segmental ischemia and reperfusion injury from disruption of radicular vasculature has also been proposed. This occurs in 4–8% of these cases.[18,19] In studies comparing the incidence of C5 palsy in cervical approaches, ventral approaches (4.3%) had a lower incidence of C5 palsy than dorsal approaches (10.9).[18] There have been studies suggesting that perioperative steroids may be of benefit, but most studies suggest that high-dose steroids may delay fusion, and the majority of these patients ultimately improve on their own.

LUMBAR DECOMPRESSION AND FUSION
Indications

Lumbar procedures have many indications but are often pursued after a lengthy workup and trial of nonoperative therapy. While there are emergent and urgent indications for surgery, such as instability secondary to trauma, epidural abscess, and cauda equina syndrome, most indications fall under criteria defined by the North American Spine Society (NASS). Indications include deformity (sagittal or coronal imbalance), lumbar stenosis, recurrent disc herniation, synovial facet cyst, discogenic low back pain, and pseudarthrosis of previous fusions. Patients often trial physical therapy, medical pain management, and pain injections with a specialist before being scheduled for surgery. This ensures the best outcome as many of these patients will do well without surgery and can be managed nonoperatively.

Procedural Highlights

Lumbar procedures are achieved through either an anterior, lateral, or posterior approach. Each has its own complications inherent to the anatomy encountered along the way to the spine. Similar to cervical surgery, the choice of approach is patient-specific. Location of pathology, vascular disease of the aorta and great vessels, and goals of surgery (such as degree of lordotic correction) all play a role in determining whether an anterior or posterior approach is more appropriate for a particular patient.

The anterior approach begins with a small, lower abdominal incision; the musculature is split longitudinally and the peritoneal cavity is pushed medially. At this point the surgeon has to retract the aorta, inferior vena cava, iliac artery, and vein to properly visualize the vertebral bodies and disc space. For this reason the approach is often performed by a general or vascular surgeon. The lumbar disc is then removed and an interbody placed with or without plate fixation, analogous to the way an anterior cervical discectomy and fusion is perform in the neck. Once completed, the access surgeon will usually assist in the closure.

Lateral approaches to the lumbar spine involve a lateral incision through which the retroperitoneal cavity is accessed and the kidney is displaced anteriorly to gain access to the lateral aspect of the lumbar spine. Using dilators, a tract is created through the retroperitoneal space, sometime right through the psoas muscle, and into the disc space for the surgery. The disc space is cleaned out, and graft and cages/spacers are placed into the disc space.

Finally, the most routinely used approach to the lumbar spine is from the back. This is achieved through a midline incision through which fascia and paraspinal muscle are separated to expose the posterior bony elements. From that point, there may be decompression of bony elements and instrumented fusion. Drains may also be left after the critical portion of surgery is completed depending on hemostasis, number of levels of surgery, and whether or not the surgery is a repeat procedure.

Perioperative Considerations

With every approach, it is important to note any neurological change in strength, sensation, and ability to void. Patients often have postoperative urinary retention secondary to Foley placement, anesthesia, and narcotics. However, a compressive lesion in lumbar surgery from bleeding can lead to urinary retention, pain, bowel/bladder incontinence, or new weakness or numbness and necessitate a return to the operating room.[20] This is especially pertinent in posterior approaches because the paraspinal musculature is very well vascularized and has a high propensity for continued bleeding.

Regarding the anterior and lateral approaches, the neurological exam is important as described earlier; however, a crucial addition here is that attention must be paid to bowel function. While any patient receiving anesthesia and narcotics is at risk for a postoperative ileus, patients undergoing an anterior or lateral approach are specifically at risk due to manipulation of the abdominal contents.[21] A clear liquid diet is usually started postoperatively and is slowly advanced once tolerated. If an ileus does develop, the patient may require nasogastric tube placement. Any signs or symptoms concerning for sepsis or peritonitis should raise suspicion for bowel injury and initiate emergent abdominal imaging as well as consultation with general surgery.[22,23]

Another component of the lateral and anterior approaches that affects postoperative care is possible injury to the iliac arteries and veins, aorta, or inferior vena cava. Broadly speaking, if a vascular injury does occur, this is usually obvious during the surgery and appropriate management begins in the operating room. Nonetheless, any new circulatory changes in the lower extremities postoperatively (e.g., swelling due to venous thrombosis or signs of limb ischemia from an arterial event) should be investigated immediately with vascular imaging.[22,23]

Finally, a complication relevant to all lumbar and cervical surgeries is CSF leak. A CSF leak occurs when the dural covering of the central nervous system is violated and may lead to complications such as intractable headaches, infections, poor wound healing, and, in severe cases, cerebral hygromas or subdural hemorrhages. Especially in revision cases, where the risk is much higher, patients may develop damage to the dura causing persistent leak which can manifest with persistent positional headache. These patients have worse symptoms when sitting up as more pressure is placed on the dural defect, and they gain relief when lying flat. They may also have leaking of spinal fluid through the incision or into Jackson-Pratt drains, causing serous output rather than serosanguineous output. If patients have a leak unable to be repaired intraoperatively, the surgeon may place a lumbar drain to drain CSF in a controlled manner that allows the dural defect to heal.[24]

CEREBRAL ANGIOGRAM
Indications

Cerebral angiography is now an indispensable part of neurosurgery, used for a wide variety of both diagnostic and therapeutic purposes. A cerebral angiogram is a dynamic vascular study that provides high-resolution temporal images of the cervical and cranial vasculature, in the arterial, capillary, and venous phases. Aneurysms, arteriovenous malformations, arteriovenous fistulas, carotid stenosis, and strokes caused by large vessel occlusion are both evaluated and routinely treated via the endovascular approach utilizing angiography. Diagnostic angiograms, carotid stents, and stroke interventions (mechanical thrombectomy) are usually performed with conscious sedation, whereas interventions such as coil embolization, intracranial stenting, or injection of a liquid embolic agent (usually Onyx) for treatment of vascular malformations is most commonly performed under general anesthesia.

Procedural Highlights

While the indications for the procedure may vary greatly, the general framework for each procedure remains largely the same. Access to the arterial system begins with a puncture of usually the femoral or radial artery, and a sheath is placed.[25] This access provides a port whereby catheters and wires can be introduced without repeated injury to the vessel. Catheters are then maneuvered under fluoroscopic guidance as contrast is injected to visualize the vasculature. A simple diagnostic angiogram consists of only obtaining the x-ray images—taking pictures—and, in almost all instances, the catheter does not have to be advanced beyond the level of the neck. For interventions, more sophisticated catheters, balloons, and wires are employed to treat pathology throughout the cervical and cranial vasculature.

Once the procedure is completed, catheters and wires are removed and a closure device is used for hemostasis where the sheath had been placed. For radial access this consists of a bracelet that contains an inflatable pressure dressing. Several different closure devices are used for femoral closure and apply a subcutaneous stitch or collagen plug to the arteriotomy.

Perioperative Considerations

As with most neurosurgical procedures, neurological status should be monitored closely after any diagnostic angiogram or intervention. An acute embolic event during the procedure should be immediately recognized by the interventionalist who, at that time, can potentially attempt a mechanical or chemical thrombectomy while the patient is still in the angio suite. For the patient who has left the angio suite and is on the floor, neurological changes must be promptly recognized and worked up. Arterial dissection or stent thrombosis may cause sudden changes consistent with an ischemic stroke. Vessel injury leading to hemorrhage or hemorrhage into a stroke will usually present as a rapid progression toward coma. For straightforward diagnostic angiograms the risk of a hemorrhagic or ischemic complication is generally felt to be less than 1%. This risk is higher in more complicated interventions.[26]

Physicians caring for patients undergoing a cerebral angiogram must also have a strong understanding of the patient's renal function. While patients are hydrated before and after the procedure with intravenous fluids, they are at risk of contrast-induced nephropathy given the large bolus of contrast used for the procedure. In addition, heart failure and other comorbidities may limit the ability to fully hydrate the patient. As a result, it is important to note markers of kidney function, urine production, and electrolytes pre- and postoperatively. Renal disease is *not* a direct contraindication to the procedure but may require discontinuation of nephrotoxic medications (e.g., metformin) and administration of renal protective agents such as sodium bicarbonate and volume expansion.[27,28]

Lastly, the other perioperative issue to monitor for in this patient population is vascular complications related to puncture of the artery. If the patient has poor vascular status, this may compromise the artery and result in distal limb ischemia.[28,29] Patients will note excruciating pain distally and have a poor pulse and low pulse oximetry in the affected leg or arm. One must have a low threshold to consult vascular surgery for any concern of limb ischemia.

For patients who have had femoral access, hypotension, a drop in the hemoglobin level, or back pain should alert the practitioner to the possibility of a retroperitoneal hematoma. These patients should be watched very carefully because a patient with a large retroperitoneal bleed can suffer significant blood lose into the retroperitoneal cavity with minimal groin swelling/hematoma.[29] If there is concern for this complication, an immediate hemoglobin study and a CT of the abdomen and pelvis should be obtained to evaluate for a large bleed. This can usually be managed with blood transfusions and observation in the ICU; however, again, there should be a low threshold for consulting trauma or vascular surgery.

While it is common to avoid blood thinning medications in neurosurgical patients, endovascular procedures are often the exception to this rule. It is important to note that this is the case when flow diversion or stenting techniques are used. In these procedures, patients must strictly adhere to dual antiplatelet therapy postoperatively or risk thrombosis of the device and cerebral infarction. It is not unusual to follow lab values such as the P2Y12 to ensure adequate response to the antiplatelet agent of choice.

CONCLUSION

While neurosurgical procedures are specific to the central nervous system, a multisystem approach is required by physicians caring for these patients to ensure recognition of complications of the procedure and ensure the best outcome for the patient. Whether a craniotomy, spinal surgery, or cerebral angiogram is being performed, understanding the surgeon's goals, surgical approach, and potential pitfalls will help guide the treatment and evaluation of these patients perioperatively. Finally, it is worth stressing that there is no substitute for direct communication between the surgeon who performs the operation and the physician involved in caring for the patient in the postoperative period. A brief clarifying phone call between these two practitioners will undoubtedly save both time and energy in the long run and, more importantly, result in better patient care.

REFERENCES

1. Stagno V, Navarrete EA, Mirone G, Esposito F. Management of hydrocephalus around the world. *World Neurosurg.* 2013;79(23):17–20. doi: 10.1016/j.wneu.2012.02.004.

2. Lind C, Tsai A, Law A, Lau H, Muthiah K. Ventricular catheter trajectories from traditional shunt approaches: a morphometric study in adults with hydrocephalus. *J Neurosurg.* 2008;108:930–933.

3. Moza K, McMenomey SO, Delashaw JB. Indications for cerebrospinal fluid drainage and avoidance of complications. *Otolaryngol Clin N Am.* 2005;38:577–582. doi: 10.1016/j.otc.2005.01.001.

4. Hou K, Suo S, Gao X, Shu X, Zhang Y, Li G. Symptomatic intracerebral hemorrhage secondary to ventriculperitoneal shunt in adults without bleeding tendency. *World Neurosurg.* 2017;07(005):388–373. doi: 10.1016/J.WNEU.2017.07.005.

5. Chung J, Yu JS, Kim JH, Nam SJ, Kim MJ. Intraabdominal complications secondary to ventriculoperitoneal shunts: CT findings and review of the literature. *Am J Roentgenol.* 2009;193:1311–1317. doi: 10.2214/AJR.09.2463.

6. Spiegelman L, Asija R, Da Silva S, Krieger M, McComb JG. What is the risk of infecting a cerebrospinal fluid-diverting shunt with percutaneous tapping? *J Neurosurg Pediatrics.* 2014;14:336–339. doi: 10.3171/2014.7.PEDS13612.

7. Vahedi K, Hofmeijer J, Juettler E, et al. Early decompressive surgery in malignant infarction of the middle cerebral artery: a pooled analysis of three randomized controlled trials. *Lancet Neurol.* 2007;6:215–222. doi: 10.1016/S1474-4422(07)70036-4.

8. Bullock MR, Chesnut R, Ghajar J, et al. Surgical management of acute subdural hematomas. *Neurosurgery.* 2006;58(3 Suppl):S16–S24.

9. Witsch J, Neugebauer H, Zweckberger K, Juttler E. Primary cerebellar haemorrhage: complications, treatment and outcome. *Clin Neurol Neurosurg.* 2013;115:863–869. doi: 10.1016/j.clineuro.2013.04.009.

10. Prabhakar H, Singh GP, Anand V, Kalavani M. Mannitol versus hypertonic saline for brain relaxation in patients undergoing craniotomy. *Cochrane Database Syst Rev.* 2014;7:CD010026. doi: 10.1002/14651858.CD010026.pub2.

11. Seo H, Ki E, Jung H, et al. A prospective randomized trial of the optimal dose of mannitol for intraoperative brain relaxation in patients undergoing craniotomy for supratentorial brain tumor resection. *J Neurosurg.* 2017;126(6):1839–1846. doi: 10.3171/2016.6.JNS16537.

12. Chiang HY, Kamath AS, Pottinger JM, et al. Risk factors and outcomes associated with surgical site infections after craniotomy or craniectomy. *J Neurosurg.* 2014;120(1):509–521. doi: 10.3171/2013.9.JNS13843.

13. Dasenbrock HH, Liu KX, Chavakula V, et al. Body habitus, serum albumin, and the outcomes after craniotomy for tumor: a National Surgical Quality Improvement Program analysis. *J Neurosurg.* 2017;126(3):677–689. doi: 10.3171/2016.2.JNS152345.

14. Tasiou A, Giannis T, Brotis AG, et al. Anterior cervical spine surgery-associated complications in a retrospective case-control study. *J Spine Surg.* 2017 Sep;3(3):444–459. doi: 10.21037/jss.2017.08.03.

15. Staartjes VE, de Wispelaere MP, Schroder ML. Recurrent laryngeal nerve palsy is more frequent after secondary than after primary anterior cervical discectomy and fusion: insights from a registry of 525 patients. *World Neurosurg.* 2018 Aug;116:e1047–e1053. doi: 10.1016/j.wneu.2018.05.16.

16. Mallur PS, Rosen CA. Vocal fold injection: review of indications, techniques, and materials for augmentation. *Clin Exp Otorhinolaryngol.* 2010 Dec;3(4):177–182. doi: 10.3342/ceo.2010.3.4.177.

17. Goldstein CL, Bains I, Hurlbert RJ. Symptomatic spinal epidural hematoma after posterior cervical surgery: incidence and risk factors. *Spine J.* 2015 Jun 1;15(6):1179–1187. doi: 0.1016/j.spinee.2013.11.043.

18. Kratzig T, Mohme M, Mende KC, Eicker SO, Floeth FW. Impact of the surgical strategy on the incidence of C5 nerve root palsy in decompressive cervical surgery. *PLoS One.* 2017 Nov 16;12(11):e0188338. doi: 10.1371/journal.pone.0188338.

19. Pan F, Wang S, Ma B, Wu D. C5 nerve root palsy after posterior cervical spine surgery: A review of the literature. *J Orthop Surg.* 2017 Jan;25(1):2309499016684502. doi: 10.1177/2309499016684502.

20. Aono H, Ohwada T, Hosono N, et al. Incidence of postoperative symptomatic epidural hematoma in spinal decompression surgery. *J Neurosurg Spine.* 2001 Aug;15(2):202–205. doi: 0.3171/2011.3.SPINE10716.

21. Fineberg SJ, Nandyala SV, Kurd MF, et al. Incidence and risk factors for postoperative ileus following anterior, posterior, and circumferential lumbar fusion. *Spine J.* 2014 Aug 1;14(8):1680–1685. doi: 10.1016/j.spinee.2013.10.015.

22. Samudrala S, Khoo LT, Rhim SC, Fessler RG. Complications during anterior surgery of the lumbar spine: an anatomically based study and review. *Neurosurg Focus.* 1999 Dec 15;7(6):e9. doi: 0.3171/foc.1999.7.6.10.

23. Mobbs RJ, Phan K, Daly D, Rao PJ, Lennox A. Approach-related complications of anterior lumbar interbody fusion: results of a combined spine and vascular surgical team. *Global Spine J.* 2016 Mar;6(2):147–154.

24. Epstein NE. A review article on the diagnosis and treatment of cerebrospinal fluid fistulas and dural tears occurring during spinal surgery. *Surg Neurol Int.* 2013 May 6;49(Suppl 5):S301–S317. doi: 10.4103/2152-7806.111427.

25. Oselkin M, Satti SR, Sundararajan SH, Kung D, Hurst HW, Pukenas BA. Endovascular treatment for acute basilar thrombosis via a transradial approach: Initial experience and future considerations. *Interv Neuroradiol.* 2018 Feb;24(1):64–69. doi: 10.1177/1591019917733709.

26. Deek H, Newton P, Sheerin N, Noureddine S, Davidson PM. Contrast media induced nephropathy: a literature review of the available evidence and recommendations for practice. *Aust Crit Care.* 2014 Nov;27(4):166–171. doi: 10.1016/j.aucc.2013.12.002.

27. Sharma J, Nanda A, Jung RS, Mehta S, Pooria J, Hsu DP. Risk of contrast-induced nephropathy in patients undergoing endovascular treatment of acute ischemic stroke. *J Neurointerv Surg.* 2013 Nov;5(6):543–545. doi: 10.1136/neurintsurg-2012-010520.

28. Choudhri O, Schoen M, Mantha A, et al. Increased risk for complications following diagnostic cerebral angiography in older patients: trends from Nationwide Inpatient Sample (1999–2009). *J Clin Neurosci.* 2016 Oct;32:109–114. doi: 0.1016/j.jocn.2016.04.007.

29. Fifi JT, Meyers PM, Lavine SD, et al. Complications of modern diagnostic cerebral angiography in an academic medical center. *J Vasc Interv Radiol.* 2009 Apr;20(4):442–447. doi: 10.1016/j.jvir.2009.01.012.

2 Preoperative Evaluation of Neurosurgical Patients

Aditya Munshi and Geno Merli

INTRODUCTION

Traditionally, preoperative evaluation has consisted mainly of assessing a patient's cardiac risk and determining the need for cardiac testing before surgery. However, patients undergoing noncardiac surgery are at risk for a multitude of complications involving different organ systems. Patients undergoing surgery are at risk for cardiac complications as well as risks from the procedure being performed. Procedural risks are grouped, first, into risks arising from the surgery itself and from anesthesia; these are usually nonmodifiable and are not addressed in this chapter. The second group is that of medical complications, the risk of which is determined by the patient's overall condition, comorbidities, and nutritional and functional status. These factors are modifiable up to a certain degree, and the aim of this chapter is to address the approach to stratify these risks in a neurosurgical patient.

Neurosurgical patients are often chronically ill, having other comorbid conditions affecting their surgical outcomes.[1,2] Additionally, bleeding events within the small confines of the central nervous system can have catastrophic consequences, making identification of coagulation abnormalities imperative. Many neurosurgical procedures are performed urgently or emergently, making them inherently high risk from the cardiac standpoint.[3] These patients also tend to have longer hospital stays with prolonged periods of immobilization, making thrombosis prevention critical.

This chapter covers a broad approach from the perspective of a hospitalist physician evaluating a patient prior to surgery; here, we review current guidelines, recommendations, and future directions on stratification of cardiac, thrombotic, and bleeding risk, as well as the role of placing inferior vena cava (IVC) filters preoperatively. We also cover the use of risk assessment scores to aid in decision-making and how to combine their use with diagnostic testing such as electrocardiograms or echocardiograms in selected patients.

CARDIOVASCULAR RISK STRATIFICATION OF THE NEUROSURGICAL PATIENT

Cardiovascular events account for one of the largest causes of intra- and postoperative morbidity and mortality.[3] A significant number of patients have asymptomatic coronary artery disease and an even larger number have risk factors predisposing to coronary disease. Careful and systematic assessment of these patients is therefore an imperative step of the presurgical encounter. Per guidelines of the American College of Cardiology and the American Heart Association (ACC/AHA),[3] risk stratification should be based on the combined risk of the procedure itself, urgency of the procedure, and clinical factors. The ACC/AHA guidelines define a low-risk procedure as one that has less than 1% risk of major adverse cardiac events (MACE) based on the combined patient and surgical characteristics. A risk of 1% or more for MACE for a procedure is considered elevated risk. The most recent guidelines (2014) stratify procedures into two groups only—low risk and elevated risk.[3] In addition, many neurological surgeries fall under the urgent or emergent categories, thereby adding to the combined risk. A retrospective study based on the American College of Surgeons–Surgeons National Surgical Quality Improvement Program (ACS–NSQIP) looked at factors associated with perioperative cardiac arrest in craniotomy and spine surgery.[1] The results suggested that the risk for cardiac arrest was significantly higher with craniotomies compared to spine surgery and concluded that American Society of Anesthesiology (ASA) class 4 and 5 patients, totally dependent patients, and Asian and black patients were at higher risk of having a cardiac arrest in the perioperative period. These findings highlight the importance of including functional capacity and comorbid conditions, and they favor an overall comprehensive approach for each neurosurgical patient. In this chapter, we review existing guidelines and aim to provide a comprehensive approach incorporating the use of risk indices, functional status, procedural risk, and urgency of surgery.

Risk Indices

Risk indices provide an easily accessible and standardized approach to estimating each patient's risk for perioperative complications. There are several scales in use today.

The first preoperative risk index was published by Goldman et al.[4] in 1977; it used a point-based system assigned to nine factors found to have independent correlation to cardiac outcomes. Indices have evolved a lot since this first one was published. Here, we review some of the most widely used ones and provide a brief overview of the differences between them.

Lee's Revised Cardiac Risk Index

In 1999, Lee et al.[5] developed a risk assessment tool based on a patient cohort aged older than 50 years with an expected length of stay (LOS) of 2 days or longer: the

Revised Cardiac Risk Index (RCRI). It was validated against the existing risk assessment indices available at the time. Lee's risk index is one of the simplest risk assessment tools available; it uses six factors—high-risk surgery (intrathoracic, intraperitoneal supra-inguinal vascular); history of ischemic heart disease; history of congestive heart failure; history of stroke or transient ischemic attack (TIA); preop treatment with insulin; or creatinine greater than 2 mg/dL at baseline. The usefulness of the RCRI in predicting MACE has been tested on several other datasets and was found to perform satisfactorily on patients undergoing mixed noncardiac surgery.[6] It underperformed in predicting cardiac complications after vascular surgery.[6,7] Close to two decades after it was published, it remains one of the most widely used risk indices today. With time, it will require modification to include new evidence and data, as is the case with all such indices.

ACS NSQIP Surgical Risk Calculator

The ACS NSQIP database was created in the Veterans Health Administration with the aim to improve surgical outcomes. It now includes more than 600 hospitals and over time has been shown to have improved surgical quality and reduced mortality.[8,9] In 2013, Bilimoria et al.[10,11] developed an online tool using this dataset; it was based on nearly 1.5 million patients from more than 350 hospitals in the ACS NSQIP database. The tool uses 21 factors to predict 8 complications of surgery, making it far more extensive than other risk indices. It has been shown to perform well for all eight outcomes. It includes a surgeon adjustment score to incorporate the subjective component based on a surgeon's assessment. Despite being based only on hospitals included in the NSQIP database, it provides a useful tool to predict mortality as well as other postsurgical complications in patients undergoing a wide range of procedures.

Gupta Scale

In 2011, Gupta et al.[12] used the ACS NSQIP data to publish a risk calculator to predict the risk of myocardial infarction (MI) or cardiac arrest intra- and postoperatively. It was validated against the RCRI and performed better overall. Five factors were used in the final calculator; these include American Stroke Association (ASA) class, dependent functional status, creatinine level of 1.5 mg/dL or greater, type of surgery, and increasing age. Limitations of the NSQIP database have carried forward to the Gupta scale. These include lack of data on preop cardiac testing, limited endpoints (MI and cardiac arrest only), no consideration of beta-blocker use, and no accounting for the presence of aortic stenosis.

Use of Risk Scales in Estimating Perioperative Risk

Although several risk assessment tools are available to the physician performing a preoperative evaluation, it is recommended that one of the preceding tools be used. The Gupta and Bilimoria scales based on ACS NSQIP data include high-risk patients and have been shown to estimate risk accurately. On the other hand, the RCRI is simple to use and performed moderately well in distinguishing high-risk from low-risk patients. We recommend using a risk index to determine if a patient's risk for MACE is 1% or higher (as noted earlier, patients are considered low risk if the risk for MACE is <1% and elevated risk if the risk is ≥1%). However, it must be kept in mind that risk indices are not a substitute for clinical judgment or a physical exam. An approach to the patients at elevated risk is discussed later in this chapter.

Functional Status

Exercise capacity or functional status has long been considered a marker of cardiovascular health and, indirectly, a metric for predicting operative cardiovascular risk. The 2014 ACC/AHA clinical practice guidelines recommend using functional capacity to aid in the decision-making process for ordering cardiac testing preoperatively.[3] The most commonly used method of quantifying functional status is a subjective approach in which patients are asked what level of activity they can routinely perform without symptoms. Predefined activities are correlated to metabolic equivalents (METs). For example, 1 MET is equivalent to the resting oxygen consumption of a 40-year-old male weighing 70 kg; less than 4 METS is equivalent to slow walking; and more than 4 METS is equivalent to climbing up a flight of steps, or walking uphill, or performing heavy work around the house. Any patient unable to tolerate 4 METS of physical activity is considered to be at elevated risk.[13] Standardized tools for measurement of functional capacity also exist, such as the Duke Activity Status Index (DASI)[14] or cardiopulmonary exercise testing (CPET). In 2018, Wijeysundera et al.[15] published data comparing outcomes in patients who underwent functional capacity assessment by DASI, self-reported subjective assessment, and CPET. It was reported that only DASI scores correlated to postoperative cardiac events, whereas subjective assessment and CPET did not (patients doing poorly on CPET had a higher rate of pulmonary and other noncardiac complications but there was no correlation with cardiac events). Additionally, the same study showed that a higher level of N-terminal pro b-type natriuretic peptide (NT-proBNP) correlated with a higher risk of 30-day myocardial injury and death as well as 1-year death.[15] These findings are significant because they highlight the limited role of self-reported functional status and show that a lab test could potentially be a substitute for it. CPET was not shown to be useful in predicting cardiac events but did predict other adverse outcomes; more data are needed to show how it can be incorporated into the assessment algorithm.

Canadian Cardiovascular Society Guidelines

Of the published preoperative guidelines, the recently released Canadian guidelines were one of the earliest to place emphasis on changing the existing approach to preop assessment; therefore we incorporate a detailed overview of these guidelines here.

In 2017, the Canadian Cardiovascular Society updated their preoperative cardiac risk assessment guidelines.[16] These guidelines introduced several changes to established practice. They recommend a change in focus from preoperative noninvasive testing to biomarker measurement and postoperative troponin level measurement. The main points from the paper are summarized here:

- Recommend measuring NT-proBNP or BNP in patients who are 65 years of age or older or 45–64 years of age with a cardiac history or have an RCRI of 1 or greater.[17–21]
- Recommend against performing resting echocardiography, CT coronary angiography, CPET, exercise stress testing, or nuclear stress testing for preoperative risk assessment.
- Do not recommend initiating or continuing aspirin for cardiac prevention (unless the patient has a recently placed coronary stent or had a recent carotid endarterectomy).
- Do no recommend starting beta-blockers or alpha-2 agonists in the day prior to surgery.
- Recommend holding angiotensin converting enzyme (ACE) inhibitors or angiotensin receptor blockers for 24 hours prior to surgery.
- Recommend smoking cessation to be encouraged prior to surgery.
- Recommend daily troponin measurement in the first 48–72 hours postop for patients who have a significant cardiac history or are 65 years old or older.
- Recommend that patients who develop postop MI or myocardial injury be started on long-term statin and aspirin therapy.

These updates change established practices in several ways. Measurement of NT-pro-BNP or BNP for high-risk patients is recommended instead of noninvasive cardiac imaging or stress testing, which have long been the approach to stratifying high-risk patients. The recommendation to measure NT-proBNP or BNP was based on several meta-analyses showing a correlation between elevated NT-proBNP/BNP levels and MI or death in the postoperative period.[17–21] In addition, there was evidence suggesting that biomarker measurement was superior to echocardiography in predicting adverse perioperative outcomes.[22] The other significant recommendation is to measure daily troponin for 48–72 hours in patients deemed at high risk on the initial assessment (patients ≥65 years or older or those with elevated biomarkers). This addresses the problem of many postoperative MIs being asymptomatic or "silent." The routine surveillance of troponin levels ensures that perioperative myocardial injury does not remain undetected. There is evidence showing that an elevated postoperative troponin level is a strong predictor of mortality at 30 days and 1 year.[23,24]

In summary, the 2017 Canadian Cardiovascular Society guidelines cover important updates to the preop assessment approach. These recommendations are based on high quality evidence, and it is our recommendation that a gradual transition be made from established practices to those recommended in these guidelines.[22]

Who Should Undergo a Preoperative Cardiovascular Evaluation?

Choosing patients who require a preoperative cardiovascular evaluation for neurosurgery requires that certain specific considerations be taken into account. If we consider a preoperative evaluation covering all organ systems, all patients except those requiring emergent surgery should have a thorough history and physical exam. This includes a history of bleeding events, thrombosis, serious drug reactions, and signs indicating poor respiratory or cardiac function. Surgeries that are emergently indicated should not be delayed to perform a preoperative evaluation. In almost all these cases, the risks of delaying surgery outweigh the benefits from identifying any modifiable condition. Examples of emergent neurosurgeries would include spine surgery for neurological compromise arising from cord compression or epidural abscess and urgent craniotomy for intracranial hemorrhage where even a short delay can lead to irreversible neurologic damage.

All other patients should have a risk assessment performed using a risk index. Based on this score, they are classified into a low-risk or elevated-risk group. Our approach to stratifying cardiac risk in patients is outlined here.

Very-high-risk patients: Patients who have ongoing or decompensated cardiac conditions are at a very high risk for intra- and postoperative cardiac complications. Examples include patients with severe or symptomatic valvular heart disease, recent MI with or without revascularization, unstable angina, decompensated heart failure, high-grade conduction abnormalities, or malignant ventricular arrhythmias. These patients should be referred to a cardiologist before proceeding with surgery.

Low-risk patients: Patients with a less than 1% risk for cardiac complications on a risk assessment scale are considered low risk and do not need further testing prior to noncardiac surgery.[3,16]

Elevated-risk patients: Patients with a 1% risk or higher are considered elevated risk. The Canadian guidelines recommend that all patients older than 65 years of age and those between 18 and 64 with significant heart disease also be included in this category.[16] If a patient is found to be at elevated risk, it is recommended that further testing be carried out. The choice of test should be determined by the patient's functional capacity and overall clinical presentation. The Canadian guidelines recommend biomarker testing in every patient who is at elevated risk and troponin monitoring 48–72 hours postoperatively.[16] Patients with poor functional capacity (<4 METS) need to undergo further cardiac testing. We recommend selecting a testing modality based on a patient's individual clinical presentation. The different modalities are discussed in brief here.

Stress testing: In routine practice, noninvasive stress testing is used to detect asymptomatic coronary artery disease (CAD) in patients with specific clinical indications. Preoperative stress testing should not be performed just because a patient is undergoing surgery,[25] and it should be limited to patients in whom asymptomatic CAD is suspected. There have been several studies evaluating the usefulness of preoperative stress testing in detecting CAD.[25–29] In addition, studies have shown that a higher percent of ischemic myocardium and multiple reversible defects on myocardial perfusion imaging are associated with a higher incidence of postop cardiac death or nonfatal MI.[30,31] Stress testing has a very high negative predictive value, but the positive predictive value is not very high. Therefore, patients with a negative stress test have a very low risk of postoperative cardiac complications, but its utility in the highest risk patients is somewhat limited.[32,33]

Resting echocardiography: The use of resting echocardiography in the preoperative setting should be primarily limited to evaluation of left ventricular ejection fraction in patients who are suspected of having systolic heart failure on the preliminary assessment or workup of suspected severe valvular disease in a patient undergoing semi-urgent or elective surgery. Resting echocardiography has not been shown to be superior to biomarker testing and is not recommended as a substitute to stress testing or BNP testing for elevated risk patients. This was discussed in detail earlier.

Role of preoperative electrocardiography: A 12-lead ECG is performed in a significant number of patients undergoing a preoperative evaluation. Its utility is well-defined in patients with arrhythmias, ischemic heart disease, and known CAD. However, the ECG may be normal or nonspecific even in patients with ischemic heart disease. Moreover, nonspecific, common baseline abnormalities make it less useful as a tool to diagnose asymptomatic CAD. It has been shown that bundle branch blocks, ST depressions, pathologic Q-waves, and left ventricular hypertrophy on preop ECGs were predictive of postoperative MIs.[34] However, the findings from different studies have not been consistent in defining which abnormalities correlate to higher risk of postoperative cardiac complications nor was this correlation found to be superior to using risk factors obtained from the patient's history.[3,35] Our recommendation is to use preoperative ECGs to aid decision-making in patients undergoing intermediate- or high-risk surgery.[3] Routine ECGs for every patient undergoing surgery are not recommended, and age cutoffs should not be used as this has not shown to be of benefit in predicting adverse cardiac outcomes from surgery.[34,36]

The proposed algorithm for preoperative cardiovascular risk stratification of neurosurgical patients is outlined in Figure 2.1.

PREOPERATIVE HEMOSTASIS RISK ASSESSMENT

An assessment of bleeding risk and identification of coagulation abnormalities is a vital step in all preoperative evaluations. Surgeries to the brain and spine, if complicated by bleeding, can have devastating consequences given the small confines of the central nervous system. If these are not detected and addressed in time, the patient may be left with permanent neurological deficits. Historically, an approach combining history and judicious lab testing has been favored.[37] Thorough history-taking can identify most coagulation abnormalities.[38,39] However, lab tests have the advantage of overcoming inconsistencies in the patient's memory in providing a history or a physician who does not obtain a proper history. Sometimes patients have a coagulation defect that has not yet presented itself or have an acquired coagulation defect that was not present at the time the patient last had surgery.[40] Therefore, we favor the combined approach outlined here.

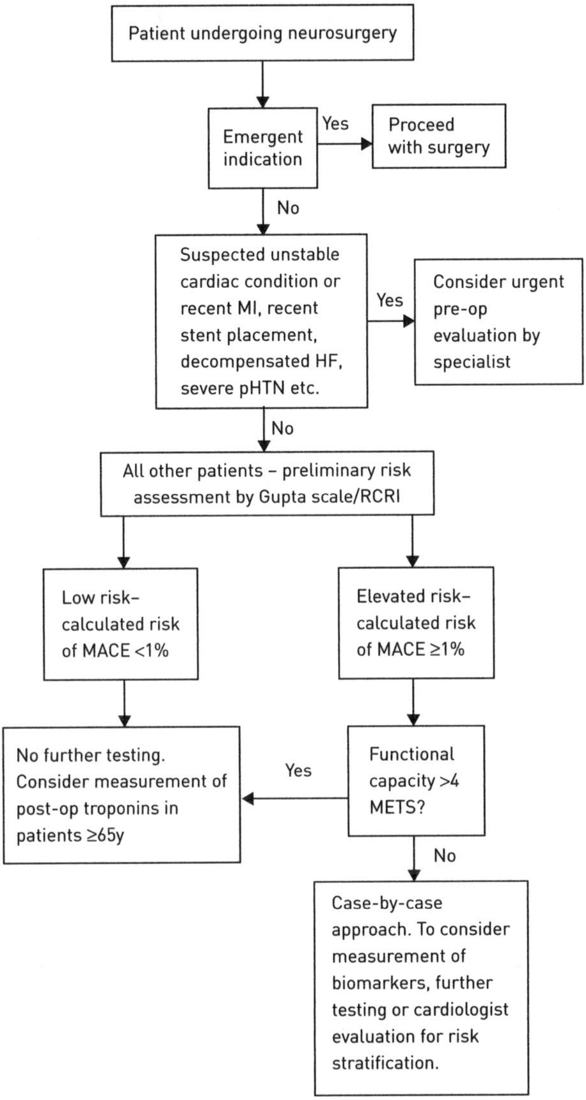

FIGURE 2.1 Cardiovascular risk stratification of patients undergoing neurosurgery.

Rapaport published a review in 1983 to guide physicians ordering lab tests for preop hemostasis assessment; most recommendations covered in his paper are still followed today. Detection of coagulation abnormalities requires a thorough and standardized approach to avoid missing any relevant information and to provide consistent results between different providers. We recommend using a questionnaire based on that published by Rapaport[37]; a slightly modified version is outlined here.

- Have you had prolonged bleeding after a minor injury such as biting your tongue or lip?
- Do you develop large bruises without any obvious injury?
- Have you had any tooth extractions? And if yes, for how long did you bleed after the extraction?

- Have you had any surgeries or procedures? Was bleeding difficult to control during or after these surgeries?
- What medications do you take? Do you take any anticoagulants or aspirin?
- Have any blood relatives had bleeding problems? If yes, what led to the bleeding event?

In addition to this questionnaire, a physical examination must be performed to look for signs such as petechiae, bruises, spider angiomas, joint deformities, hematomas, and the like. Routine laboratory testing of every patient undergoing surgery is not recommended.[37,39,41]

If the history and physical exam indicate that a coagulation abnormality is present, a prothrombin time (PT), activated partial thromboplastin time (aPTT), and platelet count should be checked.[41] A patient with a history of serious bleeding or a clinical condition such as liver disease requires a more comprehensive assessment and possibly referral to a specialist. For more details regarding management of bleeding disorders in the neurosurgical patients, please see Chapter 7.

VENOUS THROMBOEMBOLISM RISK IN THE NEUROSURGICAL PATIENT

Deep venous thrombosis (DVT) and pulmonary embolism (PE) are causes of significant morbidity and mortality in hospitalized patients and even more so in postoperative patients.[42] Moreover, neurosurgical patients are at high risk for DVT/PE, including patients with brain tumors, spine surgery, and patients undergoing craniotomy for indications other than tumors.[43-48] This makes the assessment and reduction of thromboembolism risk critical in all patients undergoing neurosurgery.

The modified Caprini index is a widely used scoring system based on the Caprini index modified by the American College of Chest Physicians (ACCP).[49] It has been validated in patients undergoing surgery. Points are assigned for various VTE risk factors and added up. Based on the total score, patients are grouped into very low risk, low risk, moderate risk and high risk (Figure 2.2). This provides a simple and easy-to-use method of estimating a surgical patient's VTE risk. The ACCP recommends prophylaxis based on estimated baseline risk; the recommendations are summarized in Figure 2.2.

Moreover, the ACCP guidelines provide recommendations for specific surgical procedures. We summarize those relevant to neurosurgeries here[49]:

- *Patients undergoing craniotomy*: Recommend mechanical prophylaxis versus no prophylaxis or pharmacological prophylaxis. For craniotomy patients at very high risk for VTE (undergoing surgery for malignancy) the addition of pharmacological prophylaxis (low-dose unfractionated heparin [UFH] 5,000 units SC q12h or q8h *or* low-molecular weight heparin [LMWH] 40 mg/d SC) to

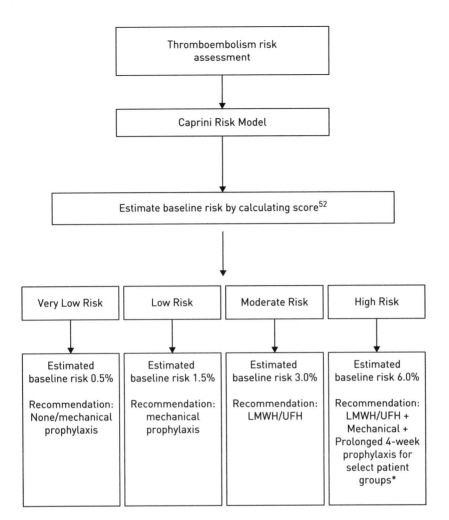

LMWH: low molecular weight heparin; UFH: unfractionated heparin.

*A Prolonged 4-week course of VTE prophylaxis is recommended for patients with cancer, and those undergoing abdominal and pelvis surgery.

FIGURE 2.2 Algorithm describing estimation of venous thromboembolic (VTE) baseline risk and prophylaxis recommendations.

mechanical is recommended once adequate hemostasis has been achieved and bleeding risk is deemed to be lowered.

- *Patients undergoing spine surgery*: Recommend mechanical prophylaxis over no prophylaxis, LMWH, or UFH. If a spine surgery patient is at high VTE risk (malignancy or anterior-posterior approach surgeries), then the addition of low-dose UFH 5,000 units SC q12h or q8h *or* LMWH 40 mg/d SC to mechanical prophylaxis is recommended after adequate hemostasis has been achieved and bleeding risk decreased as far as possible.

IVC filters were developed to prevent PE arising from the deep veins of the lower extremities when full-dose anticoagulation cannot be administered. However, use of IVC filters is also associated with complications arising from the presence of the device. In general, the ACCP guidelines do not recommend the use of IVC filters for VTE prophylaxis.[49] The development of retrievable filters has made it possible to decrease or, in theory, eliminate the occurrence of DVT associated with the long-term presence of an IVC filter. But, in practice, there are immediate complications after filter placement, and many retrievable filters are never removed.[50,51] Given that IVC filter placement is not widely recommended and that the decision for patient selection involves consideration of several complex clinical factors, we recommend that high-risk patients who have an acute proximal DVT with contraindications to anticoagulation be evaluated by a specialist for IVC filter placement. These patients should also have close follow-up in the postoperative period to coordinate retrieval of the filter with resumption of anticoagulation postoperatively.

CONCLUSION

In this chapter, we address the overall approach that a hospitalist physician should follow while risk stratifying a neurosurgical patient preoperatively. We review some of the relevant recent guidelines and recommendations, highlighting nuances specific to neurosurgical patients. Therefore, in addition to what is covered in this chapter, other general preoperative considerations common to the evaluation of patients undergoing noncardiac surgery should be followed. In conclusion, our current approach combines the recommendations from the ACC/AHA guidelines while incorporating new data and guidelines from the recently published Canadian guidelines for certain patients, and we recommend this approach until more data are available in support of the changes recommended in the Canadian update of 2017.

REFERENCES

1. Quinn TD, Brovman EY, Aglio LS, Urman RD. Factors associated with an increased risk of perioperative cardiac arrest in emergent and elective craniotomy and spine surgery. *Clin Neurol Neurosurg.* 2017;161:6–13.

2. Bapat S, Luoma AM. Current UK practice of preoperative risk assessment prior to neurosurgery. *Br J Neurosurg.* 2016;30:195–199.

3. Fleisher LA, Fleischmann KE, Auerbach AD, et al. 2014 ACC/AHA guideline on perioperative cardiovascular evaluation and management of patients undergoing noncardiac surgery: executive summary: a report of the American College of Cardiology/American Heart Association Task Force on practice guidelines. Developed in collaboration with the American College of Surgeons, American Society of Anesthesiologists, American Society of Echocardiography, American Society of Nuclear Cardiology, Heart Rhythm Society, Society for Cardiovascular Angiography and Interventions, Society of Cardiovascular Anesthesiologists, and Society of Vascular Medicine Endorsed by the Society of Hospital Medicine. *J Nucl Cardiol.* 2015;22:162–215.

4. Goldman L, Caldera DL, Nussbaum SR, et al. Multifactorial index of cardiac risk in noncardiac surgical procedures. *N Engl J Med.* 1977;297:845–850.

5. Lee TH, Marcantonio ER, Mangione CM, et al. Derivation and prospective validation of a simple index for prediction of cardiac risk of major noncardiac surgery. *Circulation.* 1999;100:1043–1049.

6. Goldman L. The revised cardiac risk index delivers what it promised. *Ann Intern Med.* 2010;152:57–58.

7. Ford MK, Beattie WS, Wijeysundera DN. Systematic review: prediction of perioperative cardiac complications and mortality by the revised cardiac risk index. *Ann Intern Med.* 2010;152:26–35.

8. Hall BL, Hamilton BH, Richards K, Bilimoria KY, Cohen ME, Ko CY. Does surgical quality improve in the American College of Surgeons National Surgical Quality Improvement Program: an evaluation of all participating hospitals. *Ann Surg.* 2009;250:363–376.

9. Khuri SF, Daley J, Henderson W, et al. The Department of Veterans Affairs' NSQIP: the first national, validated, outcome-based, risk-adjusted, and peer-controlled program for the measurement and enhancement of the quality of surgical care. National VA Surgical Quality Improvement Program. *Ann Surg.* 1998;228:491–507.

10. Bilimoria KY, Liu Y, Paruch JL, et al. Development and evaluation of the universal ACS NSQIP surgical risk calculator: a decision aid and informed consent tool for patients and surgeons. *J Am Coll Surg.* 2013;217:833–842 e1–e3.

11. Cohn SL, Subramanian S. Estimation of cardiac risk before noncardiac surgery: the evolution of cardiac risk indices. *Hosp Pract (1995).* 2014;42:46–57.

12. Gupta PK, Gupta H, Sundaram A, et al. Development and validation of a risk calculator for prediction of cardiac risk after surgery. *Circulation.* 2011;124:381–387.

13. Reilly DF, McNeely MJ, Doerner D, et al. Self-reported exercise tolerance and the risk of serious perioperative complications. *Arch Intern Med.* 1999;159:2185–2192.

14. Hlatky MA, Boineau RE, Higginbotham MB, et al. A brief self-administered questionnaire to determine functional capacity (the Duke Activity Status Index). *Am J Cardiol.* 1989;64:651–654.

15. Wijeysundera DN, Pearse RM, Shulman MA, et al. Assessment of functional capacity before major non-cardiac surgery: an international, prospective cohort study. *Lancet.* 2018;391:2631–2640.

16. Duceppe E, Parlow J, MacDonald P, et al. Canadian Cardiovascular Society Guidelines on Perioperative Cardiac Risk Assessment and Management for Patients Who Undergo Noncardiac Surgery. *Can J Cardiol.* 2017;33:17–32.

17. Karthikeyan G, Moncur RA, Levine O, et al. Is a preoperative brain natriuretic peptide or N-terminal pro-B-type natriuretic peptide measurement an independent predictor of adverse cardiovascular outcomes within 30 days of noncardiac surgery? A systematic review and meta-analysis of observational studies. *J Am Coll Cardiol.* 2009;54:1599–1606.

18. Rodseth RN, Biccard BM, Le Manach Y, et al. The prognostic value of preoperative and postoperative B-type natriuretic peptides in patients undergoing noncardiac surgery: B-type natriuretic peptide and N-terminal fragment of pro-B-type natriuretic peptide: a systematic review and individual patient data meta-analysis. *J Am Coll Cardiol.* 2014;63:170–180.

19. Rodseth RN, Padayachee L, Biccard BM. A meta-analysis of the utility of preoperative brain natriuretic peptide in predicting early and intermediate-term mortality and major adverse cardiac events in vascular surgical patients. *Anaesthesia.* 2008;63:1226–1233.

20. Ryding AD, Kumar S, Worthington AM, Burgess D. Prognostic value of brain natriuretic peptide in noncardiac surgery: a meta-analysis. *Anesthesiology.* 2009;111:311–319.

21. Young YR, Sheu BF, Li WC, et al. Predictive value of plasma brain natriuretic peptide for postoperative cardiac complications—a systemic review and meta-analysis. *J Crit Care.* 2014;29:696 e1–e10.

22. Park SJ, Choi JH, Cho SJ, et al. Comparison of transthoracic echocardiography with N-terminal pro-brain natriuretic peptide as a tool for risk stratification of patients undergoing major noncardiac surgery. *Korean Circ J.* 2011;41:505–511.

23. Levy M, Heels-Ansdell D, Hiralal R, et al. Prognostic value of troponin and creatine kinase muscle and brain isoenzyme measurement after noncardiac surgery: a systematic review and meta-analysis. *Anesthesiology.* 2011;114:796–806.

24. Vascular Events in Noncardiac Surgery Patients Cohort Evaluation Study I, Devereaux PJ, Chan MT, et al. Association between postoperative troponin levels and 30-day mortality among patients undergoing noncardiac surgery. *JAMA.* 2012;307:2295–2304.

25. Carliner NH, Fisher ML, Plotnick GD, et al. Routine preoperative exercise testing in patients undergoing major noncardiac surgery. *Am J Cardiol.* 1985;56:51–58.

26. Leppo J, Plaja J, Gionet M, Tumolo J, Paraskos JA, Cutler BS. Noninvasive evaluation of cardiac risk before elective vascular surgery. *J Am Coll Cardiol.* 1987;9:269–276.

27. Mangano DT, London MJ, Tubau JF, et al. Dipyridamole thallium-201 scintigraphy as a preoperative screening test. A reexamination of its predictive potential. Study of Perioperative Ischemia Research Group. *Circulation.* 1991;84:493–502.

28. McPhail N, Calvin JE, Shariatmadar A, Barber GG, Scobie TK. The use of preoperative exercise testing to predict cardiac complications after arterial reconstruction. *J Vasc Surg.* 1988;7:60–68.

29. Arous EJ, Baum PL, Cutler BS. The ischemic exercise test in patients with peripheral vascular disease. Implications for management. *Arch Surg.* 1984;119:780–783.

30. Etchells E, Meade M, Tomlinson G, Cook D. Semiquantitative dipyridamole myocardial stress perfusion imaging for cardiac risk assessment before noncardiac vascular surgery: a meta-analysis. *J Vasc Surg.* 2002;36:534–540.

31. Shaw LJ, Eagle KA, Gersh BJ, Miller DD. Meta-analysis of intravenous dipyridamole-thallium-201 imaging (1985 to 1994) and dobutamine echocardiography (1991 to 1994) for risk stratification before vascular surgery. *J Am Coll Cardiol.* 1996;27:787–798.

32. Kertai MD, Boersma E, Bax JJ, et al. A meta-analysis comparing the prognostic accuracy of six diagnostic tests for predicting perioperative cardiac risk in patients undergoing major vascular surgery. *Heart.* 2003;89:1327–1334.

33. Picano E, Bedetti G, Varga A, Cseh E. The comparable diagnostic accuracies of dobutamine-stress and dipyridamole-stress echocardiographies: a meta-analysis. *Coron Artery Dis.* 2000;11:151–159.

34. Noordzij PG, Boersma E, Bax JJ, et al. Prognostic value of routine preoperative electrocardiography in patients undergoing noncardiac surgery. *Am J Cardiol.* 2006;97:1103–1106.

35. van Klei WA, Bryson GL, Yang H, Kalkman CJ, Wells GA, Beattie WS. The value of routine preoperative electrocardiography in predicting myocardial infarction after noncardiac surgery. *Ann Surg.* 2007;246:165–170.

36. Liu LL, Dzankic S, Leung JM. Preoperative electrocardiogram abnormalities do not predict postoperative cardiac complications in geriatric surgical patients. *J Am Geriatr Soc.* 2002;50:1186–1191.

37. Rapaport SI. Preoperative hemostatic evaluation: which tests, if any? *Blood.* 1983;61:229–231.

38. Laine C, Williams SV, Wilson JF. In the clinic. Preoperative evaluation. *Ann Intern Med.* 2009;151:ITC1–15, quiz ITC6.

39. Eisenberg JM, Clarke JR, Sussman SA. Prothrombin and partial thromboplastin times as preoperative screening tests. *Arch Surg.* 1982;117:48–51.

40. Akamatsu Y, Hayashi T, Yamamoto J, Karibe H, Kameyama M, Tominaga T. Newly diagnosed acquired hemophilia a manifesting as massive intracranial hemorrhage following a neurosurgical procedure. *World Neurosurg.* 2018;111:175–180.

41. Chee YL, Crawford JC, Watson HG, Greaves M. Guidelines on the assessment of bleeding risk prior to surgery or invasive procedures. British Committee for Standards in Haematology. *Br J Haematol.* 2008;140:496–504.

42. Stubbs JM, Assareh H, Curnow J, Hitos K, Achat HM. Incidence of in-hospital and post-discharge diagnosed hospital-associated venous thromboembolism using linked administrative data. *Intern Med J.* 2018;48:157–165.

43. Chan AT, Atiemo A, Diran LK, et al. Venous thromboembolism occurs frequently in patients undergoing brain tumor surgery despite prophylaxis. *J Thromb Thrombolysis.* 1999;8:139–142.

44. Cote DJ, Smith TR. Venous thromboembolism in brain tumor patients. *J Clin Neurosci.* 2016;25:13–18.

45. Geerts WH, Bergqvist D, Pineo GF, et al. Prevention of venous thromboembolism: American College of Chest Physicians Evidence-Based Clinical Practice Guidelines (8th edition). *Chest.* 2008;133:381S–453S.

46. Hamilton MG, Hull RD, Pineo GF. Prophylaxis of venous thromboembolism in brain tumor patients. *J Neurooncol.* 1994;22:111–126.

47. Jeraq M, Cote DJ, Smith TR. Venous thromboembolism in brain tumor patients. *Adv Exp Med Biol.* 2017;906:215–228.

48. White RH, Zhou H, Romano PS. Incidence of symptomatic venous thromboembolism after different elective or urgent surgical procedures. *Thromb Haemost.* 2003;90:446–455.

49. Gould MK, Garcia DA, Wren SM, et al. Prevention of VTE in nonorthopedic surgical patients: Antithrombotic Therapy and Prevention of Thrombosis, 9th ed: American College of Chest Physicians Evidence-Based Clinical Practice Guidelines. *Chest.* 2012;141:e227S–e77S.

50. Dabbagh O, Nagam N, Chitima-Matsiga R, Bearelly S, Bearelly D. Retrievable inferior vena cava filters are not getting retrieved: where is the gap? *Thromb Res.* 2010;126:493–497.

51. Mismetti P, Rivron-Guillot K, Quenet S, et al. A prospective long-term study of 220 patients with a retrievable vena cava filter for secondary prevention of venous thromboembolism. *Chest.* 2007;131:223–229.

52. Gould MK, Garcia DA, et al. Prevention of VTE in nonorthopedic surgical patients: Antithrombotic Therapy and Prevention of Thrombosis, 9th ed: American College of Chest Physicians Evidence-Based Clinical Practice Guidelines. *Chest.* 2012 Feb; 141:e227S–e277S. Erratum in: *Chest.* 2012;141:1369

3 Medical Management of Patients with Subarachnoid or Intracranial Hemorrhage and Increased Intracranial Pressure

Ahmad Sweid, Pascal M. Jabbour,
Sage P. Rahm, Stavropoula Tjoumakaris,
M. Reid Gooch, and
Robert H. Rosenwasser

SUBARACHNOID HEMORRHAGE

Introduction

Subarachnoid hemorrhage (SAH), bleeding into the subarachnoid space of the meninges, is often a life-altering event for patients (Figure 3.1). Nearly a quarter of patients die before arrival to the hospital,[1,2] and 45% of all SAH patients die within the first few days.[3] Half of those who survive remain neurologically compromised,[2,4] with 20% demonstrating global cognitive impairment after 1 year.[5] Many struggles to reintegrate back into their daily lives and may be unable to remain employed or live independently.[5] Early diagnosis and appropriate treatment are imperative, as patients who are misdiagnosed are four times more likely to suffer from disability and mortality than those treated appropriately.[6]

The most common cause of SAH is posttraumatic, commonly after car accidents or large falls where the head receives forceful contact. These patients will frequently present with skull fractures, traumatic brain injuries, intracerebral hemorrhage (ICH), subdural hematomas, epidural hematomas, or other systemic injuries

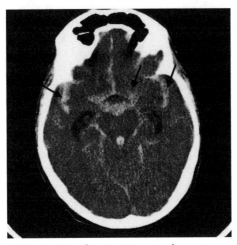

FIGURE 3.1 Subarachnoid hemorrhage (marked by arrows).

requiring intensive care. Prognosis often depends on the severity of trauma and the amount of intracranial bleeding.[7-10]

Aneurysm rupture remains the second most common cause of SAH (aSAH). An estimated 6.5 per 100,000 people a year will suffer from an aneurysmal SAH worldwide, affecting nearly 500,000 individuals annually.[11] Individuals above the age of 50 are the most affected.[12]

Significant risk factors for aSAH are a prior aSAH and the presence of an intracranial aneurysm (particularly if >7 mm).[13-15] Individuals with a family history of aSAH, autosomal dominant polycystic disease, fibromuscular dysplasia, and type IV Ehlers-Danlos syndrome carry an increased risk of aSAH. Well-known common modifiable risk factors for aSAH are hypertension, tobacco use, and sympathomimetic drugs.[2,12]

In 5% of cases, SAH is due to a cerebral arteriovenous malformation (AVM). AVMs are disorganized bundles of arteries and veins with no cerebral tissue within the tangled vessels. AVMs may be surgically resected, thrombosed with stereotactic radiosurgery, or treated endovascularly with adhesive glues, coils, or other materials to prevent blood flow through the vascular bundle.[16,17] A few other uncommon causes of SAH include vasculitis, tumors, superficial cerebral artery rupture, pituitary apoplexy, dural sinus thrombosis, and coagulation disorders.[1]

Symptoms and Diagnosis of Subarachnoid Hemorrhage

One of the most common symptoms of SAH includes a thunderclap headache ("worst headache of my life") that occurs in nearly 80% of patients.[18] Less than half of patients with aSAH may experience a sentinel headache beginning 2–8 weeks prior to aneurysm rupture. Sentinel headaches often indicate a worse prognosis due to increased risk of rebleed or rerupture of an aneurysm. Patients with aSAH are at high risk of rebleed within hours of the first episode.[19]

Box 3.1 Hunt and Hess Score[26]

0   Intact aneurysm

1   May present with no symptoms or a headache and mild neck stiffness

2   No focal neurological deficits except for a cranial nerve palsy, nuchal rigidity with moderate to a severe headache

3   Mild focal neurological deficit; confused or drowsy

4   Stuporous, may have a moderate to severe hemiparesis

5   Coma, decerebrate posturing

Blood and its breakdown products in the subarachnoid space trigger inflammation. Inflammation of the meninges and brain parenchyma can trigger nausea and vomiting, stiff neck, and photophobia. Inflammation, elevated intracranial pressure (ICP), and ischemia lead to temporary loss of consciousness or focal neurological deficits such as ocular palsies. On examination of the inner eye, there may be evidence of ocular hemorrhage in some patients.[2,20]

The severity of an SAH should be graded. The two most common scales used to grade SAH are the Hunt and Hess (H&H) Score and the World Federation of Neurological Surgeons (WFNS) grading scale (Boxes 3.1 and 3.2). Higher grade H&H scores (IV and V) require more intensive care and have significantly higher mortality rates and reduced long-term functional outcomes overall.[21,22]

The gold standard diagnostic imaging study for SAH is a CT scan without contrast.[2] Within the first 3 days of SAH, CT without contrast has a nearly 100% accuracy and will often reveal blood as abnormal hyperdensity in the subarachnoid space.[23,24] Traumatic SAH will often have blood in the sulci at the vertex of the brain, whereas SAH from aneurysms will often present with blood in the basal cisterns or ventricles.[24]

If a CT scan returns negative and there is still a high clinical suspicion of SAH, a lumbar puncture may be used to detect xanthochromia. A lumbar puncture is very sensitive but may result in a false positive due to a traumatic tap, so clinicians are advised to utilize the fourth vial of cerebrospinal fluid (CSF) collected. The CSF in

Box 3.2 World Federation of Neurological Surgeons Grading Scale[27]

1   No motor deficit and Glasgow Coma Scale (GCS) of 15

2   No motor deficit and GCS 13–14

3   Motor deficit and GCS 13–14

4   A motor deficit may or may not be present, GCS 7–12

5   A motor deficit may or may not be present, GCS 3–6

SAH should have normal glucose levels but elevated proteins and red blood cells (>100,000 cells per cubic meter). If there is obstructive hydrocephalus and increased ICP, lumbar puncture is contraindicated due to increased risk of cerebral herniation.

When a CT scan is inconclusive or the source of an SAH needs to be identified, CT angiography (CTA), digital subtraction angiography (DSA), or magnetic resonance angiography (MRA) may be ordered.[2,25,26]

If an aneurysm is identified as the culprit of the SAH and the patient is hemodynamically stable, he or she may be eligible for aneurysm repair treatments. Neurological surgeons and interventional neuroradiologists can secure aneurysms endovascularly by either filling the aneurysm with coils or inserting a flow diverter inducing aneurysm thrombosis.[27,28] A patient may also undergo microsurgical clipping, where a clip is placed across the aneurysm neck. These treatment options all aim to prevent blood flow within the aneurysm sac and significantly reduce the risk of aneurysmal rupture.

Admitting and Managing Subarachnoid Hemorrhage Patients

A patient suffering from acute SAH may develop hemodynamic instability and respiratory failure. The patient's airway must be secured. Following a traumatic incident, the cervical spine must be stabilized. The patient should be admitted to the ICU for at least 14 days with vital signs and neurological exams taken every hour. A complete blood count (CBC), blood metabolic panel, arterial blood gas, and coagulation studies should be ordered daily. Blood glucose should be monitored closely. A cardiac event recorder should be started on admission as arrhythmias are common in SAH patients.[1,29-32]

A CT scan without contrast should be ordered to diagnose SAH. Once diagnosed, a CTA or DSA may be indicated to identify whether an aneurysm is the culprit. High-grade patients may require a ventriculostomy and placement of an intraventricular catheter (IVC), mainly if there is significant hemorrhage on the CT scan. The IVC in high-grade patients allows for monitoring of ICP.

In patients with a decreased level of consciousness, an arterial line is recommended to monitor blood pressure. Systolic blood pressure (SBP) goals are between 120 and 160 mm Hg.[2] If SBP is above 160 mm Hg, nicardipine or labetalol administration is recommended.[33,34] Decreasing SBP below 120 mm Hg may cause insufficient blood flow to the brain and exacerbate complications.

The overall goal in these patients is to ensure consistent cerebral blood flow (CBF) by maintaining euvolemia and appropriate cerebral perfusion.[1] Volume loss is common in SAH patients—the clinician must ensure that the patient does not become volume depleted by monitoring the patient's "ins and outs" (I&Os) along with the patient's daily weight. Hypovolemia is often exacerbated by a patient's NPO diet placed in preparation for aneurysm treatment.

Not uncommonly, SAH patients may experience hyponatremia due to the syndrome of inappropriate antidiuretic hormone secretion (SIADH) or cerebral salt wasting (CSW).[35,36] Electrolytes should be ordered daily. Tracking urine and serum osmolality may enable differentiation of SIADH from the CSW profile. Patients who develop hyponatremia should not receive hypotonic fluids. Sodium levels can be stabilized with normal saline (NS) and potassium chloride (20 mg/L at 2 mL/kg/h). Hyponatremia may also be treated with intravenous 3% saline; electrolytes should be checked every 4–6 hours in this case.[37,38] If the hematocrit values are below 40% on admission, 4% albumin (500 mL over 4 hours) may be administered.[2]

The patient room should be set up appropriately. These patients may experience photophobia and should be placed in a quiet, low-stimulation environment with no visitors. The bed should be tilted to a 30-degree angle. Intravenous ondansetron (4 mg q8h hours) reduces the risk of vomiting and aspiration pneumonia. If the patient is nonambulatory or unconscious, insert a Foley catheter. Order pneumatic compression boots to decrease the risk of deep vein thrombosis (DVT). To avoid constipation due to the lack of mobility and hospital diet, docusate (100 mg twice a day) may be given prophylactically. Proton pump inhibitors (PPIs) such as lansoprazole and H$_2$ receptor blockers are given to reduce the risk of stress ulcers.

If the patient has a history of seizures or is at risk of developing seizures, short-term antiepileptic drug (AED) administration (levetiracetam 500 mg PO or IV q12h) may be provided.[2] Occupational therapy, physical therapy, and speech and language pathology should be consulted to improve recovery and to recommend appropriate rehabilitation therapy at discharge.[1]

The initial management is essential as it can significantly decrease the risk of morbidity and mortality in these patients.

Complications of Subarachnoid Hemorrhage
Fever

Fever affects nearly 70% of individuals with aSAH and is associated with worse clinical outcomes.[39–43] Elevated temperatures should be treated aggressively with cooling blankets and antipyretic medications such as acetaminophen or ibuprofen.[44,45] The goal is normothermia. It is essential to distinguish inflammatory fever from infectious fever to avoid unnecessary antibiotic administration.

Rebleed

An aneurysmal SAH carries a 4–22% risk of rebleeding, particularly within the first 24 hours.[19,46–49] Close to half of the rebleeds will occur within the first 6 hours of the original aSAH.[50] If an aneurysm is not secured after an SAH, there is a 50% risk of rebleed in the following 6 months.[51] Rebleeds are associated with higher mortality and worse long-term outcomes.[52] Treat early and maintain systolic blood pressure between 120 and 160 mm Hg.[2] When choosing an appropriate antihypertensive, nicardipine has shown significant benefit. An alternative to nicardipine is clevidipine, which has a more rapid onset of action.[2] Labetalol and sodium nitroprusside may be considered but do not lower blood pressure as evenly as nicardipine.[33,34]

If an aneurysm is suitable for treatment and the patient is hemodynamically stable, the optimal method of preventing a rebleed is to secure the aneurysm endovascularly or surgically. Since most rebleeds occur within the first 24 hours, rapid obliteration of an aneurysm is recommended.[2,19]

Hydrocephalus

Hydrocephalus is estimated to occur in 15–20% of SAH patient.[53-57] New-onset hydrocephalus often presents with headaches, nausea, blurred vision, unsteady gait, drowsiness, behavioral changes, and potentially seizures.

In those who develop hydrocephalus, 30–60% will show no changes in mental status.[58,59] Generally, half of those affected will improve spontaneously.[58] Ventriculostomy is recommended in those with decreased levels of consciousness since it is difficult to monitor changes in their neurological function.

Acute hydrocephalus may be managed temporarily with acetazolamide or mannitol, although, eventually, these patients will require drain placement. An extraventricular drain (EVD) may be placed for short-term management and a ventriculoperitoneal shunt (VPS) for long-term management.[58,60,61] The goal is to maintain ICPs around 15–25 mm Hg.[62]

Delayed Cerebral Ischemia and Vasospasm

After an SAH, patients are prone to cerebral artery vasospasm, a narrowing of a cerebral artery. When a cerebral artery vasospasms, it may cut off the blood supply to the downstream tissue causing delayed cerebral ischemia (DCI). Patients are at highest risk of developing vasospasms between day 7 and day 21 post-SAH, but in some cases as early as day 4.[2] When small arteries are affected, there may be no noticeable neurological changes, but when a large artery is affected, symptoms may mimic those of a thromboembolic stroke (middle cerebral artery [MCA] syndrome) and lead to significant morbidity and mortality.[52,63] Generally, 30–70% of patients who suffer from SAH will develop vasospasms on angiography.[64]

Vasospasm may lead to altered mental status, focal neurological deficits, and a decreased Glasgow Coma Score (GCS). A CT without contrast is often necessary along with arterial blood gas, CBC, and electrolytes to rule out other potential causes such as stroke, rebleed, hydrocephalus, and hyponatremia.[65]

The modified Fisher Grading Scale may aid in predicting the likelihood of developing vasospasms (Box 3.3). The higher the score, the increased the risk of developing vasospasm.

Frequent neurological exams may help identify DCI in patients who are responsive and with high GCS.[1] Transcranial Doppler ultrasound (TCD) may detect presymptomatic vasospasms. Perfusion imaging with either a CT scan or an MRI may also diagnose vasospasm.[2]

Early administration of nimodipine (60 mg q4h for 21 days; 30 mg q2h if hypotension occurs)[66] and maintenance of euvolemia significantly decrease the risk of vasospasm.[67-69] If a patient develops vasospasms, hemodynamic augmentation therapy (triple H therapy) may be indicated.[70,71]

> **Box 3.3** Modified Fisher Scale Determined via CT Scan Without Contrast
>
> 0   No SAH or intraventricular hemorrhage (IVH)
> 1   Thin focal or diffuse SAH (<1 mm), no IVH
> 2   Thin focal or diffuse SAH (<1 mm), IVH
> 3   Thick focal or diffuse SAH (>1 mm), no IVH
> 4   Thick focal or diffuse SAH (>1 mm), IVH
>
> *IVH, intraventricular hemorrhage; SAH, subarachnoid hemorrhage.*

Triple H therapy involves hemodilution, hypervolemia, and hypertensive therapy. Ensure that the patient does not have elevated ICP before initiating treatment. Hemodilution aims to keep hematocrit at 30–35%, although its use is controversial.[72] Hypervolemia focuses on maintaining euvolemia with crystalloid fluids (e.g., normal saline and lactated Ringer's) while avoiding a volume overloaded state.[72] Hypertensive therapy involves the use of norepinephrine, phenylephrine, and dopamine with mean arterial pressure (MAP) goals ranging from 70 to 210 mm Hg and SBP within 140–240 mm Hg (pressures should be raised in 15% SBP increments).[73-75] Hypertensives are withheld in patients already on hypertensives or with a contraindicated cardiac disease.[2] Be wary of developing signs of pulmonary edema and rebleeds.

If triple H therapy fails, endovascular therapy may be provided. Percutaneous transluminal balloon angioplasty (PTCA), an endovascular catheter-based procedure, may be used to relieve approximately 90%[76] of proximal vasospasms in large-caliber cerebral vessels.[77] Catheter-released vasodilators such as calcium channel blockers, nitric oxide (NO), and papaverine may resolve more distal cerebral vasospasms in small-caliber arteries.[78,79]

Seizures

Recent studies suggest that 1–10%[80-82] of individuals with SAH may develop seizures; whether they are of epileptic origin is unclear. Seizures predominantly appear within the first 24 hours and may be an indicator of increased ICP, inflammation, and tissue hypoxia.[83,84] Appropriate prophylactic AED treatment remains controversial, as extensive research has not been conducted on the topic.

Current guidelines recommend AED use posthemorrhagic SAH immediately if deemed necessary, particularly in patients with prior seizures, intracerebral hematomas, intractable hypertension, infarction, and an MCA aneurysm.[2] Interestingly, a recent propensity score-matched analysis of 350 patients with spontaneous SAH demonstrated that AEDs do not adequately prevent seizures in SAH patients.[80] Insufficient evidence supports the routine use of prophylactic AEDs.[2] Chapter 5 covers antiseizure drugs in more detail.

Hyponatremia

Hyponatremia occurs in 10–30% of cases of SAH with an average duration of 4 days.[2,85-87] One cause of hyponatremia is the natriuretic peptide release that triggers salt wasting and water loss in the kidney.[35,36] Another cause of hyponatremia is SIADH, which leads to water retention due to increased release of ADH.[35,36]

Significant hyponatremia to treat has been suggested recently as sodium of 130 mEq/L or less.[88] Do not induce volume contraction or administer hypotonic fluids. In patients with high-grade SAH, volume status should be monitored via central venous pressures and pulmonary wedge pressure. Administer intravenous 3% saline and check electrolytes every 4–6 hours.[37,38] Crystalloid fluids may also be utilized to maintain euvolemia in these patients.

SIADH hyponatremic patients may be fluid-restricted to less than 500 mL/day,[89] but current guidelines generally do not recommend fluid restriction.[86] If SIADH patients become hypovolemic, treat with crystalloids or packed red blood cells to ensure adequate blood flow to the brain.[2] Please see Chapter 9 for more details on the management of hyponatremia.

Hyperglycemia

The American Diabetes Association (ADA) suggests maintaining glucose levels below 180 mg/dL in noncritical patients and between 110 and 140 mg/dL in selective critical patients.[90] In patients with SAH, hyperglycemia is associated with worse outcomes, increased risk of stroke within the first 72 hours, and an increased risk of vasospasm.[91-93] Hyperglycemia on admission, along with blood glucose variations during the hospital stay, are correlated with increased 1-year mortality.[94,95]

Management of hyperglycemia is described in detail in Chapter 10.

Anemia

To date, there is no common optimal goal for hemoglobin level. It is known that increased hemoglobin improves oxygen delivery to the brain and is associated with positive outcomes and decreased incidence of vasospasm.[96-99] Current guidelines do not recommend packed red blood cell (RBC) transfusions in all patients who are anemic.[2,100] The Neurocritical Care Society (NCS) advises maintaining hemoglobin above 8–10 g/dL.[71] Patients maintained with a hemoglobin of greater than 10 g/dL demonstrated improved outcomes, although patients who were anemic before hemorrhage did not show significant improvement.[101]

In-Hospital Venous Thromboembolism

SAH patients have a 4.4% risk of developing a VTE.[102] VTE encompasses DVT and pulmonary embolism (PE).[103]

Prophylactic therapy such as pneumatic compression boots and anticoagulants such as low-molecular-weight heparin (LMWH) alternatives (enoxaparin sodium) are recommended.[104,105] Subcutaneous injection of heparin is an appropriate option as well, but it confers a higher risk of heparin-induced thrombocytopenia (HIT) type II.

Pulmonary Complications

Some institutions stipulate that pulmonary complications in SAH patients such as pneumonia, PEs, neurogenic pulmonary edema, and acute respiratory distress (ARDS) may account for nearly 50% of the fatal complications in the first 3 months after SAH.[106–109]

Ventilator-associated pneumonia may be one of the most common complications and must be treated with antibiotics. Transitioning from a ventilator to a tracheostomy has shown to reduce pulmonary complications significantly, as has maintaining normoglycemia, improving the patient's oral hygiene, and administering cefuroxime at the time of initial intubation (two 1,500 mg doses).[110,111]

Neurogenic pulmonary edema (NPE) is associated with increased catecholamine release due to increased ICP. NPE often resolves within the first 72 hours when managed conservatively with positive pressure ventilation (low PEEP) and reduction of elevated ICP.

Cardiac Complications

Cardiac complications may occur in up to 50% of SAH patients and often present as arrhythmias, subclinical troponin release (<2.8 ng/mL),[112] ECG abnormalities, and stress-induced cardiomyopathy.[30–32,113–116]

Monitoring cardiac function with ECG is recommended. Any evidence of stress-induced cardiomyopathy or ST-T changes should receive a cardiac workup,[1,114] An echocardiogram may be indicated in patients with an increased troponin level or a high-grade SAH.[29,114] Patients with reduced ejection fractions, particularly if they are showing signs of hypotension or congestive heart failure, may be given dobutamine (with SBP <90 mm Hg and decreased SVR) or milrinone (with SBP >90 mm Hg or patients on long-term beta blockers).[117]

Pregnancy-Related Subarachnoid Hemorrhage

SAH is associated with 4.1% of pregnancy-related deaths.[118,119] Women with hypertensive disorders, coagulopathy, increased maternal age, aneurysms, or AVMs are at increased risk.[119,120] Peripartum SAH is frequently nonaneurysmal and is due to a venous bleed from an intracranial venous thrombosis or a pial vessel rupture due to hypertension.[119,120]

Managing pregnant SAH patients requires consideration of the fetus. Noncontrast CT must have shielding of the fetus. Agents such as AEDs should be used carefully. Mannitol and nitroprusside should be avoided. Nimodipine must be used cautiously as it may be teratogenic.[1] The fetus may be delivered vaginally or via C-section if it is older than 24 weeks. Generally, obstetrician-gynecologists should be consulted before the neurosurgical intervention.

INTRACEREBRAL HEMORRHAGE
Introduction

ICH is defined as blood localized within brain parenchyma (Figure 3.2). Primary ICH and SAH account for 10–20% of stroke subtypes.[121] The incidence has been stable over the recent decades at 24.6 per 100,000 person-years,[122] however, the case mortality has fallen over the past four decades from 47% to 29%.[123] ICH may be a consequence of different etiologies; however, 60% are due to a rupture of a small arteriole secondary to chronic hypertension. A most common location is in the basal ganglia, thalamus, pons (brainstem), and cerebellum. Other etiologies include cerebral amyloid angiopathy, coagulopathy, sympathomimetic drugs such as cocaine, and underlying vascular anomalies such as AVMs or cavernous malformations.[124] Acute ICH is not only complex and etiologically diverse, but also the most serious, least treatable, and more variable in incidence and management compared to other stroke subtypes.[125] Most importantly, its consequence concerning "loss of productive life years" is disproportionately greater on a global scale than is acute ischemic stroke because ICH is severe and tends to affect people at earlier ages.[126] Patients who make it to the hospital still face a 30-day fatality risk of up to 45% in some studies.[127] There is good evidence that, similar to an ischemic stroke, management of ICH patients on specialized multidisciplinary stroke or neurocritical care units improves outcome.[128] Management of ICH includes both medical and surgical components. The initial management during the golden hour has a drastic effect on the outcome.

Initial Evaluation

The majority of fatalities occur in the first 2 days of the onset of symptoms.[129] Rapid initial diagnosis is crucial in the early management of ICH.[130]

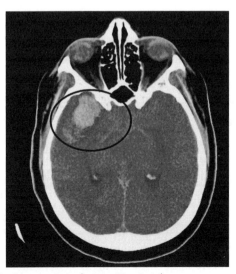

FIGURE 3.2 Intracerebral hemorrhage (marked by circle).

- Patients with ICH need to be immediately evaluated for airway protection, breathing, and circulation. If the patient has a depressed level of consciousness and a GCS of 8 or lower, endotracheal intubation should follow.
- Next, the clinical severity should be scored and documented using the National Institutes of Health (NIH) Stroke Scale (NIHSS) and the GCS.
- Then rapid and accurate diagnosis using neuroimaging should be performed. The American Heart Association considers neuroimaging with CT (the gold standard) or MRI mandatory, with the use of contrast-enhanced CTA when available to assess for vascular pathology and likelihood of further clot expansion.[131,132]
- After having the diagnosis of ICH, immediate consideration should be given to the need for[124]
  - Acute control of elevated blood pressure
  - Correction of coagulopathy due to medications or underlying medical conditions
  - The need for urgent surgical hematoma evacuation
- Laboratory testing in cases suggestive of ICH should include CBC including platelets, an INR, a partial thromboplastin time (PTT) for hematologic disorders, a toxicology screen for sympathomimetic drug use, and serum glucose, as elevated levels have been associated with hematoma expansion and worse outcomes.
- The anticipation of specific patient care needs such as:
  - Specific treatment aspects related to underlying ICH cause
  - Risk for early clinical deterioration and hematoma expansion; Hematoma expansion occurs in up to one-third of patients and generally occurs within 24 hours although delayed expansion is described.[133] The expansion, regardless of definition, is significantly associated with clinical deterioration and worse outcomes, especially when resulting in midline shift or cerebral herniation.[131] Volume status should be assessed along with routine monitoring of electrolytes.
  - Need for ICP or other neuromonitoring

Managing Intracerebral Hemorrhage Patients
Hemostasis and Coagulopathy, Antiplatelet Agents

Patients with platelet abnormality, coagulation factor deficiency, or who are taking anticoagulants have an increased likelihood of intraparenchymal hemorrhage (IPH) expansion, higher mortality, and worse outcome.[134] The immediate reversal of anticoagulation is a must to decrease the risk of mortality.

Heparin acts by inactivating thrombin through binding to antithrombin, leading to thrombolysis. Heparin-induced ICH can be easily treated by reversal of heparin action. Protamine sulfate reverses the action of heparin given at a rate of 1 mg per 100 units of heparin received in the prior 2 hours, with a maximum dose of 50 mg.[135] If the last dose of heparin was given more than 4 hours earlier, then reversal with protamine sulfate is likely unnecessary due to the short half-life of heparin. LMWH follows the same process; however its half-life is up to 8 hours, and incomplete reversal might happen with protamine.[124]

The current guideline recommends that patients taking vitamin K antagonist (VKA) should receive a rapid-acting agent for an immediate effect in addition to the administration of 5–10 mg of vitamin K intravenously by slow push because vitamin K typically takes hours after administration to reverse VKA, but it has a more long-lasting effect.[136] Although for years the rapid-acting agent used was fresh frozen plasma (FFP), recently more effective alternatives have been used such as prothrombin complex concentrates (PCC), activated PCC factor VIII inhibitor bypassing activity (FEIBA), and recombinant activated factor VIIa (rFVIIa).[131] Recently the Neurocritical Care Society recommended weight-based dosing for PCC, with the dose adjusted based on INR.[137] In contrast to FFP, PCC is readily available, does not need compatibility testing before transfusion, and the smaller volume allows infusion over a shorter period with the lower risk of fluid overload.[136,138] Large-volume FFP (10–15 mg/kg) is often required, which places ICH patients at risk of fluid overload and brain edema.[139] PCCs contains a higher concentration of clotting factors in smaller amounts of volume than FFP.[138] The time range for a complete reversal of anticoagulation and the value of INR are two essential factors necessary in reducing early hematoma expansion. The INR should be dropped to lower than 1.3 in less than 4 hours after admission.[140]

Novel anticoagulants are increasingly used due to their advantages over warfarin in that they do not need frequent dose calibration and have less interaction with food and other drugs. Also, they carry about a 50% lower risk of intracranial hemorrhage compared to VKA.[141] They compromise direct thrombin inhibitors (DTIs) dabigatran and factor Xa inhibitors (FXa-Is) apixaban, edoxaban, and rivaroxaban. The activity level of novel anticoagulants can be estimated based on the half-life of each drug used and the patient's renal function.[142] A coagulation assay can be performed to estimate the presence and concentration of the drug level in the body.

Dabigatran effect can be monitored by activated partial thromboplastin time (aPTT). A high aPTT at trough may be associated with a higher risk of bleeding. A normal aPTT has been used in emergencies to exclude any residual anticoagulant effect. Among the novel anticoagulants, only dabigatran has a reversal agent, idarucizumab, a humanized monoclonal antibody fragment against dabigatran. Bolus injection of idarucizumab rapidly reverses the anticoagulant effect of dabigatran in healthy volunteers[143] and even patients with renal failure.[144] Also, activated charcoal (50 g) should also be given if ICH occurs within 2 hours of the most recent dabigatran dose;[131] as a last resort, hemodialysis can be used.[125]

As for factor Xa inhibitors, reversal agents are still in phase III trials such as Andexanet alfa, are not available for clinical use.[145] Most hospital protocols include the administration of PCC for the reversal of FXa-Is; although there is currently no randomized prospective data to base this decision on, there are case series and some animal experiments to support its use.[136]

As the optimal timing for resuming anticoagulation after ICH is unknown, physicians should balance the risk of stroke versus ICH recurrence when deciding when to resume anticoagulation.[140] In general, resuming VKA within the first month is associated with a high risk of recurrent ICH.[146]

Other than anticoagulation, a significant number of patients presenting with ICH are on antiplatelet medication. Cyclooxygenase inhibitors such as aspirin and P2Y12 inhibitors such as clopidogrel, prasugrel, and ticagrelor irreversibly block their targets in platelets and thereby decrease platelet aggregation. Although theoretically ICH patients taking antiplatelet agents are at an increased risk of worse clinical outcomes and increased hematoma expansion, there is considerable controversy surrounding this stance.[147–149] A randomized phase III trial (PATCH) was recently completed 2 years ago to assess whether platelet transfusion in IPH patients improved outcomes. The study revealed that platelet transfusions increased mortality or dependence at 3 months (odds ratio [OR] 2.1).[150] Thus the Neurocritical Care Society recommends against platelet transfusion for ICH occurring while on an antiplatelet agent, and administration can only be considered as a risk reduction measure in patients planned for urgent neurosurgical intervention. They also recommend considering a single intravenous dose of 0.4 μg/kg of desmopressin (DDAVP) in antiplatelet medication–related ICH.[137]

DVT Prophylaxis

VTE occurs in up to one-fifth of patients with ICH, with an incidence of DVT ranging from 0.5% to 13% while that of PE ranges from 0.7% to 5%.[151] Thromboprophylaxis remains a complicated problem: the risk of VTE in these patients is high, while the risk of bleeding is not low, especially early on.[131] Three different trials (CLOTS trials I–III) aimed to determine appropriate thromboprophylaxis in ICH patients.[152] Based on their results the American Stroke Association (ASA) and the Neurocritical Care Society recommended that intermittent pneumatic compression starting as early as the day of hospitalization could reduce the occurrence of proximal DVT and that subcutaneous UFH or LMWH be given in those ICH patients with lack of mobility who have stable hematomas after 1–4 days from onset. If anticoagulation therapy is contraindicated, an inferior vena cava filter can be used instead.[131,153,154]

Managing Increased Intracranial Pressure

Intracranial hypertension following ICH is common, and this can complicate the situation. It occurs more commonly in younger patients with supratentorial hemorrhage, large-volume hematoma, extensive perihematomal edema, intraventricular hemorrhage (IVH), and new-onset hydrocephalus.[155] The ICP should be maintained at less than 20 mm Hg with a minimal cerebral perfusion pressure (CPP) of 60 mm Hg.[131] An ICP of higher than 30 mm Hg has been shown to be associated with poor outcome.[156] Hence the American Heart Association (AHA) and ASA recommend[131] that ICP monitoring and management should be considered in

- Patients with large hematomas or
- Those at high risk for hydrocephalus, such as patients with a

1. GCS score of 8 or lower,
2. Clinical evidence of transtentorial herniation, or
3. Significant IVH or hydrocephalus.

ICP can be measured using a catheter placed either in the ventricles or brain parenchyma. The advantage of the ventriculostomy is that it can drain CSF when needed; however, the risk of infection and hemorrhage are higher compared to intraparenchymal devices.[131] Managing elevated ICP should be undertaken in a stepwise approach, considering less invasive methods first, followed by more invasive procedures if deemed necessary.[131]

Medical management of increased ICP includes elevating the head of the bed to 30 degrees and a neutral head position, hyperventilation, and diuresis using hyperosmolar therapy with mannitol or hypertonic saline to drain CSF.[129,130] Hyperventilation is most effective in rapidly lowering intracranial hypertension, usually within minutes of achieving levels of hypocapnia in the range of 25–30 mm Hg. Intravenous mannitol (0.25–1 g/kg), a rapid and reliable way of lowering ICP, may be used along with hyperventilation in situations of neurological deterioration with impending herniation.[157]

Blood Pressure

Elevated blood pressure is prevalent in patients with ICH. While it seems reasonable that elevated blood pressure may predispose to hematoma expansion, clinical studies have produced conflicting results, as shown by the neutral result of the ATASH trial 2.[2,125] The relation between elevated blood pressure and hematoma expansion is strongest for systolic blood pressure at greater than 175 mm Hg.[158] The potential benefit of acute intensive reduction in blood pressure must be balanced against the possible harmful effects of hypotension leading to cerebral ischemia.[125] Additionally, the therapeutic target of blood pressure reduction is not clearly defined.[125,157] Based on the INTERACT-2 trial, the current AHA/ASA guideline states that blood pressure lowering to 140 mm Hg or lower is safe and can be useful to improve functional outcome.[131] The target blood pressure should be reached quickly, with minimal potential for overshoot. Intravenous beta-blockers and calcium channel blockers are the most commonly used medications for this indication. Labetalol is rapid acting, has mixed alpha- and beta-adrenergic antagonism, and is commonly used in an initial bolus dose of 5–20 mg. Nicardipine is a calcium channel blocker of the dihydropyridine family that is more selective for coronary and cerebral vascular beds. A standard initial nicardipine dose of 5 mg/h is often used, with up-titration every 15 minutes as needed. Clevidipine is another calcium channel blocker that acts even more rapidly than nicardipine.[124,157]

General Monitoring and Nursing Care

The first 24–48 hours are crucial in the management of the patient with ICH. Expansion of the hematoma, increase in blood pressure, increase perihematomal edema, development of seizure, an increase in ICP, IVH, and any medical complication such as hyponatremia and hyperthermia warrant close monitoring. Hence, patients in the acute phase of ICH should be monitored and cared for in facilities in which the close monitoring of the patient's status and frequent administration of medications are possible. Fever, defined as a temperature of higher than 38°C, is relatively common and has been reported to worsen outcomes.[159] Although often related to an infection, fever can also be related to an inflammatory reaction triggered by the hematoma or related to IVH or SAH extension of the ICH. Antipyretics are typically a simple method to reduce mild fever. External cooling devices and intravascular cold saline infusion can be used in different clinical settings.[130,131]

Glucose Management

Diabetic and nondiabetic patients presenting with ICH should have their glycemia level controlled in the normoglycemic range. Both extremes, hyperglycemia and hypoglycemia, affect the outcome negatively. Analysis of the INTERCT-2 patients showed that high blood glucose in the acute phase of ICH shows a continuous relation with early deterioration, poor functional outcome, and higher mortality regardless of diabetic status.[160] Tight glucose control should not be pursued, as intensive control has been shown to increase incidence of hypoglycemia and intracranial hypertension,[161] reduce cerebral extracellular glucose availability, and increase mortality.[162]

Seizures and Antiseizure Drugs

The routine prophylactic use of antiepileptic medications for ICH patients is not recommended.[131] Seizure, a feature of lobar hemorrhage rather deep hemorrhage, is not very common and does not seem to affect mortality or neurologic outcome. The available data seem to suggest that antiepileptic prophylaxis is associated with worse outcomes and increased mortality, in particular with the use of phenytoin.[163-166] Patients are prone to two types of seizure, early and late, classified according to the pathophysiology. Early seizures do not appear to influence prognosis concerning mortality or functional outcome but may increase the risk of long-term recurrent seizures.[167,168] Late seizures, which occur in 10% of patient, are thought to result from gliotic scarring and neuronal reorganization.[169] Seizures should be treated with benzodiazepines or a loading dose of an antiepileptic drug (AED) if they are prolonged, severe, or accompanied by mental status changes.[170] Earl tonic-clonic seizures need immediate attention because they can increase the ICP.[157] AED options include levetiracetam (Keppra), which has a very favorable therapeutic/toxic profile with a dose 500 mg twice daily, or a slow intravenous phenytoin load with 17 mg/kg over 1 hour, followed by 100 mg every 8 hours.

ICH is associated with a number of medical complications that warrant aggressive management because they are responsible for 50% of mortality. Eighty-eight percent of patients had at least one complication, including (in the order of most frequent) pneumonia, PE, respiratory failure, aspiration pneumonia, sepsis, and urinary tract infection.[170,171] Other medical complications in patients with ICH include cardiac events and death caused by acute myocardial infarction, heart failure, ventricular arrhythmias, cardiac arrest, acute kidney failure, hyponatremia, gastrointestinal bleeding, and post-stroke depression.[131] Dysphagia is a risk factor for aspiration and consequent aspiration pneumonia or chemical pneumonitis. Proper bedside swallow screening has been shown to reduce the absolute risk of pneumonia from roughly 5% to 2%.[172] To prevent aspiration in patients with dysphagia, the placement of an orogastric or nasogastric feeding tube or percutaneous endoscopic gastrostomy (PEG) tube placement reduces treatment failures and GI bleeding while increasing food delivery.[173] Ventilated patients are at risk for in-hospital mortality as high as 48% and should be surveilled for ventilator-associated pneumonia and ARDS.[174] To reduce the risk of aspiration pneumonia, the head of the bed should be kept at 30 degrees, frequent oral care should be performed, and extubation should be performed as soon as possible.[1]

Surgical Treatment of ICH

In general surgical management usually follows a trial of failed conservative medical therapy. Patients with cerebellar hemorrhage usually require hematoma evacuation due to the small compact space of the posterior fossa and the potential for sudden deterioration to coma and death in up to 75% of patients.[175] Early signs that warrant emergent surgical intervention are pontine tegmental compressions, such as ipsilateral gaze palsy and facial palsy, and development of obtundation and extensor plantar responses. Imaging criteria for early selection of surgical candidates are a large hematoma (>3 cm), the presence of hydrocephalus, and obliteration of the quadrigeminal cistern. Superficial hematoma, in contrast to deep hematomas, such as in the caudate, thalamic, brainstem, are accessible to surgical evacuation. Patients with primary IVH and hydrocephalus benefit from ventricular drainage as well. The adjunctive thrombolytic agents can overcome the drawback of catheter occlusion by the hematoma. Currently they are not recommended for routine use, but their effectiveness and safety have been documented by a randomized trial (CLEAR-III).[176] Open surgical evacuation is a life-saving procedure, but it does not hold a significant advantage over medical therapy. The Minimally Invasive Surgery and rtTPA for Intracerebral Hemorrhage Evacuation (MISTIE) trials I and II showed that hematoma clot could be targeted and drained safely using serial alteplase injections through a stereotactically targeted catheter.[177] A meta-analysis of four randomized controlled trials showed that aspiration of the hematoma decreased the likelihood of death or dependence significantly when compared to open craniotomy.[178]

REFERENCES

1. Greenberg MS. Treatment of hydrocephalus. *Handbook of neurosurgery 8th ed New York: Thieme.* 2016:414–437.

2. Connolly ES, Jr., Rabinstein AA, Carhuapoma JR, et al. Guidelines for the management of aneurysmal subarachnoid hemorrhage: a guideline for healthcare professionals from the American Heart Association/american Stroke Association. *Stroke.* 2012; 43(6):1711–1737.

3. Qureshi AI, Tuhrim S, Broderick JP, Batjer HH, Hondo H, Hanley DF. Spontaneous intracerebral hemorrhage. *New England Journal of Medicine.* 2001;344(19):1450–1460.

4. Hackett ML, Anderson CS. Health outcomes 1 year after subarachnoid hemorrhage: An international population-based study. The Australian Cooperative Research on Subarachnoid Hemorrhage Study Group. *Neurology.* 2000;55(5):658–662.

5. Springer MV, Schmidt JM, Wartenberg KE, Frontera JA, Badjatia N, Mayer SA. Predictors of global cognitive impairment 1 year after subarachnoid hemorrhage. *Neurosurgery.* 2009;65(6):1043–1050; discussion 1050–1041.

6. Kowalski RG, Claassen J, Kreiter KT, et al. Initial misdiagnosis and outcome after subarachnoid hemorrhage. *JAMA.* 2004;291(7):866–869.

7. Servadei F, Murray GD, Teasdale GM, et al. Traumatic Subarachnoid Hemorrhage: Demographic and Clinical Study of 750 Patients from the European Brain Injury Consortium Survey of Head Injuries. *Neurosurgery.* 2002;50(2):261–269.

8. Chieregato A, Fainardi E, Morselli-Labate AM, et al. Factors Associated with Neurological Outcome and Lesion Progression in Traumatic Subarachnoid Hemorrhage Patients. *Neurosurgery.* 2005;56(4):671–680.

9. Kakarieka A. Review on traumatic subarachnoid hemorrhage. *Neurological Research.* 1997;19(3):230–232.

10. León-Carrión J, del Rosario Domínguez-Morales M, y Martín JMB, Murillo-Cabezas F. Epidemiology of traumatic brain injury and subarachnoid hemorrhage. *Pituitary.* 2005;8(3-4):197–202.

11. Hughes JD, Bond KM, Mekary RA, et al. Estimating the Global Incidence of Aneurysmal Subarachnoid Hemorrhage: A Systematic Review for Central Nervous System Vascular Lesions and Meta-Analysis of Ruptured Aneurysms. *World neurosurgery.* 2018;115:430–447.e437.

12. Ingall T, Asplund K, Mähönen M, Bonita R. A multinational comparison of subarachnoid hemorrhage epidemiology in the WHO MONICA stroke study. *Stroke.* 2000;31(5):1054–1061.

13. Lall RR, Eddleman CS, Bendok BR, Batjer HH. Unruptured intracranial aneurysms and the assessment of rupture risk based on anatomical and morphological factors: sifting through the sands of data. *Neurosurgical focus.* 2009;26(5):E2.

14. Bor ASE, Koffijberg H, Wermer MJ, Rinkel GJ. Optimal screening strategy for familial intracranial aneurysms A cost-effectiveness analysis. *Neurology.* 2010;74(21): 1671–1679.

15. Broderick JP, Brown Jr RD, Sauerbeck L, et al. Greater rupture risk for familial as compared to sporadic unruptured intracranial aneurysms. *Stroke.* 2009;40(6):1952–1957.

16. Mohr J, Parides MK, Stapf C, et al. Medical management with or without interventional therapy for unruptured brain arteriovenous malformations (ARUBA): a multicentre, non-blinded, randomised trial. *The Lancet.* 2014;383(9917):614–621.

17. van Beijnum J, van der Worp HB, Buis DR, et al. Treatment of brain arteriovenous malformations: a systematic review and meta-analysis. *Jama.* 2011;306(18).

18. Bassi P, Bandera R, Loiero M, Tognoni G, Mangoni A. Warning signs in subarachnoid hemorrhage: a cooperative study. *Acta neurologica scandinavica.* 1991;84(4):277–281.

19. Germans M, Coert B, Vandertop W, Verbaan D. Time intervals from subarachnoid hemorrhage to rebleed. *Journal of neurology.* 2014;261(7):1425–1431.

20. Manschot W. Subarachnoid hemorrhage: intraocular symptoms and their pathogenesis. *American journal of ophthalmology.* 1954;38(4):501–505.

21. Seifert V, Trost HA, Stolke D. Management morbidity and mortality in grade IV and V patients with aneurysmal subarachnoid haemorrhage. *Acta neurochirurgica.* 1990;103(1-2):5–10.

22. Szklener S, Melges A, Korchut A, et al. Predictive model for patients with poor-grade subarachnoid haemorrhage in 30-day observation: a 9-year cohort study. *BMJ Open.* 2015;5(6).

23. Cortnum S, Sørensen P, Jørgensen J. Determining the sensitivity of computed tomography scanning in early detection of subarachnoid hemorrhage. *Neurosurgery.* 2010;66(5):900–903.

24. Perry JJ, Stiell IG, Sivilotti ML, et al. Sensitivity of computed tomography performed within six hours of onset of headache for diagnosis of subarachnoid haemorrhage: prospective cohort study. *BMJ (Clinical research ed).* 2011;343:d4277.

25. Agid R, Andersson T, Almqvist H, et al. Negative CT angiography findings in patients with spontaneous subarachnoid hemorrhage: when is digital subtraction angiography still needed? *American Journal of Neuroradiology.* 2010;31(4):696–705.

26. Donmez H, Serifov E, Kahriman G, Mavili E, Durak AC, Menkü A. Comparison of 16-row multislice CT angiography with conventional angiography for detection and evaluation of intracranial aneurysms. *European journal of radiology.* 2011;80(2):455–461.

27. Molyneux AJ, Kerr RS, Yu L-M, et al. International subarachnoid aneurysm trial (ISAT) of neurosurgical clipping versus endovascular coiling in 2143 patients with ruptured intracranial aneurysms: a randomised comparison of effects on survival, dependency, seizures, rebleeding, subgroups, and aneurysm occlusion. *The Lancet.* 2005;366(9488):809–817.

28. Brasiliense LB, Aguilar-Salinas P, Lopes DK, et al. Multicenter Study of Pipeline Flex for Intracranial Aneurysms. *Neurosurgery.* 2018.

29. Oras J, Grivans C, Bartley A, Rydenhag B, Ricksten S-E, Seeman-Lodding H. Elevated high-sensitive troponin T on admission is an indicator of poor long-term outcome in patients with subarachnoid haemorrhage: a prospective observational study. *Critical Care.* 2015;20(1):11.

30. Zaroff JG, Rordorf GA, Newell JB, Ogilvy CS, Levinson JR. Cardiac outcome in patients with subarachnoid hemorrhage and electrocardiographic abnormalities. *Neurosurgery.* 1999;44(1):34–39.

31. Tung P, Kopelnik A, Banki N, et al. Predictors of neurocardiogenic injury after subarachnoid hemorrhage. *Stroke.* 2004;35(2):548–551.

32. Van der Bilt I, Hasan D, Vandertop W, et al. Impact of cardiac complications on outcome after aneurysmal subarachnoid hemorrhage: a meta-analysis. *Neurology.* 2009;72(7):635–642.

33. Roitberg BZ, Hardman J, Urbaniak K, et al. Prospective randomized comparison of safety and efficacy of nicardipine and nitroprusside drip for control of hypertension in the neurosurgical intensive care unit. *Neurosurgery.* 2008;63(1):115–121.

34. Narotam PK, Puri V, Roberts JM, Taylon C, Vora Y, Nathoo N. Management of hypertensive emergencies in acute brain disease: evaluation of the treatment effects of intravenous nicardipine on cerebral oxygenation. *Journal of neurosurgery.* 2008;109(6):1065–1074.

35. Yee AH, Burns JD, Wijdicks EF. Cerebral salt wasting: pathophysiology, diagnosis, and treatment. *Neurosurgery Clinics.* 2010;21(2):339–352.

36. Rahman M, Friedman WA. Hyponatremia in neurosurgical patients: clinical guidelines development. *Neurosurgery.* 2009;65(5):925–936.

37. Suarez J, Qureshi A, Parekh P, et al. Administration of hypertonic (3%) sodium chloride/acetate in hyponatremic patients with symptomatic vasospasm following subarachnoid hemorrhage. *Journal of neurosurgical anesthesiology.* 1999;11(3):178–184.

38. Al-Rawi PG, Tseng M-Y, Richards HK, et al. Hypertonic saline in patients with poor-grade subarachnoid hemorrhage improves cerebral blood flow, brain tissue oxygen, and pH. *Stroke.* 2010;41(1):122–128.

39. Albrecht II RF, Wass CT, Lanier WL. Occurrence of potentially detrimental temperature alterations in hospitalized patients at risk for brain injury. Paper presented at: Mayo Clinic Proceedings 1998.

40. Hocker SE, Tian L, Li G, Steckelberg JM, Mandrekar JN, Rabinstein AA. Indicators of central fever in the neurologic intensive care unit. *JAMA Neurology.* 2013;70(12):1499–1504.

41. Fernandez A, Schmidt J, Claassen J, et al. Fever after subarachnoid hemorrhage: risk factors and impact on outcome. *Neurology.* 2007;68(13):1013–1019.

42. Greer DM, Funk SE, Reaven NL, Ouzounelli M, Uman GC. Impact of fever on outcome in patients with stroke and neurologic injury: a comprehensive meta-analysis. *Stroke.* 2008;39(11):3029–3035.

43. Naidech AM, Bendok BR, Bernstein RA, et al. Fever burden and functional recovery after subarachnoid hemorrhage. *Neurosurgery.* 2008;63(2):212–218.

44. Badjatia N, Fernandez L, Schmidt JM, et al. Impact of induced normothermia on outcome after subarachnoid hemorrhage: a case-control study. *Neurosurgery.* 2010;66(4):696–701.

45. Oddo M, Frangos S, Milby A, et al. Induced normothermia attenuates cerebral metabolic distress in patients with aneurysmal subarachnoid hemorrhage and refractory fever. *Stroke.* 2009;40(5):1913–1916.

46. Jane JA, Kassell NF, Torner JC, Winn HR. The natural history of aneurysms and arteriovenous malformations. *Journal of neurosurgery.* 1985;62(3):321–323.

47. Cha KC, Kim JH, Kang HI, Moon BG, Lee SJ, Kim JS. Aneurysmal rebleeding: factors associated with clinical outcome in the rebleeding patients. *Journal of Korean Neurosurgical Society.* 2010;47(2):119.

48. Guo L-m, Zhou H-y, Xu J-w, Wang Y, Qiu Y-m, Jiang J-y. Risk factors related to aneurysmal rebleeding. *World neurosurgery.* 2011;76(3-4):292–298.

49. Starke R, Connolly E. Rebleeding after aneurysmal subarachnoid hemorrhage. *Neurocritical care.* 2011;15(2):241.

50. Tanno Y, Homma M, Oinuma M, Kodama N, Ymamoto T. Rebleeding from ruptured intracranial aneurysms in North Eastern Province of Japan. A cooperative study. *Journal of the neurological sciences.* 2007;258(1-2):11–16.

51. Winn HR, Richardson AE, Jane JA. The long-term prognosis in untreated cerebral aneurysms: I. The incidence of late hemorrhage in cerebral aneurysm: A 10-year evaluation of 364 patients. *Annals of Neurology.* 1977;1(4):358–370.

52. Rahmanian A, Derakhshan N, Mohsenian Sisakht A, Karamzade Ziarati N, Raeisi Shahraki H, Motamed S. Risk Factors for Unfavorable Outcome in Aneurysmal Subarachnoid Hemorrhage Revisited; Odds and Ends. *Bulletin of emergency and trauma.* 2018;6(2):133–140.

53. Little AS, Zabramski JM, Peterson M, et al. Ventriculoperitoneal shunting after aneurysmal subarachnoid hemorrhage: analysis of the indications, complications, and outcome with a focus on patients with borderline ventriculomegaly. *Neurosurgery.* 2008;62(3):618–627; discussion 618–627.

54. Quigley M. Risk of shunt-dependent hydrocephalus after occlusion of ruptured intracranial aneurysms by surgical clipping or endovascular coiling: a single-institution series and meta-analysis. *Neurosurgery.* 2008;63(6):E1209; author reply E1209.

55. Kwon JH, Sung SK, Song YJ, Choi HJ, Huh JT, Kim HD. Predisposing factors related to shunt-dependent chronic hydrocephalus after aneurysmal subarachnoid hemorrhage. *J Korean Neurosurg Soc.* 2008;43(4):177–181.

56. Chen S, Luo J, Reis C, Manaenko A, Zhang J. Hydrocephalus after Subarachnoid Hemorrhage: Pathophysiology, Diagnosis, and Treatment. *BioMed research international.* 2017;2017:8584753.

57. Garton T, Keep RF, Wilkinson DA, et al. Intraventricular Hemorrhage: the Role of Blood Components in Secondary Injury and Hydrocephalus. *Translational stroke research.* 2016;7(6):447–451.

58. Hasan D. Management Problems in Acute Hydrocephalus After Subarachnoid Hemorrhage. 1993; Berlin, Heidelberg.

59. Graff-Radford NR, Torner J, Adams HP, Jr., Kassell NF. Factors associated with hydrocephalus after subarachnoid hemorrhage. A report of the Cooperative Aneurysm Study. *Arch Neurol.* 1989;46(7):744–752.

60. Rajshekhar V, Harbaugh RE. Results of routine ventriculostomy with external ventricular drainage for acute hydrocephalus following subarachnoid haemorrhage. *Acta neurochirurgica.* 1992;115(1-2):8–14.

61. Ransom ER, Mocco J, Komotar RJ, et al. External ventricular drainage response in poor grade aneurysmal subarachnoid hemorrhage: effect on preoperative grading and prognosis. *Neurocrit Care.* 2007;6(3):174–180.

62. Voldby B, Enevoldsen EM. Intracranial pressure changes following aneurysm rupture. Part 1: clinical and angiographic correlations. *J Neurosurg.* 1982;56(2):186–196.

63. De Marchis GM, Lantigua H, Schmidt JM, et al. Impact of premorbid hypertension on haemorrhage severity and aneurysm rebleeding risk after subarachnoid haemorrhage. *J Neurol Neurosurg Psychiatry.* 2014;85(1):56–59.

64. Heros RC, Zervas NT, Varsos V. Cerebral vasospasm after subarachnoid hemorrhage: An update. *Annals of Neurology.* 1983;14(6):599–608.

65. Francoeur CL, Mayer SA. Management of delayed cerebral ischemia after subarachnoid hemorrhage. *Critical care (London, England).* 2016;20(1):277.

66. Pickard JD, Murray GD, Illingworth R, et al. Effect of oral nimodipine on cerebral infarction and outcome after subarachnoid haemorrhage: British aneurysm nimodipine trial. *BMJ (Clinical research ed).* 1989;298(6674):636–642.

67. Petruk KC, West M, Mohr G, et al. Nimodipine treatment in poor-grade aneurysm patients. Results of a multicenter double-blind placebo-controlled trial. *J Neurosurg.* 1988;68(4):505–517.

68. Allen GS, Ahn HS, Preziosi TJ, et al. Cerebral arterial spasm--a controlled trial of nimodipine in patients with subarachnoid hemorrhage. *The New England journal of medicine.* 1983;308(11):619–624.

69. Dorhout Mees S, Rinkel GJE, Feigin VL, et al. Calcium antagonists for aneurysmal subarachnoid haemorrhage. *Cochrane Database of Systematic Reviews.* 2007(3).

70. Lennihan L, Mayer SA, Fink ME, et al. Effect of hypervolemic therapy on cerebral blood flow after subarachnoid hemorrhage : a randomized controlled trial. *Stroke*. 2000;31(2):383–391.

71. Diringer MN, Bleck TP, Claude Hemphill J, et al. Critical Care Management of Patients Following Aneurysmal Subarachnoid Hemorrhage: Recommendations from the Neurocritical Care Society's Multidisciplinary Consensus Conference. *Neurocritical Care*. 2011;15(2):211.

72. Sen J, Belli A, Albon H, Morgan L, Petzold A, Kitchen N. Triple-H therapy in the management of aneurysmal subarachnoid haemorrhage. *The Lancet Neurology*. 2003;2(10):614–621.

73. Al-Mufti F, Amuluru K, Damodara N, et al. Novel management strategies for medically-refractory vasospasm following aneurysmal subarachnoid hemorrhage. *Journal of the Neurological Sciences*. 2018;390:44–51.

74. Darby JM, Yonas H, Marks EC, Durham S, Snyder RW, Nemoto EM. Acute cerebral blood flow response to dopamine-induced hypertension after subarachnoid hemorrhage. *J Neurosurg*. 1994;80(5):857–864.

75. Kim DH, Joseph M, Ziadi S, Nates J, Dannenbaum M, Malkoff M. Increases in Cardiac Output Can Reverse Flow Deficits from Vasospasm Independent of Blood Pressure: A Study Using Xenon Computed Tomographic Measurement of Cerebral Blood Flow. *Neurosurgery*. 2003;53(5):1044–1052.

76. Chalouhi N, Tjoumakaris S, Thakkar V, et al. Endovascular management of cerebral vasospasm following aneurysm rupture: outcomes and predictors in 116 patients. *Clinical neurology and neurosurgery*. 2014;118:26–31.

77. Zubkov YN, Nikiforov BM, Shustin VA. Balloon catheter technique for dilatation of constricted cerebral arteries after aneurysmal SAH. *Acta neurochirurgica*. 1984;70(1-2):65–79.

78. Albanese E, Russo A, Quiroga M, Willis RN, Jr., Mericle RA, Ulm AJ. Ultrahigh-dose intraarterial infusion of verapamil through an indwelling microcatheter for medically refractory severe vasospasm: initial experience. Clinical article. *J Neurosurg*. 2010; 113(4):913–922.

79. Numaguchi Y, Zoarski GH, Clouston JE, et al. Repeat intra-arterial papaverine for recurrent cerebral vasospasm after subarachnoid haemorrhage. *Neuroradiology*. 1997;39(10):751–759.

80. Panczykowski D, Pease M, Zhao Y, et al. Prophylactic Antiepileptics and Seizure Incidence Following Subarachnoid Hemorrhage. *Stroke*. 2016;47(7): 1754–1760.

81. Chumnanvej S, Dunn IF, Kim DH. Three-day phenytoin prophylaxis is adequate after subarachnoid hemorrhage. *Neurosurgery*. 2007;60(1):99–103.

82. Rosengart AJ, Huo D, Tolentino J, et al. Outcome in patients with subarachnoid hemorrhage treated with antiepileptic drugs. 2007.

83. Choi K-S, Chun H-J, Yi H-J, Ko Y, Kim Y-S, Kim J-M. Seizures and epilepsy following aneurysmal subarachnoid hemorrhage: incidence and risk factors. *Journal of Korean Neurosurgical Society*. 2009;46(2):93.

84. Rhoney D, Tipps L, Murry K, Basham M, Michael D, Coplin W. Anticonvulsant prophylaxis and timing of seizures after aneurysmal subarachnoid hemorrhage. *Neurology*. 2000;55(2):258–265.

85. Sherlock M, O'Sullivan E, Agha A, et al. The incidence and pathophysiology of hyponatraemia after subarachnoid haemorrhage. *Clinical Endocrinology*. 2006; 64(3):250–254.

86. Mapa B, Taylor BE, Appelboom G, Bruce EM, Claassen J, Connolly ES. Impact of hyponatremia on morbidity, mortality, and complications after aneurysmal subarachnoid hemorrhage: a systematic review. *World neurosurgery*. 2016;85:305–314.

87. Saramma P, Menon RG, Srivastava A, Sarma PS. Hyponatremia after aneurysmal subarachnoid hemorrhage: Implications and outcomes. *Journal of neurosciences in rural practice*. 2013;4(1):24–28.

88. Shah K, Turgeon R, Gooderham PA, Ensom MH. Prevention and Treatment for Hyponatremia in Patients with Subarachnoid Hemorrhage: A Systematic Review. *World neurosurgery*. 2017.

89. Marupudi N, Mittal S. Diagnosis and management of hyponatremia in patients with aneurysmal subarachnoid hemorrhage. *Journal of clinical medicine*. 2015;4(4):756–767.

90. Association AD. 13. Diabetes care in the hospital. *Diabetes Care*. 2016;39(Supplement 1):S99–S104.

91. Lanzino G, Kassell NF, Germanson T, Truskowski L, Alves W. Plasma glucose levels and outcome after aneurysmal subarachnoid hemorrhage. *Journal of neurosurgery*. 1993;79(6):885–891.

92. Alberti O, Becker R, Benes L, Wallenfang T, Bertalanffy H. Initial hyperglycemia as an indicator of severity of the ictus in poor-grade patients with spontaneous subarachnoid hemorrhage. *Clinical neurology and neurosurgery*. 2000;102(2):78–83.

93. Kruyt ND, Biessels GJ, Haan RJd, et al. Hyperglycemia and Clinical Outcome in Aneurysmal Subarachnoid Hemorrhage. *Stroke*. 2009;40(6):e424–e430.

94. Aydın MD, Kanat A, Aydın N, et al. New Evidence for Causal Central Mechanism of Hyperglycemia in Subarachnoid Hemorrhage Secondary to Ischemic Degenerative Disruption of Circuitry Among Insular Cortex, Nodose Ganglion, and Pancreas: Experimental Study. *World neurosurgery*. 2017;106:570–577.

95. Baird TA, Parsons MW, Barber PA, et al. The influence of diabetes mellitus and hyperglycaemia on stroke incidence and outcome. *Journal of clinical neuroscience*. 2002;9(6):618–626.

96. Kramer AH, Gurka MJ, Nathan B, Dumont AS, Kassell NF, Bleck TP. Complications associated with anemia and blood transfusion in patients with aneurysmal subarachnoid hemorrhage. *Critical care medicine*. 2008;36(7):2070–2075.

97. Kramer AH, Zygun DA, Bleck TP, Dumont AS, Kassell NF, Nathan B. Relationship between hemoglobin concentrations and outcomes across subgroups of patients with aneurysmal subarachnoid hemorrhage. *Neurocritical care*. 2009;10(2):157.

98. Naidech AM, Drescher J, Ault ML, Shaibani A, Batjer HH, Alberts MJ. Higher hemoglobin is associated with less cerebral infarction, poor outcome, and death after subarachnoid hemorrhage. *Neurosurgery*. 2006;59(4):775–780.

99. Stein M, Brokmeier L, Herrmann J, et al. Mean hemoglobin concentration after acute subarachnoid hemorrhage and the relation to outcome, mortality, vasospasm, and brain infarction. *Journal of Clinical Neuroscience*. 2015;22(3):530–534.

100. Smith MJ, Le Roux PD, Elliott JP, Winn HR. Blood transfusion and increased risk for vasospasm and poor outcome after subarachnoid hemorrhage. *Journal of neurosurgery*. 2004;101(1):1–7.

101. Ayling OGS, Ibrahim GM, Alotaibi NM, Gooderham PA, Macdonald RL. Anemia After Aneurysmal Subarachnoid Hemorrhage Is Associated With Poor Outcome and Death. *Stroke*. 2018;49(8):1859–1865.

102. Kshettry VR, Rosenbaum BP, Seicean A, Kelly ML, Schiltz NK, Weil RJ. Incidence and risk factors associated with in-hospital venous thromboembolism after aneurysmal subarachnoid hemorrhage. *Journal of Clinical Neuroscience*. 2014;21(2):282–286.

103. Ray WZ, Strom RG, Blackburn SL, Ashley Jr WW, Sicard GA, Rich KM. Incidence of deep venous thrombosis after subarachnoid hemorrhage. *Journal of neurosurgery.* 2009;110(5):1010–1014.

104. Samama MM, Cohen AT, Darmon JY, et al. A comparison of enoxaparin with placebo for the prevention of venous thromboembolism in acutely ill medical patients. Prophylaxis in Medical Patients with Enoxaparin Study Group. *The New England journal of medicine.* 1999;341(11):793–800.

105. Agnelli G, Piovella F, Buoncristiani P, et al. Enoxaparin plus compression stockings compared with compression stockings alone in the prevention of venous thromboembolism after elective neurosurgery. *The New England journal of medicine.* 1998;339(2):80–85.

106. Cavallo C, Safavi-Abbasi S, Kalani MYS, et al. Pulmonary Complications After Spontaneous Aneurysmal Subarachnoid Hemorrhage: Experience from Barrow Neurological Institute. *World neurosurgery.* 2018;119:e366–e373.

107. Solenski NJ, Haley EC, Jr., Kassell NF, et al. Medical complications of aneurysmal subarachnoid hemorrhage: a report of the multicenter, cooperative aneurysm study. Participants of the Multicenter Cooperative Aneurysm Study. *Crit Care Med.* 1995;23(6):1007–1017.

108. Busl KM, Bleck TP. Neurogenic Pulmonary Edema. *Crit Care Med.* 2015;43(8):1710–1715.

109. Friedman JA, Pichelmann MA, Piepgras DG, et al. Pulmonary complications of aneurysmal subarachnoid hemorrhage. *Neurosurgery.* 2003;52(5):1025–1031; discussion 1031–1022.

110. Bouderka MA, Fakhir B, Bouaggad A, Hmamouchi B, Hamoudi D, Harti A. Early tracheostomy versus prolonged endotracheal intubation in severe head injury. *The Journal of trauma.* 2004;57(2):251–254.

111. Teoh WH, Goh KY, Chan C. The role of early tracheostomy in critically ill neurosurgical patients. *Annals of the Academy of Medicine, Singapore.* 2001;30(3):234–238.

112. Bulsara KR, McGirt MJ, Liao L, et al. Use of the peak troponin value to differentiate myocardial infarction from reversible neurogenic left ventricular dysfunction associated with aneurysmal subarachnoid hemorrhage. *J Neurosurg.* 2003;98(3):524–528.

113. Oras J, Grivans C, Dalla K, et al. High-Sensitive Troponin T and N-Terminal Pro B-Type Natriuretic Peptide for Early Detection of Stress-Induced Cardiomyopathy in Patients with Subarachnoid Hemorrhage. *Neurocritical Care.* 2015;23(2):233–242.

114. Norberg E, Odenstedt-Herges H, Rydenhag B, Oras J. Impact of Acute Cardiac Complications After Subarachnoid Hemorrhage on Long-Term Mortality and Cardiovascular Events. *Neurocrit Care.* 2018.

115. van der Bilt I, Hasan D, van den Brink R, et al. Cardiac dysfunction after aneurysmal subarachnoid hemorrhage: relationship with outcome. *Neurology.* 2014;82(4):351–358.

116. Mayer SA, Lin J, Homma S, et al. Myocardial injury and left ventricular performance after subarachnoid hemorrhage. *Stroke.* 1999;30(4):780–786.

117. Naidech A, Du Y, Kreiter KT, et al. Dobutamine versus Milrinone after Subarachnoid Hemorrhage. *Neurosurgery.* 2005;56(1):21–27.

118. Dias MS, Sekhar LN. Intracranial hemorrhage from aneurysms and arteriovenous malformations during pregnancy and the puerperium. *Neurosurgery.* 1990;27(6):855–865; discussion 865–856.

119. Bateman BT, Olbrecht VA, Berman MF, Minehart RD, Schwamm LH, Leffert LR. Peripartum subarachnoid hemorrhage: nationwide data and institutional experience. *Anesthesiology.* 2012;116(2):324–333.

120. Kanani N, Goldszmidt E. Postpartum rupture of an intracranial aneurysm. *Obstetrics and gynecology.* 2007;109(2 Pt 2):572–574.

121. Feigin VL, Lawes CM, Bennett DA, Barker-Collo SL, Parag V. Worldwide stroke incidence and early case fatality reported in 56 population-based studies: a systematic review. *The Lancet Neurology.* 2009;8(4):355–369.

122. van Asch CJ, Luitse MJ, Rinkel GJ, van der Tweel I, Algra A, Klijn CJ. Incidence, case fatality, and functional outcome of intracerebral haemorrhage over time, according to age, sex, and ethnic origin: a systematic review and meta-analysis. *The Lancet Neurology.* 2010;9(2):167–176.

123. Rincon F, Mayer SA. The epidemiology of intracerebral hemorrhage in the United States from 1979 to 2008. *Neurocritical care.* 2013;19(1):95–102.

124. Hemphill JC, Lam A. Emergency Neurological Life Support: Intracerebral Hemorrhage. *Neurocritical care.* 2017;27(1):89–101.

125. Schreuder FH, Sato S, Klijn CJ, Anderson CS. Medical management of intracerebral haemorrhage. *J Neurol Neurosurg Psychiatry.* 2017;88(1):76–84.

126. Krishnamurthi RV, Feigin VL, Forouzanfar MH, et al. Global and regional burden of first-ever ischaemic and haemorrhagic stroke during 1990–2010: findings from the Global Burden of Disease Study 2010. *The Lancet Global Health.* 2013;1(5): e259–e281.

127. Zahuranec DB, Lisabeth LD, Sánchez BN, et al. Intracerebral hemorrhage mortality is not changing despite declining incidence. *Neurology.* 2014;82(24):2180–2186.

128. Langhorne P, Fearon P, Ronning OM, et al. Stroke unit care benefits patients with intracerebral hemorrhage: systematic review and meta-analysis. *Stroke.* 2013;44(11):3044–3049.

129. Mayer SA, Rincon F. Treatment of intracerebral haemorrhage. *The Lancet Neurology.* 2005;4(10):662–672.

130. Kim JY, Bae H-J. Spontaneous intracerebral hemorrhage: management. *Journal of stroke.* 2017;19(1):28.

131. Hemphill III JC, Greenberg SM, Anderson CS, et al. Guidelines for the management of spontaneous intracerebral hemorrhage: a guideline for healthcare professionals from the American Heart Association/American Stroke Association. *Stroke.* 2015;46(7):2032–2060.

132. Halpin S, Britton J, Byrne J, Clifton A, Hart G, Moore A. Prospective evaluation of cerebral angiography and computed tomography in cerebral haematoma. *Journal of Neurology, Neurosurgery & Psychiatry.* 1994;57(10):1180–1186.

133. Dowlatshahi D, Demchuk A, Flaherty M, Ali M, Lyden P, Smith E. Defining hematoma expansion in intracerebral hemorrhage relationship with patient outcomes. *Neurology.* 2011:WNL. 0b013e3182143317.

134. Hanger HC, Fletcher VJ, Wilkinson TJ, Brown AJ, Frampton CM, Sainsbury R. Effect of aspirin and warfarin on early survival after intracerebral haemorrhage. *Journal of neurology.* 2008;255(3):347–352.

135. Schulman S, Bijsterveld NR. Anticoagulants and their reversal. *Transfusion medicine reviews.* 2007;21(1):37–48.

136. Veltkamp R, Purrucker J. Management of Spontaneous Intracerebral Hemorrhage. *Current neurology and neuroscience reports.* 2017;17(10):80.

137. Frontera JA, Lewin III JJ, Rabinstein AA, et al. Guideline for reversal of antithrombotics in intracranial hemorrhage: executive summary. A statement for healthcare professionals from the Neurocritical Care Society and the Society of Critical Care Medicine. *Critical care medicine.* 2016;44(12):2251–2257.

138. Sarode R, Milling TJ, Refaai MA, et al. Efficacy and safety of a four-factor prothrombin complex concentrate (4F-PCC) in patients on vitamin K antagonists presenting with major bleeding: a randomized, plasma-controlled, phase IIIb study. *Circulation.* 2013:CIRCULATIONAHA. 113.002283.

139. Hanley J. Warfarin reversal. *Journal of Clinical Pathology.* 2004;57(11):1132–1139.

140. Kuramatsu JB, Gerner ST, Schellinger PD, et al. Anticoagulant reversal, blood pressure levels, and anticoagulant resumption in patients with anticoagulation-related intracerebral hemorrhage. *Jama.* 2015;313(8):824–836.

141. Ruff CT, Giugliano RP, Braunwald E, et al. Comparison of the efficacy and safety of new oral anticoagulants with warfarin in patients with atrial fibrillation: a meta-analysis of randomised trials. *The Lancet.* 2014;383(9921):955–962.

142. Tran H, Joseph J, Young L, et al. New oral anticoagulants: a practical guide on prescription, laboratory testing and peri-procedural/bleeding management. *Internal medicine journal.* 2014;44(6):525–536.

143. Glund S, Stangier J, Schmohl M, et al. Safety, tolerability, and efficacy of idarucizumab for the reversal of the anticoagulant effect of dabigatran in healthy male volunteers: a randomised, placebo-controlled, double-blind phase 1 trial. *The Lancet.* 2015;386(9994):680–690.

144. Glund S, Stangier J, van Ryn J, et al. Effect of age and renal function on idarucizumab pharmacokinetics and idarucizumab-mediated reversal of dabigatran anticoagulant activity in a randomized, double-blind, crossover phase Ib study. *Clinical pharmacokinetics.* 2017;56(1):41–54.

145. Tummala R, Kavtaradze A, Gupta A, Ghosh RK. Specific antidotes against direct oral anticoagulants: a comprehensive review of clinical trials data. *International journal of cardiology.* 2016;214:292–298.

146. Majeed A, Kim Y-K, Roberts RS, Holmström M, Schulman S. Optimal timing of resumption of warfarin after intracranial hemorrhage. *Stroke.* 2010;41(12): 2860–2866.

147. Naidech AM, Bernstein RA, Levasseur K, et al. Platelet activity and outcome after intracerebral hemorrhage. *Annals of Neurology: Official Journal of the American Neurological Association and the Child Neurology Society.* 2009;65(3):352–356.

148. Naidech AM, Jovanovic B, Liebling S, et al. Reduced platelet activity is associated with early clot growth and worse 3-month outcome after intracerebral hemorrhage. *Stroke.* 2009;40(7):2398–2401.

149. Sansing L, Messe S, Cucchiara B, et al. Prior antiplatelet use does not affect hemorrhage growth or outcome after ICH. *Neurology.* 2009;72(16):1397–1402.

150. Baharoglu MI, Cordonnier C, Salman RA-S, et al. Platelet transfusion versus standard care after acute stroke due to spontaneous cerebral haemorrhage associated with antiplatelet therapy (PATCH): a randomised, open-label, phase 3 trial. *The Lancet.* 2016;387(10038):2605–2613.

151. Huge V. Critical care management of intracerebral hemorrhage. *Medizinische Klinik, Intensivmedizin und Notfallmedizin.* 2018;113(3):164–173.

152. Collaboration CT. Effectiveness of thigh-length graduated compression stockings to reduce the risk of deep vein thrombosis after stroke (CLOTS trial 1): a multicentre, randomised controlled trial. *The Lancet.* 2009;373(9679):1958–1965.

153. Guyatt GH, Akl EA, Crowther M, Gutterman DD, Schünemann HJ. Executive summary: antithrombotic therapy and prevention of thrombosis: American College of Chest Physicians evidence-based clinical practice guidelines. *Chest.* 2012;141(2 Suppl):7S.

154. Nyquist P, Bautista C, Jichici D, et al. Prophylaxis of venous thrombosis in neurocritical care patients: an evidence-based guideline: A Statement for Healthcare Professionals from the Neurocritical Care Society. *Neurocritical care.* 2016;24(1):47–60.

155. Kamel H, Hemphill JC. Characteristics and sequelae of intracranial hypertension after intracerebral hemorrhage. *Neurocritical care.* 2012;17(2):172–176.

156. Ziai WC, Melnychuk E, Thompson CB, Awad I, Lane K, Hanley DF. Occurrence and impact of intracranial pressure elevation during treatment of severe intraventricular hemorrhage. *Critical care medicine.* 2012;40(5):1601.

157. Daroff RB, Jankovic J, Mazziotta JC, Pomeroy SL. *Bradley's Neurology in Clinical Practice E-Book.* Elsevier Health Sciences; 2015.

158. Fujii Y, Takeuchi S, Sasaki O, Minakawa T, Tanaka R. Multivariate analysis of predictors of hematoma enlargement in spontaneous intracerebral hemorrhage. *Stroke.* 1998;29(6):1160–1166.

159. Schwarz S, Häfner K, Aschoff A, Schwab S. Incidence and prognostic significance of fever following intracerebral hemorrhage. *Neurology.* 2000;54(2):354–361.

160. Saxena A, Anderson CS, Wang X, et al. Prognostic significance of hyperglycemia in acute intracerebral hemorrhage: the INTERACT2 study. *Stroke.* 2016;47(3):682–688.

161. Meier R, Béchir M, Ludwig S, et al. Differential temporal profile of lowered blood glucose levels (3.5 to 6.5 mmol/l versus 5 to 8 mmol/l) in patients with severe traumatic brain injury. *Critical Care.* 2008;12(4):R98.

162. Vespa P, Boonyaputthikul R, McArthur DL, et al. Intensive insulin therapy reduces microdialysis glucose values without altering glucose utilization or improving the lactate/pyruvate ratio after traumatic brain injury. *Critical care medicine.* 2006;34(3):850–856.

163. Battey TW, Falcone GJ, Ayres AM, et al. Confounding by indication in retrospective studies of intracerebral hemorrhage: antiepileptic treatment and mortality. *Neurocritical care.* 2012;17(3):361–366.

164. Messé SR, Sansing LH, Cucchiara BL, Herman ST, Lyden PD, Kasner SE. Prophylactic antiepileptic drug use is associated with poor outcome following ICH. *Neurocritical care.* 2009;11(1):38–44.

165. Mullen MT, Kasner SE, Messé SR. Seizures do not increase in-hospital mortality after intracerebral hemorrhage in the nationwide inpatient sample. *Neurocritical care.* 2013;19(1):19–24.

166. Zandieh A, Messé SR, Cucchiara B, Mullen MT, Kasner SE, Collaborators V-I. Prophylactic use of antiepileptic drugs in patients with spontaneous intracerebral hemorrhage. *Journal of Stroke and Cerebrovascular Diseases.* 2016;25(9):2159–2166.

167. De Herdt V, Dumont F, Henon H, et al. Early seizures in intracerebral hemorrhage Incidence, associated factors, and outcome. *Neurology.* 2011:WNL. 0b013e31823648a31823646.

168. Serafini A, Gigli GL, Gregoraci G, et al. Are early seizures predictive of epilepsy after a stroke? Results of a population-based study. *Neuroepidemiology.* 2015;45(1):50–58.

169. de Greef BT, Schreuder FH, Vlooswijk MC, et al. Early seizures after intracerebral hemorrhage predict drug-resistant epilepsy. *Journal of neurology.* 2015;262(3):541–546.

170. Cusack TJ, Carhuapoma JR, Ziai WC. Update on the Treatment of Spontaneous Intraparenchymal Hemorrhage: Medical and Interventional Management. *Current treatment options in neurology.* 2018;20(1):1.

171. Lyden PD, Shuaib A, Lees KR, et al. Safety and tolerability of NXY-059 for acute intracerebral hemorrhage: the CHANT Trial. *Stroke.* 2007;38(8):2262–2269.

172. Hinchey JA, Shephard T, Furie K, Smith D, Wang D, Tonn S. Formal dysphagia screening protocols prevent pneumonia. *Stroke.* 2005;36(9):1972–1976.

173. Geeganage C, Beavan J, Ellender S, Bath PM. Interventions for dysphagia and nutritional support in acute and subacute stroke. *Cochrane Database of Systematic Reviews*. 2012(10).

174. Elmer J, Hou P, Wilcox SR, et al. Acute respiratory distress syndrome after spontaneous intracerebral hemorrhage. *Critical care medicine*. 2013;41(8):1992.

175. Luney M, English S, Longworth A, et al. Acute posterior cranial fossa hemorrhage—is surgical decompression better than expectant medical management? *Neurocritical care*. 2016;25(3):365–370.

176. Hanley DF, Lane K, McBee N, et al. Thrombolytic removal of intraventricular haemorrhage in treatment of severe stroke: results of the randomised, multicentre, multiregion, placebo-controlled CLEAR III trial. *The Lancet*. 2017;389(10069):603–611.

177. Mould WA, Carhuapoma JR, Muschelli J, et al. Minimally invasive surgery plus recombinant tissue-type plasminogen activator for intracerebral hemorrhage evacuation decreases perihematomal edema. *Stroke*. 2013;44(3):627–634.

178. Wang J-W, Li J-P, Song Y-L, et al. Stereotactic aspiration versus craniotomy for primary intracerebral hemorrhage: a meta-analysis of randomized controlled trials. *PloS one*. 2014;9(9):e107614.

4 Role of Hospital Medicine in Management of Intracranial Brain Tumors

Donald Y. Ye, Thana Theofanis,
Tomas Garzon-Muvdi, and James J. Evans

INTRODUCTION

The co-management of patients admitted to the hospital for evaluation of intracranial tumors is a unique challenge with several special considerations during preoperative evaluation and postoperative management. The neurosurgeon relies on a multidisciplinary team including hospitalists for management of systemic comorbidities that are often exacerbated during the treatment of brain tumor–related symptoms.[1-3] In addition, the hospitalist must also be cognizant of the outpatient oncology team that has or will have a considerable input into the patient's ongoing care. Ultimately, recommendations for these patients can vary significantly based on the nature of the patient's primary diagnosis, their baseline functional status, and their expected outcomes.

The neurosurgical treatment of brain tumors depends significantly on the primary diagnosis, extent of disease, and the patient's functional status with the risks of surgery weighed against the potential benefits. Relatively benign diseases such as meningiomas and pituitary adenoma usually become symptomatic slowly. Surgery for these conditions is aimed at decompression of affected neurological structures but is rarely emergent in nature. Thus, ample time should be afforded for optimization of as many surgical risk factors as possible prior to proceeding to the operating room. On the other hand, glioblastoma, a malignant primary brain tumor, progresses rapidly, with significantly worse long-term outcomes. It is essential to confirm the pathological diagnosis rapidly and initiate adjuvant chemoradiation therapy sooner.[4,5] The surgical plan to biopsy or resect in a subtotal or gross total fashion will often be negotiated on an expedited timeline which is dictated by the patient's preoperative medical conditions, functional status, and the anticipated surgical risk. The hospitalist plays a vital role in elucidating these risks, assisting both neurosurgeon and patient to arrive at a consensus treatment plan.

Last, patients with brain tumors have elevated risk for many perioperative complications including infection, adrenal axis abnormalities, and thrombotic events such as deep vein thrombosis (DVT) and pulmonary embolism (PE) because of the nature of their disease and the side effects of common treatment options.[6] The hospitalist must be attuned to these risk factors to help coordinate perioperative management of medications and provide appropriate recommendations regarding screening tests.

EPIDEMIOLOGY OF INTRACRANIAL TUMORS

Intracranial primary central nervous system (CNS) tumors account for approximately 1% of all cancer diagnoses and 2–3% of cancer-related deaths.[7-9] Between 2010 and 2014, the age-adjusted incidence of primary CNS tumors was reported to be 22.64 cases tumors per 100,000 people in the United States. Metastatic disease to the CNS accounts for an additional 2.8–14.3 cases per 100,000.[10] The vast majority of newly diagnosed intracranial tumors occur in patients older than 40, with a median age of 59 years. A similar pattern exists for patients with other primary cancers with metastasis to the CNS, with a peak incidence occurring between 50–69 years for most other cancers.[11]

Primary CNS tumors consist of both benign and malignant histologic phenotypes and confer dramatically different prognoses and management strategies. The vast majority of newly diagnosed CNS tumors fall within the spectrum of benign tumors (WHO grade I/II) which include meningiomas (36.3%), pituitary adenomas (16.2%), schwannomas (8.4%), and low-grade gliomas (1.1%).[7] Glioblastoma represents the most common malignant CNS tumor (14.9%) with a median overall survival of approximately 16 months and a 5-year survival rate of less than 5%.

Metastatic disease to the brain most commonly arises from primary lung, breast, skin, kidney, and GI tract cancers in descending order.[11] Lung cancer has the highest overall prevalence and is the leading primary source of metastatic brain tumors in both males and females. Breast cancer represents one of the leading primary sources in women, accounting for up to 30% of all metastatic brain tumors and occurs in up to 30% of all patients with breast cancer. Skin cancers, specifically malignant melanoma, accounts for 5–21% of all metastatic brain tumors and is the most likely primary tumor to metastasize to the brain.

SYSTEMIC COMORBIDITIES AND FUNCTIONAL STATUS

Patients who present to the hospital with intracranial tumors represent a patient population that is preferentially older and more likely to have significant systemic comorbidities that increases surgical risk and perioperative complications. These patients may also have neurological deficits with diminished alertness, cognitive impairments, or focal hemiparesis or hemiplegia that significantly limits their ability to care for themselves.

100	Normal, no complaints, no evidence of disease
90	Able to carry on normal activity; minor signs or symptoms of disease
80	Normal activity with effort; some signs or symptoms of disease
70	Cares for self; unable to carry on normal activity or do active work
60	Requires occasional assistance, able to care for most personal needs
50	Requires considerable assistance and frequent medical care
40	Disabled; requires special care and assistance
30	Severely disable; hospital admission is indicated although death not imminent
20	Very sick; hospital admission necessary; active supportive treatment necessary
10	Moribund, fatal processes progressing rapidly
0	Dead

The Karnofsky Performance Status Scale (KPS) is an often-utilized tool to quantify baseline function and serves as a predictor of long-term outcomes related to brain tumor pathology (see Table 4.1). A KPS score of greater than 70 serves as a threshold for patients who are able to care for themselves independently and predicts perioperative complications.[12,13]

Other metrics have also been utilized to incorporate systemic comorbidities that are likely to be prevalent in brain tumor patients. Cardiovascular and pulmonary diseases are common in metastatic brain tumor populations and primary glioblastoma.[14] In addition, hyperglycemia from preexisting diabetes mellitus or provoked by chronic glucocorticoid use is common and contributes to perioperative infections. The Charlson Comorbidity Index has been used in some instances to predict postoperative mortality and morbidity after surgery for metastatic brain tumors and benign meningiomas in elderly patients.[15,16] The Charlson Comorbidity Index incorporates factors such as cardiovascular health (previous myocardial infarction, congestive heart failure, peripheral vascular disease, strokes), neurological health (dementia, hemiplegia), and other systemic disease (chronic obstructive pulmonary disease [COPD], gastroesophageal reflux disease [GERD], diabetes, cancer, liver dysfunction) and provides correction for increased age to provide a holistic patient-disease severity score (see Table 4.2).

The Revised Cardiac Risk Index (RCRI) provides an additional metric for assessing perioperative risk in noncardiac surgeries and has been widely validated outside of craniotomy for tumors to predict 30-day cardiac-cause mortality (Table 4.3).[17,18] The RCRI accounts for previous history of cardiovascular events, preoperative insulin requirements suggesting poorly controlled diabetes, and elevated serum creatinine reflecting poor renal function. Calculators exist to correlate the total score with percentage risk of 30-day cardiac-cause mortality. A limitation of the RCRI is that it does not take into consideration the patient's neurological condition or burden of intracranial disease. However, in combination with the KPS, the RCRI can often guide surgical decision-making by determining high-risk patients

Table 4.2 Charlson Comorbidity Index

Comorbidity component (one point, unless noted)	Myocardial infarction	
	Congestive heart failure	
	Peripheral vascular disease	
	Dementia	
	COPD	
	Connective tissue disease	
	Peptic ulcer disease	
	Diabetes mellitus (uncomplicated, +2 points if end-organ damage)	
	Moderate to severe chronic kidney disease (2 points)	
	Hemiplegia (2 points)	
	Leukemia (2 points)	
	Malignant lymphoma (2 points)	
	Solid tumor (2 points, +6 points in metastatic)	
	Liver disease (mild, +3 points in moderate to severe)	
	AIDS (6 points)	
Age correction	Age < 50 years	0 points
	Age 50–59 years	1 point
	Age 60–69	2 points
	Age 60–79 years	3 points

and guiding surgeons toward safer procedures with lower expected blood loss or shorter exposure to anesthetics.[19]

APPROACHES TO SURGERY AND RELEVANCE TO PERIOPERATIVE MANAGEMENT

Brain tumors represent a wide array of intracranial pathology and can be treated with a variety of operative approaches. The hospitalist should be familiar with these approaches as the associated risk profiles can be dramatically different depending on the goals of the procedure and the location of the tumor. The important considerations are the number of tumors, the expected extent of resection, and the location of the tumors in relation to eloquent structures and critical vascular structures such as the major cerebral arteries and draining sinuses and veins. These aspects of a patient's intracranial tumor burden will then dictate the possible operative plans.

Most brain tumors are supratentorial and can be approached with standard open craniotomy through the frontal, temporal, or parietal bone.[20] The patient is positioned supine with few constraints on ventilation. If gross total resection is unrealistic due to the location of the tumor in or near an eloquent cortical structure, then stereotactic needle biopsy is often employed, reducing the exposure of critical neurovascular structures, reducing the risk of neurological deficits due to aggressive

High-risk surgical procedure (+ 1 point)	Intraperitoneal
	Intrathoracic
	Suprainguinal vascular
History of ischemic heart disease (+1 point)	Myocardial infarction
	Positive exercise test
	Current chest pain secondary to myocardial ischemia
	Use of nitrate therapy
	ECG with pathological Q waves
History of congestive heart failure (+1 point)	History of congestive heart failure
	Pulmonary edema
	Paroxysmal nocturnal dyspnea
	Bilateral rales or S3 gallop
	Chest radiograph with pulmonary vascular redistribution
History of cerebrovascular disease (+1 point)	History of transient ischemic attack or stroke
Preoperative treatment with insulin (+1 point)	
Preoperative serum creatinine > 2.0 mg/dL (+1 point)	

Points	Risk of Major Cardiac Event
0	0.4%
1	0.9%
2	6.6%
3 or more	11%

resection of the tumor and surrounding brain tissue, and reducing the duration of surgery and exposure to anesthesia.

If there are multiple tumors, as can often be the case in metastatic disease, it is important to note the locations of all of the brain tumors that are expected to be treated by surgery. For example, two tumors within the same hemisphere may be addressed through a single large craniotomy, affording a relatively similar duration of surgery. On the other hand, if two or more tumors are on opposite hemispheres or one is anterior and one more posterior—such as in the occipital lobe or cerebellum—then the surgical approach may represent two craniotomies with two separate positions, multiplying the anesthesia and cardiac risk.

The location of the tumor also determines that patient's positioning. Although most brain tumors can be approached through standard frontotemporoparietal craniotomies in a supine position, some require positioning the patient in varying degrees of a lateral position or require the patient to be prone.[21,22] In these situations, it is important to recognize any potential cardiopulmonary risks and consider body habitus to identify potential challenges in ventilation. In rare circumstances, for example pineal region and some posterior fossa tumors, a surgeon may choose to place a patient in a sitting position, which can induce additional cardiopulmonary stress due to impaired ventilation and reduced venous return.[23,24] Operations of the posterior fossa and middle fossa near the transverse and sigmoid sinuses also increase the risk of intraoperative complications associated with venous sinus injury. These complications can lead to excessive blood loss and venous air embolus, which are typically monitored and managed by the anesthesiologist; however, they should be factored into any preoperative risk assessment and optimization strategy.

Pituitary and parasellar tumors, as well as some anterior cranial base tumors, can also be treated through various approaches through the aerated nasal sinuses. Recent developments in endoscopic techniques enable surgeons to reach the anterior cranial base and parasellar region through an endonasal transsphenoidal approach that minimizes blood loss, disruption of normal structures, and anesthesia time compared to previous transcranial approaches.[25,26] Although the endocrinopathies associated with macroadenomas and secretory adenomas contribute to other perioperative medical risks, the surgical approach itself has few intrinsic factors that place patients at greater risk.

NEOADJUVANT TREATMENTS AND ALTERNATIVES TO SURGERY

Not all patients with brain tumors necessarily need brain surgery. Management of benign intracranial pathologies like meningiomas, schwannomas, and pituitary adenomas can often be deferred until the patient has all required perioperative testing complete and is optimized from a medical perspective. Serial observation at 3- to 6-month intervals is not an unreasonable approach in asymptomatic or mildly symptomatic benign tumors that are newly diagnosed if the surgical risk is very high. Stereotactic radiosurgery (SRS)—which includes gamma knife, cyberknife, and other linear accelerator (LINAC)–based machines—or fractionated radiotherapy are alternatives to surgery that convey less cardiovascular risk in the elderly or significantly comorbid patient.[27–32] Although radiation-based treatments do not typically reverse symptomatic mass effect in the short term, they can provide durable clinical benefit in a well-selected patient population.

Metastatic disease can also be treated with systemic chemotherapy or radiation alone in the appropriately selected patient. Those with a known primary cancer diagnosis with new brain metastases will often not need additional tissue diagnosis from the site of distant metastasis and have similar local control rates with SRS as with tumor resection.[33] Avoiding surgery can often accelerate a patient toward initiating systemic chemotherapy earlier as the oncologists no longer have to consider postoperative bleeding or complications with tissue healing. In some instances, larger tumors are not amenable to standard SRS, and single metastases may be neurologically symptomatic despite their favorable profiles. In these instances, oncologists and radiation oncologists along with the neurosurgeon may opt to proceed with preoperative SRS followed by short-interval resection.[34] Although this is a decision often left to the specialists involved in the patient's care team, it is important to recognize these nuances to help coordinate the patient's care.

POSTOPERATIVE CARE AND COMMON COMPLICATIONS AND MANAGEMENT

In the postoperative care of the brain tumor patient, complication avoidance is key. Nearly every patient requires steroids peri- and postoperatively, and this is not without consequence. New seizures may arise in the setting of recently having undergone a craniotomy. These patients are also at high risk for postoperative surgical site and systemic infections, electrolyte disturbances, and thromboembolic events.[6,20]

Role and Risks of Glucocorticoids

Glucocorticoid steroids such as dexamethasone are arguably the most common medication added to the regimen of patients with a newly diagnosed brain tumor.[35] It is important for any treating clinician to understand the rationale behind initiating steroids for symptom relief or for symptom prophylaxis. Most commonly, patients are placed on a taper over 1–2 weeks after surgery to assist with perioperative edema.[36] Factors that often influence the dose and duration of steroids include extent of preoperative cerebral edema, extent of resection, and the location of the tumor. If a patient has a subtotal resection due to an eloquent location in the brain, the neurosurgeon may opt to maintain the patient on a low dose of steroid for a longer period of time to avoid complications secondary to worsening edema.

In the case of a pituitary or parasellar tumor, other steroids are often used for temporary or permanent dysfunction of the hypothalamic-pituitary axis and cortisol production. Postoperative cortisol levels can be useful in determining the need for steroids, and, if warranted, patients can be maintained on a low dose of hydrocortisone, prednisone, or dexamethasone until outpatient follow-up with an endocrinologist.[37] Patients may also present in a delayed fashion with lethargy, headaches, and electrolyte abnormalities such as hyponatremia. The treating physician should have a high suspicion for cortisol insufficiency, and urgent steroid administration often will result in resolution of symptoms.[38]

Patients may develop extremely poor glycemic control while on steroids; this is often seen in patients with preexisting diabetes.[39] Without adequate monitoring and titration of steroids, there is a significant risk of ketoacidosis. Poor postoperative glycemic control also increases the risk of systemic infections such as urinary tract infections and local surgical site infections. In severe cases, the addition of an insulin regimen may be necessary while the patient is on steroids; however, it is important to communicate with the treating neurosurgeon or oncologists to determine the need for prolonged steroid use and attempt to taper the patient off steroids sooner rather than later. More details on glucose control can be found in Chapter 5.

Perhaps one of the most concerning side effects of steroids is that they can result in a state of confusion, rage, or outright delirium,[40] particularly in older patients. This can pose significant risk for both the patient and his or her caregivers. In this case, it may be prudent to stop any type of steroid altogether to ensure patient safety. If this occurs, the clinician should also provide clear documentation of such side effects in the patient's electronic medical records as a courtesy to other clinicians who may treat the patient in the future.

Finally, chronic glucocorticoid use can also result in steroid-induced myopathy characterized by severe proximal muscle weakness.[41] This can often be confounded by disease progression, postradiation pseudo-progression, or radiation necrosis. In those cases, typical approaches would be to increase steroids in order to reduce symptomatic cerebral edema. However, recognizing steroid-induced myopathy allows an earlier recovery of function and can reduce other complications related to immobility such as DVT and pneumonias. Patients usually recover over the course of 3–4 weeks after discontinuing steroids.

SEIZURE PROPHYLAXIS

Both benign and malignant intracranial disease can cause cortical irritation that predisposes patients to seizures.[42–46] These can be subtle auras or focal seizures— twitches, tingling, flashes of light—or gross alterations of consciousness. In the most severe cases, seizures can generalize into tonic-clonic convulsions and persist, resulting in status epilepticus. Unrecognized and unaddressed, status epilepticus has a high risk of permanent neurological injury and mortality.[47]

In the setting of new-onset seizures, it is often appropriate to seek consultation from expert neurologists to help recommend appropriate antiepileptic drugs (AEDs) and to titrate them until symptom resolution.[48] Typical agents include levetiracetam, lacosamide, phenytoin, and valproate, and which medication is utilized often depends on the patient's comorbidities and the expected side-effect profile.[49] For example, levetiracetam is commonly used as a first-line agent due to its generally well-tolerated side-effect profile.[50] However, it must be dose-adjusted in the setting of kidney disease and must be used cautiously in elderly patients and patients with cognitive impairment due to its potential to cause cognitive depression and behavioral changes. Thorough evaluation with CT and MRI should also be used to assess for new intracranial pathology or progression of known intracranial disease. A bedside EEG or continuous EEG may be warranted if seizures persist or the patient does not return to his or her neurological baseline. More details on antiseizure medications can be found in Chapter 5.

For patients who do not have active seizures from their intracranial disease, recommendations regarding seizure prophylaxis depend on the tumor type, location, and extent of cortical involvement. Tumors involving the frontal, temporal, and parietal lobes are most commonly associated with seizures.[51] Lesions in the occipital lobes as well as infratentorial locations are less likely and rarely cause seizures.

Intractable epilepsy is more commonplace in tumors involving the mesiotemporal and insular structures. Additionally, cortical tumors have a much higher incidence of associated epilepsy versus noncortical deeper lesions, regardless of location. Although no high-level clinical data exist to support the prophylactic use of AEDs, patients with supratentorial tumors are routinely maintained on them in the perioperative period for 1–2 weeks.

Different types of tumors can also predispose patients to heightened seizure risk. Immunohistochemical studies have suggested an intrinsic hyperexcitable neuronal component for glioneuronal tumors. Infiltrative tumors such as low-grade gliomas have a high propensity to provoke seizures, up to 80% in some studies,[45] by producing an epileptogenic environment, affecting the normal neuronal connectivity, and lowering the threshold for seizures to occur. Glioblastoma similarly has a high rate of seizure—between 30% and 50% of all patients will have a seizure during their clinical course.[52] Metastatic disease is less likely than infiltrative disease to cause seizures, but factors such as likelihood of hemorrhage, extent of metastatic burden, and involvement of the temporal lobe and insula are associated with higher seizure risk. Choriocarcinoma, melanoma, papillary thyroid carcinoma, and renal cell carcinoma all demonstrate a high propensity for hemorrhage and may be more likely to benefit from seizure prophylaxis. Large metastatic lesions are also more likely to cause seizures due to metabolic alterations secondary to mass effect, with local ischemia leading to hypoxia and acidosis of glial tissue.

Despite these considerations, the American Academy of Neurology provided recommendations in 2000 against routine prophylaxis based on a meta-analysis of limited studies that had not demonstrated a significant benefit from routine prophylactic AED use in a generic population of patients with brain tumors.[53,54] Additional retrospective and prospective cohorts have also suggested that the perioperative seizure rates are relatively low (2–10%),[55,56] without significant differences between groups given prophylaxis and those that have not. However, many of these earlier studies examined patients maintained on phenytoin rather than newer AEDs such as levetiracetam or lacosamide, both of which were better tolerated with fewer systemic side effects and drug–drug interactions than phenytoin,[57] and the studies examined only perioperative seizure risk related to craniotomy. Given the morbidity of late-onset epilepsy related to disease progression and the risk of status epilepticus, it is not inappropriate to initiate seizure prophylaxis in some brain tumors. Ultimately, careful deliberation and discussion with the surgery and oncology teams is crucial to providing the appropriate recommendations for the patient.

ELECTROLYTE DISTURBANCES

Electrolyte disturbances with sodium—and, accordingly, free water shifts in the body—are most commonly seen in patients who have had surgery for pituitary pathology.[58–62] Involvement of the vascular supply to the pituitary gland and manipulation of the infundibulum (pituitary stalk) should be conveyed by the neurosurgeon to the medical teams in order to properly assess the risk of potential endocrine and electrolyte imbalances. For example, craniopharyngiomas are tumors that arise from the neurohypophysis or pituitary stalk. The stalk is frequently transected during surgery to achieve gross total resection. Central diabetes insipidus, transient or permanent, is a near universal postoperative consequence and should be expected and managed appropriately.

In most patients, the observed changes in water-electrolyte metabolism are often transient and secondary to manipulation of but not inherent damage to the neurohypophysis. Secretion of antidiuretic hormone (ADH)—also referred to as vasopressin—is impaired and the kidneys are unable to hold free water.[58,59] Initial increases in urine output with associated increases in serum sodium will occur, resulting in central diabetes insipidus (CDI). Initial workup may include serum chemistry studies and osmolality paired with urine electrolytes and osmolality. Elevated serum values with low urine sodium and osmolality are indicative of CDI. A variety of management strategies exist for postoperative CDI, including the administration of exogenous desmopressin (DDAVP) as an ADH analog. However, CDI follows an unpredictable triphasic response. Initial hypernatremia due to a lack of appropriate ADH secretion is followed by the lysis of neurohypophyseal cells, resulting in a surge of inappropriate ADH secretion and hyponatremia until the cells are exhausted of the ADH reserve and the patient returns to the picture of CDI with hypernatremia. DDAVP administration during the second phase can exacerbate hyponatremia and result in fatigue, lethargy, alterations in mental status, seizures, coma, and death. For this reason, a more conservative approach is often employed. Since CDI does not affect thirst, patients are encouraged to drink free water ad lib to replete their free water deficit until the course of their CDI is better understood. If the free water requirements exceed a patient's ability to drink, particularly if the need to urinate leads to an inability to sleep at night, intranasal or oral DDAVP can be initiated and titrated until serum sodium levels stabilize and water intake is appropriate.

On the opposite end of the spectrum is hyponatremia. This is the most common electrolyte imbalance in hospital inpatients and can be particularly troublesome in patients with brain tumors.[63-65] In the setting of acute hyponatremia, patients may suffer from worsening cerebral edema, impaired consciousness, seizures, or even death due to cerebral herniation. Therefore, it is important that this be recognized and treated appropriately. The most common cause is the syndrome of inappropriate ADH secretion (SIADH). Diagnostic criteria include serum osmolality less than 280 mOsm/kg; inappropriately high urine osmolality, greater than 100 mOsm/kg; and elevated urinary sodium greater than 20-40 mEq/L. It is important to exclude other endocrine disorders such as hypothyroidism and adrenal insufficiency and to ensure that patients are euvolemic without deficiencies in water or salt intake. SIADH is typically treated by simple fluid restriction; however, loop diuretics, hypertonic saline, and vaptans can also be utilized.[66] More details on treatment of SIADH can be found in Chapter 9.

INFECTIONS AND FEVERS

Fevers are incredibly common in the postoperative setting. In patients with brain tumors, many aspects of their history can help narrow causes of fevers and lead to appropriate testing and treatment. Patient comorbidities, the type of surgery, the type of tumor, and the time course of the fever are important distinguishing features. Early fevers are often associated with physiological responses to surgical stress but pneumonia and pneumonitis, urinary tract infections, and thrombophlebitis occur in postoperative craniotomies just as in any other surgery. Subacute fevers should be more alarming for surgical site infections. Hospitalists who frequently see neurosurgical patients should become familiar with inspecting cranial incisions and identifying poor wound healing and surgical site infections. Visual cues include superficial dehiscence, erythema, or distinct purulent discharge. Persistent fluid collection can also represent an infected cranial flap, and tenderness to palpation suggests persistent inflammation due to local infection. Patients with multiple surgeries, recent chemotherapy treatments, chronic steroid use, or a history of diabetes are at higher risk of having an infection.[67]

Patient hygiene is incredibly important. Prior to discharge, all members of the patient's care team—including surgeon and hospitalist—should emphasize basic but often overlooked good hygiene practices with his or her patients. This includes regular hair washing, using a gentle or even a baby shampoo, initially. During the months of warmer weather, sun protection is critical—patients should wear a loose fitted hat or cap to keep their incision covered. With surgeries involving the posterior fossa, it is important to monitor for clear fluid drainage from the ear or nose that may represent a persistent spinal fluid leak or the development of a fluid-filled collection—a pseudomeningocele—which may portend poor tissue healing and may result in a spinal fluid leak that will become infected and result in meningitis.

In cases of suspected wound infection, the workup should also include a complete blood count with differential and blood cultures, as well as cerebrospinal fluid cultures in certain cases of suspected meningitis. An erythrocyte sedimentation rate (ESR) and C-reactive protein (CRP) can often be used to verify systemic inflammation and trend response to therapy. Superficial wound cultures can be obtained, but should be done only after adequate preparation of the site in order to decontaminate surrounding skin flora. In the event that a wound infection is confirmed and deeper infection is suspected, a patient should have an MRI brain with and without contrast to assess for any concerning findings to suggest that the infection is involving the meninges or even the parenchyma. A subdural empyema or cerebral abscess is a worrying finding that may necessitate rapid surgical consultation and early debridement for source control. It is usually appropriate to withhold initiation of antibiotic therapy until tissue cultures are obtained to identify the infectious organism and to initiate appropriately narrow antibiotics. An exception should be made if the patient is hemodynamically unstable due to sepsis or presenting with severe meningitis.

VENOUS THROMBOSIS AND PULMONARY EMBOLUS

Venous thromboembolism is a common occurrence in patients with brain tumors. Patients are at high risk because the malignancy pushes the milieu of the body to a prothrombotic state.[6,68] Patient with brain tumors may also be less mobile due to a neurological deficit. All patients who are hospitalized or at a facility where their mobility may be restricted should be maintained on prophylaxis with subcutaneous injection of heparin, low-molecular-weight heparin, or fondaparinaux.[69] Intermittent compression devices should be utilized to reduce inpatient venous thrombosis. However, lower extremity edema or acute-onset pain should trigger further investigation of lower limb DVT. Similarly, chest pain, shortness of breath, tachypnea, and tachycardia should warrant evaluation for PE.

If a patient is diagnosed with a DVT and/or PE, is important for the hospitalist to know when the patient last had surgery. A recent craniotomy is a relative contraindication for typical anticoagulation, and early discussion with the neurosurgeon is critical to determine the risk and benefit of anticoagulation. For DVTs without PE, an inferior vena cava filter (IVC filter) can be deployed to prevent catastrophic cardiopulmonary complications until it is safe to initiate anticoagulation from a surgical standpoint. On the other hand, for PE with severe cardiopulmonary compromise and left heart strain, an IVC filter is ineffective, and anticoagulation may be required to prevent death. Each case should be discussed and include input from both the surgical and medical teams, and clinical decision-making should occur on an individualized basis.

If anticoagulation is necessary and there has been sufficient time since surgery, it is recommended to initiate anticoagulation after an initial baseline CT of the head to rule out new intratumoral hemorrhages. If there is residual tumor, particularly in the cases of high-grade gliomas or metastatic tumors that are prone to bleeding, the patient and family should be counseled extensively on the risks of anticoagulation, and the patient should be followed very closely when the anticoagulation is being administered. A heparin infusion without an initial bolus dose is preferred in these higher risk patients to avoid a spontaneous intracranial hemorrhage into tenuous brain parenchyma. Once the patient is appropriately anticoagulated, a repeat CT of the head can be performed to ensure no new hemorrhages have occurred and that the patient can be maintained safely in an anticoagulated state. If there is any concern of new neurological symptoms, change in mental status, or seizures, further neuroimaging is warranted and anticoagulation may need to be discontinued or reversed if a new hemorrhage is discovered. The key to preventing devastating hemorrhagic complications from anticoagulation is careful neurological exams. Even a subtle change should prompt new imaging to evaluate for early intracranial hemorrhage.

SPECIAL CONSIDERATIONS FOR ANTI-ANGIOGENESIS THERAPY

Anti-angiogenesis agents targeting the vascular endothelial growth factor (VEGF) pathway have been approved for a variety of indications and present their own challenge in perioperative management.[70,71] More patients are now started on anti-VEGF therapies for symptomatic relief of cerebral edema, especially in steroid-reducing regimens associated with immunotherapy-based clinical trials. Patients on bevacizumab typically suffer from higher blood pressure and are at higher risk for gastrointestinal hemorrhages and other bleeding complications, as well as for thromboembolic events. Given these side effects, patients should be risk profiled by screening for hypertension and hyperlipidemia prior to initiating therapy. VEGF typically phosphorylates endothelial nitric oxide (NO) synthase, which lowers plasminogen activator inhibitor-1 expression. This clinically translates to lower blood pressure. Inhibition of this pathway during bevacizumab-induced VEGF blockade leads to the hypertension associated with the drug. For this reason, angiotensin converting enzyme (ACE) inhibitors are often effective in treating bevacizumab-induced hypertension.

Importantly, patients treated with bevacizumab are at high risk for wound complications. Thus it is often important to discontinue bevacizumab for several weeks prior to the planned surgery and to hold for several weeks after a craniotomy.

REFERENCES

1. Drappatz J, Schiff D, Kesari S, Norden AD, Wen PY. Medical management of brain tumor patients. *Neurol Clin.* 2007;25(4):1035–1071. doi: 10.1016/j.ncl.2007.07.015

2. Pruitt AA. Medical management of patients with brain tumors. *Continuum.* 2015;21(2):314. doi: 10.1212/01.CON.0000464172.50638.21

3. Schiff D, Lee EQ, Nayak L, Norden AD, Reardon DA, Wen PY. Medical management of brain tumors and the sequelae of treatment. *Neuro Oncol.* 2015;17(4):488–504. doi: 10.1093/neuonc/nou304

4. Lacroix M, Abi-Said D, Fourney DR, et al. A multivariate analysis of 416 patients with glioblastoma multiforme: prognosis, extent of resection, and survival. *J Neurosurg.* 2001;95(2):190–198. doi: 10.3171/jns.2001.95.2.0190

5. Stupp R, Mason WP, van den Bent MJ, et al. Radiotherapy plus concomitant and adjuvant temozolomide for glioblastoma. *N Engl J Med.* 2005;352(10):987–996. doi: 10.1056/NEJMoa043330

6. Wong JM, Panchmatia JR, Ziewacz JE, et al. Patterns in neurosurgical adverse events: intracranial neoplasm surgery. *Neurosurg Focus.* 2012;33(5):E16. doi: 10.3171/2012.7.FOCUS12183

7. Barnholtz-Sloan JS, Ostrom QT, Cote D. Epidemiology of brain tumors. *Neurol Clin.* 2018;36(3):395–419. doi: 10.1016/j.ncl.2018.04.001

8. Ostrom QT, Gittleman H, Liao P, et al. CBTRUS statistical report: primary brain and other central nervous system tumors diagnosed in the United States in 2010–2014. *Neuro-oncology.* 2017;19(suppl_5):v1–v88. doi: 10.1093/neuonc/nox158

9. Siegel RL, Miller KD, Jemal A. Cancer statistics, 2017. *CA Cancer J Clin.* 2017;67(1):7–30. doi: 10.3322/caac.21387

10. Fox BD, Cheung VJ, Patel AJ, Suki D, Rao G. Epidemiology of metastatic brain tumors. *Neurosurg Clin N Am.* 2011;22(1):1–6, v. doi: 10.1016/j.nec.2010.08.007

11. Barnholtz-Sloan JS, Sloan AE, Davis FG, Vigneau FD, Lai P, Sawaya RE. Incidence proportions of brain metastases in patients diagnosed (1973 to 2001) in the Metropolitan Detroit Cancer Surveillance System. *J Clin Oncol.* 2004;22(14):2865–2872. doi: 10.1200/JCO.2004.12.149

12. Asano K, Nakano T, Takeda T, Ohkuma H. Risk factors for postoperative systemic complications in elderly patients with brain tumors. Clinical article. *J Neurosurg.* 2009;111(2):258–264. doi: 10.3171/2008.10.17669

13. Reponen E, Tuominen H, Korja M. Evidence for the use of preoperative risk assessment scores in elective cranial neurosurgery: a systematic review of the literature. *Anesth Analg.* 2014;119(2):420–432. doi: 10.1213/ANE.0000000000000234

14. Fisher JL, Palmisano S, Schwartzbaum JA, Svensson T, Lönn S. Comorbid conditions associated with glioblastoma. *J Neurooncol.* 2014;116(3):585–591. doi: 10.1007/s11060-013-1341-x

15. Grossman R, Mukherjee D, Chang DC, et al. Preoperative Charlson comorbidity score predicts postoperative outcomes among older intracranial meningioma patients. *World Neurosurg.* 2011;75(2):279–285. doi: 10.1016/j.wneu.2010.09.003

16. Grossman R, Mukherjee D, Chang DC, et al. Predictors of inpatient death and complications among postoperative elderly patients with metastatic brain tumors. *Ann Surg Oncol.* 2011;18(2):521–528. doi: 10.1245/s10434-010-1299-2

17. Goldman L, Caldera DL, Nussbaum SR, et al. Multifactorial index of cardiac risk in noncardiac surgical procedures. *N Engl J Med.* 1977;297(16):845–850. doi: 10.1056/NEJM197710202971601

18. Lee TH, Marcantonio ER, Mangione CM, et al. Derivation and prospective validation of a simple index for prediction of cardiac risk of major noncardiac surgery. *Circulation.* 1999;100(10):1043–1049.

19. Fleisher LA, Beckman JA, Brown KA, et al. ACC/AHA 2007 Guidelines on Perioperative Cardiovascular Evaluation and Care for Noncardiac Surgery: Executive Summary: A Report of the American College of Cardiology/American Heart Association Task Force on Practice Guidelines (Writing Committee to Revise the 2002 Guidelines on Perioperative Cardiovascular Evaluation for Noncardiac Surgery) developed in collaboration with the American Society of Echocardiography, American Society of Nuclear Cardiology, Heart Rhythm Society, Society of Cardiovascular Anesthesiologists, Society for Cardiovascular Angiography and Interventions, Society for Vascular Medicine and Biology, and Society for Vascular Surgery. *J Am Coll Cardiol.* 2007;50(17):1707–1732. doi: 10.1016/j.jacc.2007.09.001

20. Brown DA, Himes BT, Major BT, et al. Cranial tumor surgical outcomes at a high-volume academic referral center. *Mayo Clin Proc.* 2018;93(1):16–24. doi: 10.1016/j.mayocp.2017.08.023

21. Edgcombe H, Carter K, Yarrow S. Anaesthesia in the prone position. *Br J Anaesth.* 2008;100(2):165–183. doi: 10.1093/bja/aem380

22. Chui J, Craen RA. An update on the prone position: continuing professional development. *Can J Anaesth.* 2016;63(6):737–767. doi: 10.1007/s12630-016-0634-x

23. Saladino A, Lamperti M, Mangraviti A, et al. The semisitting position: analysis of the risks and surgical outcomes in a contemporary series of 425 adult patients undergoing cranial surgery. *J Neurosurg.* 2017;127(4):867–876. doi: 10.3171/2016.8.JNS16719

24. Himes BT, Mallory GW, Abcejo AS, et al. Contemporary analysis of the intraoperative and perioperative complications of neurosurgical procedures performed in the sitting position. *J Neurosurg.* 2017;127(1):182–188. doi: 10.3171/2016.5.JNS152328

25. Lobatto DJ, de Vries F, Zamanipoor Najafabadi AH, et al. Preoperative risk factors for postoperative complications in endoscopic pituitary surgery: a systematic review. *Pituitary.* September 2017. doi: 10.1007/s11102-017-0839-1

26. Kim JH, Lee JH, Lee JH, Hong AR, Kim YJ, Kim YH. Endoscopic transsphenoidal surgery outcomes in 331 nonfunctioning pituitary adenoma cases after a single surgeon learning curve. *World Neurosurg.* 2018;109:e409–e416. doi: 10.1016/j.wneu.2017.09.194

27. Kondziolka D, Madhok R, Lunsford LD, et al. Stereotactic radiosurgery for convexity meningiomas. *J Neurosurg.* 2009;111(3):458–463. doi: 10.3171/2008.8.JNS17650

28. Bloch O, Kaur G, Jian BJ, Parsa AT, Barani IJ. Stereotactic radiosurgery for benign meningiomas. *J Neurooncol.* 2012;107(1):13–20. doi: 10.1007/s11060-011-0720-4

29. Golfinos JG, Hill TC, Rokosh R, et al. A matched cohort comparison of clinical outcomes following microsurgical resection or stereotactic radiosurgery for patients with small- and medium-sized vestibular schwannomas. *J Neurosurg.* 2016;125(6):1472–1482. doi: 10.3171/2015.12.JNS151857

30. Ding D, Mehta GU, Patibandla MR, et al. Stereotactic radiosurgery for acromegaly: an international multicenter retrospective cohort study. *Neurosurgery.* May 2018. doi: 10.1093/neuros/nyy178

31. Narayan V, Mohammed N, Bir SC, et al. Long-term outcome of nonfunctioning and hormonal active pituitary adenoma after gamma knife radiosurgery. *World Neurosurg.* 2018;114:e824–e832. doi: 10.1016/j.wneu.2018.03.094

32. Snyder MH, Shepard MJ, Chen C-J, Sheehan JP. Stereotactic radiosurgery for trigeminal schwannomas: a 28-year single-center experience and review of the literature. *World Neurosurg.* 2018;119:e874–e881. doi: 10.1016/j.wneu.2018.07.289

33. Linskey ME, Andrews DW, Asher AL, et al. The role of stereotactic radiosurgery in the management of patients with newly diagnosed brain metastases: a systematic review and evidence-based clinical practice guideline. *J Neurooncol.* 2010;96(1):45–68. doi: 10.1007/s11060-009-0073-4

34. Patel KR, Burri SH, Asher AL, et al. Comparing preoperative with postoperative stereotactic radiosurgery for resectable brain metastases: a multi-institutional analysis. *Neurosurgery.* 2016;79(2):279–285. doi: 10.1227/NEU.0000000000001096

35. Nahaczewski AE, Fowler SB, Hariharan S. Dexamethasone therapy in patients with brain tumors—a focus on tapering. *J Neurosci Nurs.* 2004;36(6):340–343.

36. Kaal ECA, Vecht CJ. The management of brain edema in brain tumors. *Curr Opin Oncol.* 2004;16(6):593–600.

37. Marko NF, Gonugunta VA, Hamrahian AH, Usmani A, Mayberg MR, Weil RJ. Use of morning serum cortisol level after transsphenoidal resection of pituitary adenoma to predict the need for long-term glucocorticoid supplementation. *J Neurosurg.* 2009;111(3):540–544. doi: 10.3171/2008.12.JNS081265

38. Ausiello JC, Bruce JN, Freda PU. Postoperative assessment of the patient after transsphenoidal pituitary surgery. *Pituitary.* 2008;11(4):391–401. doi: 10.1007/s11102-008-0086-6

39. McGirt MJ, Chaichana KL, Gathinji M, et al. Persistent outpatient hyperglycemia is independently associated with decreased survival after primary resection of malignant brain astrocytomas. *Neurosurgery.* 2008;63(2):286–291; discussion 291. doi: 10.1227/01.NEU.0000315282.61035.48

40. Ismail MF, Lavelle C, Cassidy EM. Steroid-induced mental disorders in cancer patients: a systematic review. *Future Oncol.* 2017;13(29):2719–2731. doi: 10.2217/fon-2017-0306

41. Pereira RMR, Freire de Carvalho J. Glucocorticoid-induced myopathy. *Joint Bone Spine.* 2011;78(1):41–44. doi: 10.1016/j.jbspin.2010.02.025

42. Liigant A, Haldre S, Oun A, et al. Seizure disorders in patients with brain tumors. *Eur Neurol.* 2001;45(1):46–51. doi: 10.1159/000052089

43. Lynam LM, Lyons MK, Drazkowski JF, et al. Frequency of seizures in patients with newly diagnosed brain tumors: a retrospective review. *Clin Neurol Neurosurg.* 2007;109(7):634–638. doi: 10.1016/j.clineuro.2007.05.017

44. Rudà R, Trevisan E, Soffietti R. Epilepsy and brain tumors. *Curr Opin Oncol.* 2010;22(6):611–620. doi: 10.1097/CCO.0b013e32833de99d

45. Pallud J, Audureau E, Blonski M, et al. Epileptic seizures in diffuse low-grade gliomas in adults. *Brain.* 2014;137(Pt 2):449–462. doi: 10.1093/brain/awt345

46. Englot DJ, Magill ST, Han SJ, Chang EF, Berger MS, McDermott MW. Seizures in supratentorial meningioma: a systematic review and meta-analysis. *J Neurosurg.* 2016;124(6):1552–1561. doi: 10.3171/2015.4.JNS142742

47. Cavaliere R, Farace E, Schiff D. Clinical implications of status epilepticus in patients with neoplasms. *Arch Neurol.* 2006;63(12):1746–1749. doi: 10.1001/archneur.63.12.1746

48. Vecht CJ, van Breemen M. Optimizing therapy of seizures in patients with brain tumors. *Neurology.* 2006;67(12 Suppl 4):S10–S13.

49. van Breemen MSM, Wilms EB, Vecht CJ. Epilepsy in patients with brain tumours: epidemiology, mechanisms, and management. *Lancet Neurol.* 2007;6(5):421–430. doi: 10.1016/S1474-4422(07)70103-5

50. Nasr ZG, Paravattil B, Wilby KJ. Levetiracetam for seizure prevention in brain tumor patients: a systematic review. *J Neurooncol.* 2016;129(1):1–13. doi: 10.1007/s11060-016-2146-5

51. Chen DY, Chen CC, Crawford JR, Wang SG. Tumor-related epilepsy: epidemiology, pathogenesis and management. *J Neurooncol.* 2018;139(1):13–21. doi: 10.1007/s11060-018-2862-0

52. Rosati A, Tomassini A, Pollo B, et al. Epilepsy in cerebral glioma: timing of appearance and histological correlations. *J Neurooncol.* 2009;93(3):395–400. doi: 10.1007/s11060-009-9796-5

53. Glantz MJ, Cole BF, Forsyth PA, et al. Practice parameter: anticonvulsant prophylaxis in patients with newly diagnosed brain tumors. Report of the Quality Standards Subcommittee of the American Academy of Neurology. *Neurology.* 2000;54(10):1886–1893.

54. Mikkelsen T, Paleologos NA, Robinson PD, et al. The role of prophylactic anticonvulsants in the management of brain metastases: a systematic review and evidence-based clinical practice guideline. *J Neurooncol.* 2010;96(1):97–102. doi: 10.1007/s11060-009-0056-5

55. Wu AS, Trinh VT, Suki D, et al. A prospective randomized trial of perioperative seizure prophylaxis in patients with intraparenchymal brain tumors. *J Neurosurg.* 2013;118(4):873–883. doi: 10.3171/2012.12.JNS111970

56. Dewan MC, White-Dzuro GA, Brinson PR, et al. The influence of perioperative seizure prophylaxis on seizure rate and hospital quality metrics following glioma resection. *Neurosurgery.* 2017;80(4):563–570. doi: 10.1093/neuros/nyw106

57. Iuchi T, Kuwabara K, Matsumoto M, Kawasaki K, Hasegawa Y, Sakaida T. Levetiracetam versus phenytoin for seizure prophylaxis during and early after craniotomy for brain tumours: a phase II prospective, randomised study. *J Neurol Neurosurg Psychiatry.* 2015;86(10):1158–1162. doi: 10.1136/jnnp-2014-308584

58. Adams JR, Blevins LS, Allen GS, Verity DK, Devin JK. Disorders of water metabolism following transsphenoidal pituitary surgery: a single institution's experience. *Pituitary.* 2006;9(2):93–99. doi: 10.1007/s11102-006-9276-2

59. Kristof RA, Rother M, Neuloh G, Klingmüller D. Incidence, clinical manifestations, and course of water and electrolyte metabolism disturbances following transsphenoidal pituitary adenoma surgery: a prospective observational study. *J Neurosurg.* 2009;111(3):555–562. doi: 10.3171/2008.9.JNS08191

60. Hussain NS, Piper M, Ludlam WG, Ludlam WH, Fuller CJ, Mayberg MR. Delayed postoperative hyponatremia after transsphenoidal surgery: prevalence and associated factors. *J Neurosurg.* 2013;119(6):1453–1460. doi: 10.3171/2013.8.JNS13411

61. Barber SM, Liebelt BD, Baskin DS. Incidence, etiology and outcomes of hyponatremia after transsphenoidal surgery: experience with 344 consecutive patients at a single tertiary center. *J Clin Med.* 2014;3(4):1199–1219. doi: 10.3390/jcm3041199

62. Alzhrani G, Sivakumar W, Park MS, Taussky P, Couldwell WT. Delayed complications after transsphenoidal surgery for pituitary adenomas. *World Neurosurg.* 2018;109:233–241. doi: 10.1016/j.wneu.2017.09.192

63. Kelly DF, Laws ER, Fossett D. Delayed hyponatremia after transsphenoidal surgery for pituitary adenoma. Report of nine cases. *J Neurosurg.* 1995;83(2):363–367. doi: 10.3171/jns.1995.83.2.0363

64. Zada G, Liu CY, Fishback D, Singer PA, Weiss MH. Recognition and management of delayed hyponatremia following transsphenoidal pituitary surgery. *J Neurosurg.* 2007;106(1):66–71. doi: 10.3171/jns.2007.106.1.66

65. Bohl MA, Ahmad S, Jahnke H, et al. Delayed hyponatremia is the most common cause of 30-day unplanned readmission after transsphenoidal surgery for pituitary tumors. *Neurosurgery.* 2016;78(1):84–90. doi: 10.1227/NEU.0000000000001003

66. Lien Y-HH, Shapiro JI. Hyponatremia: clinical diagnosis and management. *Am J Med.* 2007;120(8):653–658. doi: 10.1016/j.amjmed.2006.09.031

67. McCutcheon BA, Ubl DS, Babu M, et al. Predictors of surgical site infection following craniotomy for intracranial neoplasms: an analysis of prospectively collected data in the American College of Surgeons National Surgical Quality Improvement Program Database. *World Neurosurg.* 2016;88:350–358. doi: 10.1016/j.wneu.2015.12.068

68. Brandes AA, Scelzi E, Salmistraro G, et al. Incidence of risk of thromboembolism during treatment high-grade gliomas: a prospective study. *Eur J Cancer.* 1997;33(10):1592–1596.

69. Alshehri N, Cote DJ, Hulou MM, et al. Venous thromboembolism prophylaxis in brain tumor patients undergoing craniotomy: a meta-analysis. *J Neurooncol.* 2016;130(3):561–570. doi: 10.1007/s11060-016-2259-x

70. Kreisl TN, Kim L, Moore K, et al. Phase II trial of single-agent bevacizumab followed by bevacizumab plus irinotecan at tumor progression in recurrent glioblastoma. *J Clin Oncol.* 2009;27(5):740–745. doi: 10.1200/JCO.2008.16.3055

71. Gilbert MR, Dignam JJ, Armstrong TS, et al. A randomized trial of bevacizumab for newly diagnosed glioblastoma. *N Engl J Med.* 2014;370(8):699–708. doi: 10.1056/NEJMoa1308573

5 Antiepileptic Medication Use in Neurosurgical Patients

Megan Margiotta and Timothy Ambrose

INDICATIONS FOR TREATMENT

Antiepileptic medication is warranted in patients who have an increased risk of recurrent seizures. This includes patients who have had two or more unprovoked seizures separated by greater than 24 hours. Generally, a patient who has had only one unprovoked seizure does not require antiepileptic medication.[1,2] However, if a patient has had only one seizure, starting medication should be considered for those patients at an increased risk of having additional seizures. Patients may have an increased risk for recurrent seizures if they have a functional or structural brain abnormality (infarct, hemorrhage, tumor) or if their EEG is abnormal (focal sharp waves or generalized spike-wave discharges).[2,3] Additionally, if the initial seizure occurs in sleep, this may be associated with an increased risk of recurrent seizure, although other supporting clinical or historical data may be needed to determine the risk of further seizures.

A common question encountered is whether antiepileptic medications are recommended prophylactically in neurosurgical patients who have never had a seizure. In review of the available literature, there is no evidence to support prophylactic antiepileptic medication use for patients with brain tumors, ischemic strokes, or traumatic brain injuries. However, most data study the use of older agents such as phenytoin, and there are less data available on newer agents such as levetiracetam and lacosamide, which are known to have better side-effect profiles overall. Neurosurgeons will often use these newer antiepileptic medications in the perioperative setting for seizure prophylaxis. The use of prophylactic antiepileptic medication in the context of subarachnoid hemorrhage with an unsecured aneurysm is a debated topic, with many experts stating that the relatively low risk of acute medication side effects is outweighed by the benefits of preventing a seizure in a compromised brain at risk for aneurysm rupture or vasospasm.[4] However, a large series studying prophylactic phenytoin use for subarachnoid hemorrhage was associated with worse cognitive and neurologic outcomes, so this medication in particular tends to be avoided. Of note, most of the available literature on this topic focuses on older antiepileptic medications, such as phenytoin, valproate, phenobarbital, and carbamazepine, all of which are known to have a number of side effects and significant interactions with other medications. For example, valproate can be associated with platelet dysfunction. Newer agents, such as levetiracetam and lacosamide, generally have a better side-effect profile but have not been studied as extensively. At this time, no rigorous evidence is available to specifically recommend their use over other antiepileptic medications. Usage of prophylactic antiepileptic medication is currently suggested for patients with acute subarachnoid hemorrhage with poor neurologic function, an unsecured aneurysm, and/or an associated intracerebral hemorrhage,[5] although the relative impact of prophylactic antiepileptic medication treatment on functional outcomes is unclear.

WHICH ANTIEPILEPTIC MEDICATION SHOULD BE STARTED?

Choosing the correct antiepileptic medication from the start is an important consideration. Subsequent providers are often reluctant to alter antiseizure treatments they perceive to be working, and patients tend to be hesitant to change therapy once it has started. Many antiepileptic medications, especially older ones, are associated with long-term effects to bone health and liver function. Newer agents tend to have fewer side effects and long-term health risks, but overall these medications have less long-term data available. Additionally, some newer mediations may not have generic formulations and can be expensive, thus prohibiting their use in the outpatient setting. If the medication is unaffordable, this can lead to noncompliance and an increased risk of seizures. If a new antiepileptic medication is started during hospitalization, the anticipated cost for prescription refills should be determined prior to discharge, and a less expensive alternative should be considered if indicated. In general, the overall goal of antiepileptic medication use is to select an appropriate medication that will prevent seizures with the least amount of side effects that could negatively affect compliance. The following text is a list of commonly prescribed antiepileptic medications, placed in alphabetical order for ease of reference. Please note that this order does not imply a preference in prescribing; in general, agents such as levetiracetam, phenytoin, and valproate may be prescribed more frequently in the inpatient setting compared to carbamazepine, oxcarbazepine, and lamotrigine, though the latter medications are commonly used in the outpatient setting. Please refer to Table 5.1 for a list of commonly prescribed antiepileptic medications; indications for use for focal epilepsy, generalized epilepsy, and/or status epilepticus; availability of oral or intravenous formulations; relative cost; and pregnancy risk categorization.

CARBAMAZEPINE (BRAND NAMES TEGRETOL, CARBATROL) AND OXCARBAZEPINE (BRAND NAMES TRILEPTAL, OXTELLAR XR)

Carbamazepine and oxcarbazepine are commonly used medications in the outpatient setting because they are generally well-tolerated and can be quickly titrated to

Table 5.1 Commonly prescribed antiepileptic medications, and usage considerations.

	Use	Formulation	Pregnancy Category	Cost
Carbamazepine	F, G[a]	Oral, IV	D	$$
Lacosamide	F, S	Oral, IV	Data not available	$$$
Lamotrigine	F, G	Oral	C	$
Levetiracetam	F, G, S	Oral, IV	C	$
Oxcarbazepine	F	Oral	C	$$
Phenobarbital	F, G, S	Oral, IV	D	$
Phenytoin	F, G, S	Oral, IV	D	$
Topiramate	F, G	Oral	D	$
Valproate	F, G, S	Oral, IV	D	$
Zonisamide	F	Oral	C	$$

[a]Not indicated for treatment of absence seizures.

F, focal seizures; G, generalized seizures; S, status epilepticus.

target doses. The most common reason that a provider may not choose to prescribe carbamazepine or oxcarbazepine is because of their frequent drug–drug interactions and the side effect of hyponatremia. Carbamazepine and oxcarbazepine work by inhibiting sodium, calcium, and potassium channels, as well as gamma-aminobutyric acid (GABA) receptors. They can be used to treat partial seizures or generalized tonic-clonic seizures. These medications are not effective for, and can actually worsen, absence or myoclonic seizures. Carbamazepine has oral (tablet, suspension, extended-release versions) and intravenous formulations, but oxcarbazepine is only available as an oral medication. When converting to an intravenous formulation of carbamazepine, the dose should be reduced to 70% of the oral dosing.[6]

Carbamazepine is usually initiated at 200 mg twice a day with increases of 200 mg/d made weekly. Target dosing is typically 800–1,200 mg/d in divided doses, which should be three times per day with standard carbamazepine or every 12 hours with an extended-release formulation. Metabolism is primarily through the liver P450 system, and the main metabolite is carbamazepine-10,11-epoxide. Carbamazepine undergoes a process where it induces its own metabolism, called *autoinduction*. This can last for 2–6 weeks after a stable dose has been initiated, and serum drug levels can drop initially when autoinduction takes place.[7] Drug level monitoring is recommended to ensure therapeutic dosing. A level should be drawn 3–4 weeks after reaching a target dose with a goal level between 4 and 12 mg/L.[8] Carbamazepine is excreted in the urine, and patients with decreased kidney function or on dialysis should receive lower doses of the medication.

Carbamazepine is an inducer of the CYP450 system and can interact with many medications. The epoxide metabolite causes many of the side effects seen with carbamazepine. The most common side effects are nausea, vomiting, dizziness, drowsiness, ataxia, headache, and diplopia. Carbamazepine can cause generalized rash, as well as rare but serious hypersensitivity reactions including Stevens-Johnson syndrome, toxic epidermal necrolysis, and DRESS syndrome. The risk of a severe rash is higher in patients with HLA-B*1502 allele (a variant of human leukocyte antigen-B gene). This is common in patients of Asian descent, and screening in this population should be performed prior to starting carbamazepine.[9] Other potential side effects of carbamazepine include elevated cholesterol levels, hyponatremia, and weight gain. Rarely hepatotoxicity, agranulocytosis, and aplastic anemia have been reported. There is unclear evidence that carbamazepine reduces bone density, but there have been associations reported with osteoporosis.[10] Carbamazepine has a relatively safer profile for use in pregnancy, with only a 3% risk of major congenital malformations (compared to 9.3% with valproate).[11,12]

Oxcarbazepine is preferred by most providers over carbamazepine because of a better pharmacokinetic and side-effect profile. Initial dosing is 600 mg/d divided into twice-daily dosing. Titrations can be made weekly with an increase of 300 mg/d to 600 mg/d. The target dose is typically 1,200–2,400 mg/d. Unlike carbamazepine, oxcarbazepine does not have properties of autoinduction. It induces the CYP450 system but to a lesser degree than carbamazepine. Oxcarbazepine is not metabolized to an epoxide and therefore has in general fewer side effects compared to carbamazepine. Potential side effects are similar to carbamazepine, including dizziness, fatigue, diplopia, headache, nausea, rash, and hyponatremia. Oxcarbazepine is also relatively safe in pregnancy compared to other antiepileptic medications.[12] However, for patients without insurance, carbamazepine is among the least expensive agents available and may be the only affordable option.

LACOSAMIDE (BRAND NAME VIMPAT)

Lacosamide has a relatively novel mechanism of action in that it prolongs inactivation of sodium channels after they fire an action potential and undergo afterhyperpolarization. It is available in oral and intravenous forms. Although it is currently approved by the US Food and Drug Administration (FDA) as an adjunctive therapy for focal onset seizures, lacosamide has shown anecdotally to be quite effective for both seizure prevention as well as acute treatment of seizures or status epilepticus. As such, it is often employed as a treatment for otherwise medically refractory seizures. Additionally, its use will be considered sooner in patients with multiple medical comorbidities and/or patients taking medications for which interactions will be a concern, such as with warfarin use. For initiation of lacosamide for medically refractory seizures, it is typically given as a bolus of 300–400 mg intravenously, followed by maintenance therapy at a strength of 100–200 mg every 12 hours. Serum drug levels are not typically checked. The potential side effects of lacosamide are typical for most antiepileptic medications, including fatigue, double vision, or imbalance, but the medication at higher dosages can also prolong the PR interval, so an ECG should be checked prior to starting the medication.[13]

The greatest barriers to lacosamide use lie not in its administration in the hospital but in the transition from the hospital setting to the outpatient setting. Since no generic equivalent exists, patients frequently will require a prior authorization to medication approval. If not approved by insurance, the medication co-pay can make the medication unaffordable, as the potential costs can be greater than $700 per month when not covered. This is especially common in patients with Medicare or Medicaid exclusively, without supplemental prescription coverage. When patients are unable to afford the medication, this can lead to noncompliance and subsequent seizures, potentially resulting in injury or death. As such, it is important for the hospitalist to address these issues prior to the patient's discharge. For patients with supplemental prescription coverage, there are several programs available online to provide assistance to make the medication affordable (such as a savings card and support program through the manufacturer's website at www.vimpat.com), but patients with Medicare or Medicaid exclusively are ineligible for this support. This financial barrier may potentially be alleviated once the medication starts to be manufactured in generic form. If lacosamide is not affordable but was started to halt seizures in the hospital setting, exchange with another medication that also affects sodium channels (such as oxcarbazepine or carbamazepine) may be reasonable, but it is recommended to discuss the plan with a neurologist. Lacosamide is currently classified as a Schedule V controlled substance and requires a Drug Enforcement Agency (DEA) license for prescribing in the United States.

LAMOTRIGINE (BRAND NAME LAMICTAL)

Lamotrigine is a commonly used antiepileptic medication in the outpatient setting. It acts on sodium channels to inhibit excitatory activity at the neuronal membrane. Many patients with previously established epilepsy will be taking lamotrigine as an inpatient, but it only rarely will be initiated in the inpatient setting because it requires a slow titration schedule. Rapid initiation of lamotrigine is associated with an increased risk of developing Stevens-Johnson syndrome, a severe and potentially deadly drug rash. This rash commonly affects the palms of the hands, soles of the feet, and the mucous membranes of the mouth or genitals, though it potentially can affect part of the skin. There can be sloughing of the skin, sores, and potentially systemic illness such as sepsis. With a slow, deliberate titration schedule, the risk of Stevens-Johnson syndrome is significantly reduced. The titration schedule is typically provided in a starter pack and differs depending on whether the patient is concurrently taking valproate. In a patient who is not taking valproate, a typical titration schedule is as follows:

Weeks 1 and 2: One 25 mg pill each evening
Weeks 3 and 4: 1 pill, twice a day
Week 5: 1 pill each morning, 2 pills each evening
Week 6: 2 pills, twice per day
Week 7: 2 pills each morning, 3 pills each evening
Week 8: 3 pills, twice a day.

Further increases can be made on a weekly basis at a rate of 25 mg twice daily until the desired dosage is reached, which often will be between 100 and 200 mg every 12 hours. At that point, a serum lamotrigine level can be checked, and a higher dosage pill can be prescribed for convenience.

For a patient on valproate who is starting lamotrigine, the titration schedule is significantly slower due to a reduction of lamotrigine clearance by about 50% (14), which also necessitates a lower overall dosage of lamotrigine:

Start 25 mg pills, #150
Weeks 1 and 2: One 25 mg pill every other day
Weeks 3 and 4: 1 pill per day
Weeks 5 and 6: 1 pill twice per day
Weeks 7 and 8: 1 pill each morning, 2 pills each evening
Weeks 9 and 10: 2 pills, twice per day.

Because of the prolonged course of titrating lamotrigine, it is generally not started in the inpatient setting and is instead titrated as an outpatient. However, the same principle of reduced lamotrigine clearance should be considered if valproate is started as an inpatient for a patient already on lamotrigine. In this circumstance, the overall dosage of lamotrigine will likely need to be reduced by half, and serum lamotrigine and valproic acid levels should be monitored on a daily basis until the level is stable.

Special consideration should be made if the hospitalized patient is pregnant. Lamotrigine is a commonly used medication for patients with epilepsy if they are young women of childbearing age since it has a low rate of fetal malformations. However, the clearance of lamotrigine is significantly increased during pregnancy, requiring recurrent serum lamotrigine level checks (at least every trimester) and dose adjustments as needed.

Lamotrigine is only available in an oral form; there is no intravenous equivalent. In patients unable to swallow pills while hospitalized, temporary use of benzodiazepines or other antiepileptic medications with intravenous formulations may be preferred until the patient is able to safely have enteral access.

LEVETIRACETAM (BRAND NAME KEPPRA)

Levetiracetam is now the most widely prescribed antiepileptic medication, in part because of its affordability, ease of initiation, and minimal interactions with other medications. Levetiracetam is used to treat both focal and generalized forms of epilepsy and is available in oral and intravenous dosing. Levetiracetam is most commonly started at 500 mg every 12 hours in adults, though this can be increased in 500 mg increments to 1,500 mg every 12 hours if seizures reoccur. About 24% of the medication is metabolized into an inactive form, and both the unchanged levetiracetam and the inactive metabolite are excreted in the urine. As such, the dosage should be reduced in renal failure. The medication can also be filtered in hemodialysis and generally requires an additional 250 mg or 500 mg dose following hemodialysis. Clearance of the mediation is reduced in patients with severe hepatic impairment, but an initial dosing adjustment is typically not needed. Geriatric patients also tend to clear levetiracetam more slowly and sometimes may require reduced dosages because of side effects. Common side effects are typical of most antiepileptic drugs, including dizziness, imbalance, double vision, or fatigue. Additionally, levetiracetam is associated with causing mood changes, particularly irritability, which may not be readily recognized unless patients and family members are specifically questioned. It can also be associated with worsening concurrent depression and may not be an ideal medication for patients with known psychiatric disorders.

Because this medication does not cause metabolic derangements, periodic laboratory testing is typically not needed. The half-life is only 6–8 hours, but levetiracetam is proved to be effective with dosing every 12 hours. It likely has therapeutic benefit beyond purely its concentration in the bloodstream, so the benefit of therapeutic drug level monitoring is unclear in most patients. However, periodic drug level monitoring can potentially be useful in special circumstances, such as during pregnancy, because the concentration of levetiracetam will likely diminish as the pregnancy progresses. Levetiracetam also has an extended-release formulation which can be dosed once daily. Levetiracetam is indicated as a first-line therapy when treating status epilepticus.[15]

PHENOBARBITAL

One of the oldest antiepileptic agents, phenobarbital is a barbiturate that acts on the GABA receptor-chloride ionophore complex to increase the duration of its open activated state.[16] It is an effective medication for focal epilepsy, generalized tonic-clonic seizures, and status epilepticus. However, its use comes with several drawbacks. It has a long half-life and can cause sedative side effects. It also has long-term negative effects on bone health and liver health. Furthermore, its mechanism of action results in an increased risk of overdose and death when used concurrently with benzodiazepines or alcohol. Phenobarbital use can also increase a patient's likelihood of developing symptoms of depression. Phenobarbital is pregnancy category D. It is an active hepatic enzyme inducer and, conversely, will have its metabolism inhibited by valproate,[17] which will increase its relative serum concentration with concurrent valproate use. For these reasons, phenobarbital is generally not chosen as a first-line agent for treatment of seizures except in the developing world, where it is more readily available than other antiepileptic agents and at a minimal cost.

PHENYTOIN (BRAND NAME DILANTIN)

Phenytoin is often used for the treatment of status epilepticus; however, it is not a commonly used antiepileptic medication outside of the hospital because of its multiple drug–drug interactions and narrow therapeutic window. It can be used in the treatment of focal seizures or generalized tonic-clonic seizures. The mechanism of action of phenytoin is by inhibition of voltage-dependent sodium channels. It comes in oral (tablet, chewable tablets, suspension, extended release) and intravenous forms. Phenytoin is 90% protein-bound in the body; only the unbound (free) drug is pharmacologically active and able to cross the blood–brain barrier. In low-protein disease states (e.g., renal failure, malnutrition), a corrected or free phenytoin level rather than a total level should be monitored. Metabolism occurs by the liver

P450 system, and phenytoin has zero-order pharmacokinetic properties. A fixed amount of drug will be eliminated at a constant rate, and an overdose of medication can lead to significant toxicity. Signs of phenytoin toxicity include dysarthria, ataxia, and nystagmus. At higher phenytoin levels, more severe side effects including seizures, ophthalmoplegia, lethargy, and confusion can be seen.

Fosphenytoin is a prodrug of phenytoin that can be used for status epilepticus. It can be infused more quickly than phenytoin with a lower risk of cardiac arrhythmias or skin injection site reactions. Initial dosing of fosphenytoin in status epilepticus is 20 mg PE/kg; fosphenytoin is always expressed as phenytoin sodium equivalents ("PE") to avoid the need to calculate molecular weight-based adjustments between fosphenytoin and phenytoin doses. Patients should be monitored for arrhythmias and hypotension during infusion. Two hours after a loading dose is given, a total phenytoin level should be checked with a goal level of 15–20 μg/mL. If the patient has low protein levels, the Sheiner-Tozer algorithm should be used to calculate a corrected total phenytoin level[18,19]:

$$\text{Corrected phenytoin} = \left(\text{measured phenytoin level}\right)/\left(0.2 * \text{Albumin} + 0.1\right).$$

Another option for patients with low protein level is to monitor the free phenytoin level with a goal of 1–2 μg/mL. After an initial free level is drawn, a ratio of free to total phenytoin levels can be used to calculate an estimated free phenytoin level from the measured lab total level. This can be done to avoid regularly drawing a free phenytoin level, which can generally take much longer to result from the laboratory. Once at goal, a standard starting dose of phenytoin 100 mg every 8 hours should be prescribed. A change in dosing can take 5–10 days to reach steady state, so it is important to make dose adjustments slowly. If levels are at goal and dosing has been stable over 3–5 days, weekly drug level monitoring is adequate.

There are numerous drug–drug interactions and side effects of phenytoin, which limits its use. Phenytoin is a hepatic enzyme inducer, so any medication that is metabolized by the CYP3A4 liver enzyme can be affected. Phenytoin is highly protein-bound; it may interfere with other drugs that are protein-bound (such as valproate), rendering it very difficult to predict the levels of these medications when used concurrently. Potential adverse reactions of the medication include diplopia, nystagmus, ataxia, drowsiness, cardiac arrhythmias, hypotension, rash, Stevens-Johnson syndrome, pancytopenia, liver injury, injection site reaction ("purple-glove syndrome"), gingival hyperplasia, hirsutism, osteoporosis, and cerebellar atrophy. Phenytoin remains a first-line treatment for status epilepticus and may be considered for some patients because of the low cost. Overall, medication interactions, side effects, and risk for toxicity limit the use of phenytoin outside of the hospital.[20-22]

TOPIRAMATE (BRAND NAME TOPAMAX)

Topiramate is commonly used in the outpatient setting, particularly for patients with epilepsy and migraines. Unfortunately, the use of this medication is often limited because of fatigue and cognitive side effects. For some patients, the side effect of weight loss may be beneficial. Topiramate is approved for treating both focal seizures and generalized tonic-clonic seizures. The mechanism of action is by inhibition of sodium channels and alpha-amino-3-hydroxy-5-methyl-4-isoxazolepropionic acid (AMPA) receptors, as well as enhancement of GABA activity. It is also a weak carbonic anhydrase inhibitor and can be used to treat idiopathic intracranial hypertension. It only comes in an oral formulation. Initial dosing is 25 mg twice a day, followed by weekly dose increases of 50 mg/d until reaching 100 mg twice a day, and then increasing by 100 mg/d to an ultimate target dose of 200 mg twice daily. Topiramate undergoes hepatic metabolism but the majority (80%) remains unmetabolized. Excretion is through the urine, and those patients with kidney disease should reduce doses by 50%. Topiramate is hemodialyzed, and an extra dose after dialysis should be given. Topiramate drug levels are not routinely monitored. Possible side effects of the medication include paresthesias, fatigue, and weight loss. Memory, concentration, and word retrieval difficulties are not uncommon. Interestingly, topiramate can cause decreased sweating (oligohidrosis) and hyperthermia particularly in children. Rare but more serious side effects include glaucoma, kidney stones, and metabolic acidosis. All patients should be asked about a prior history of kidney stones. Birth control can be less effective at doses of 200 mg/d or higher due to the induction of estrogen clearance. There is an increased risk of oral clefts for babies born to women on topiramate, particularly at higher doses (200 mg/d or higher).[11,23,24]

VALPROIC ACID (VALPROATE, DIVALPROEX; BRAND NAMES DEPACON, DEPAKENE, DEPAKOTE IN THE UNITED STATES)

Valproic acid is a commonly used antiepileptic medication both in the acute and chronic setting and is indicated for both focal and generalized epilepsy syndromes. Additionally, it is a first-line therapy for treatment of status epilepticus. It comes in several forms, and the prescriber should be aware of the differences between each form since it can affect the strength and frequency of dosing to achieve the same therapeutic effect. Also, valproic acid and its related formulations are known to be CYP2C9, glucuronyl transferase, and epoxide hydrolase inhibitors; they are additionally highly protein-bound and will interact with other highly protein-bound drugs as a consequence. Valproate is largely metabolized by the liver, but its rate of metabolism and clearance from the body can be affected by numerous drugs. As such, valproate can be a complicated medication to adjust in the inpatient setting, at it will potentially affect the efficacy of other medications and vice versa. In particular, valproate will inhibit the metabolism of warfarin, potentially leading to elevated INR levels and an increased risk of bleeding. Valproate can also inhibit metabolism of certain chemotherapeutic agents, increasing the risk for toxicity. Conversely, carbapenems will decrease the serum concentration of valproate, which can increase the risk for recurrent seizure. Furthermore, valproate will interact with other commonly used antiepileptic medications, and the end result of their relative concentrations is often not predictable. For example, valproate will inhibit metabolism of carbamazepine, and carbamazepine induces the metabolism of valproate. Similarly, valproate and phenytoin are both highly protein-bound, so introducing valproate can increase the serum free phenytoin concentration, which in turn can induce the metabolism of valproate.[25] When introducing or changing valproate doses in the inpatient setting, it is usually wise to check serial valproate levels on a daily basis until a steady state is achieved, in addition to appropriate serum testing for other medications that interact with the valproate.

When loaded in an intravenous form to abort status epilepticus, the recommended dosage is 20–40 mg/kg administered at rate of 3–6 mg/kg/min. Maintenance dosing is suggested to start at 10–15 mg/kg/d, in divided doses, but can be increased up to a maximum of 60 mg/kg/d. It should be noted that because of its short half-life, valproic acid should be dosed every 8 hours, whereas the related formulation divalproex (Depakote) can be dosed every 12 hours. If transitioning from divalproex to its extended-release formulation (Depakote ER), the overall dose will need to be increased by 8–20% to maintain a stable serum concentration although this can then be given as once-daily dosing. The accepted therapeutic range for valproic acid and its derivatives is 50–100 μg/mL, although some patients will achieve seizure freedom at higher levels, and some patients will experience adverse effects within the therapeutic range. Tremor is the most common adverse effect, with symptomatic tremor seen in approximately 10% of patients.[26] Other common side effects include imbalance, fatigue, weight gain, hair loss, and double vision. Rarely, patients can experience platelet dysfunction, acute liver injury, or pancreatitis. Valproic acid is contraindicated in patients with mitochondrial DNA polymerase gamma (POLG) gene hereditary neurometabolic syndromes because of the increased risk of acute liver failure with valproic acid for these patients. Children under the age of 2 years are also at increased risk of acute liver toxicity on valproate, so extreme caution is advised in using the medication.

Valproic acid's teratogenic effects are also well-described. Among antiepileptic medications, it is the therapy associated with the highest rates of congenital fetal malformations, with 9–11% of children born to mothers taking an average of 1,000 mg total daily dose showing a malformation. In addition, there is a drop of approximately 10 IQ points compared to children of mothers taking other antiepileptic monotherapies.[27] For these reasons, other antiepileptic medications are strongly advised to be considered prior to valproic acid in women of childbearing potential. However, for some patients, especially for those with certain genetically derived generalized epilepsy syndromes, this may be the only effective option.

Cancer research has also suggested that valproate may have an impact on slowing the progression of tumors, either by slowing their mitotic rate or by inducing the expression of genes that will make cancerous cells more susceptible to chemotherapeutic agents. Combined valproic acid with the chemotherapy agent temozolomide was shown to result in 2 months longer survival than treatment with temozolomide alone.[28] However, this appears to be a relatively weak association and may be in part due to a historical bias toward older studies and studies conducted in younger participants.[29]

ZONISAMIDE (BRAND NAME ZONEGRAN)

Zonisamide was approved by the FDA in 2000 as an adjunctive therapy for focal seizures. Although there have been few studies looking at zonisamide for monotherapy, in practice it is often used alone. Zonisamide works at calcium and sodium channels to stabilize neuronal membrane. Only an oral formulation is available, and it has a long half-life (approximately 50–69 hours). Starting dose is typically 100 mg/d, which can be increased to 200 mg/d after 2 weeks. Further adjustments to 300 or 400 mg/d can be made after an additional 2 weeks. Metabolism is through the hepatic CYP3A4 system, and zonisamide is excreted in the urine. It is not recommended for patients with a creatinine clearance of less than 20 mL/min. Zonisamide should not be used for patients with an allergy to sulfa agents. Common side effects include somnolence, dizziness, ataxia, weight loss, confusion, and cognitive dysfunction. More serious side effects include kidney stones, oligohidrosis, rash, metabolic acidosis, leukopenia, abnormal liver enzymes, depression, and psychosis. Zonisamide is used more commonly in the outpatient setting than topiramate because it is generally well-tolerated with less drowsiness or cognitive side effects. Given the long half-life, it is a good choice for patients who have poor compliance or difficulty taking medication more than once a day.[30]

ADDITIONAL ANTIEPILEPTIC MEDICATIONS AND CONSIDERATION FOR THERAPEUTIC INTERCHANGE OR DISCONTINUATION WHILE ADMITTED TO THE HOSPITAL

While the preceding medications are commonly prescribed for seizures and epilepsy in both inpatient and outpatient settings, there are several other antiepileptic medications that may be encountered, especially in cases of medically refractory epilepsy where numerous other agents have been tried. These medications may or may not be available in a hospital formulary. Ideally, the patient will have his or her own supply of the medication that can be administered, but, in some instances, a backup antiepileptic regimen may need to be considered while in the inpatient setting. Most commonly, lorazepam can be given for regular dosing to mitigate the chances of breakthrough seizures while in the hospital. However, standing doses of lorazepam and most benzodiazepines in general are typically not prescribed to patients for chronic seizure management long-term due to a gradual tolerance to the medication and diminished benefit at the same dose with consistent use.

Clobazam (brand name Onfi in the United States; also marketed as Frisium, Urbanol, and Tapclob worldwide) is one benzodiazepine-class medication that is used as a standing antiepileptic drug, generally for treatment-resistant epilepsy. It is currently only available as an oral agent and has no intravenous form. Clobazam is typically used as adjunctive therapy in treatment-resistant focal epilepsy with impaired awareness. For patients taking either marijuana or its active anticonvulsant component cannabidiol (Epidiolex), there appears to be a significant increase in the serum concentration of clobazam's anticonvulsant metabolite N-desmethylclobazam with concurrent cannabidiol use.[31] In the hospital, since cannabidiol may not be readily available due to its illegality in some locations, N-desmethylclobazam levels may diminish with a prolonged hospital stay, leading to breakthrough seizures.

Gabapentin (brand name Neurontin) is commonly prescribed for neuropathic pain and other neurologic complaints, but it is also an antiepileptic medication. To see an effect in epilepsy, the dose as a monotherapy should be at least 600 mg three times per day in adults to be considered therapeutic. Despite its name and origin as a GABA analogue, gabapentin does not bind to GABA receptors and instead inhibits alpha-2-delta subunit-containing voltage-dependent calcium channels.[32] Pregabalin (brand name Lyrica) has a similar anticonvulsant mechanism of action and is also prescribed for neuropathic pain. It can be 3–10 times more potent an anticonvulsant in animal models compared to gabapentin.[32] Currently, gabapentin and pregabalin are typically not chosen as a first-line agent for management of epilepsy because of their additional sedative qualities. However, they undergo little to no metabolism and typically are excreted unchanged in the urine.[33] As a result, these medications can be helpful and relatively safe agents to use in patients who have concurrent end-stage liver disease.

Eslicarbazepine (Aptiom) and brivaracetam (Briviact) are newer antiepileptic drugs that are derived from carbamazepine and levetiracetam, respectively. These medications can provide more targeted therapies that have fewer side effects than their older counterparts. However, as of this writing, both of these medications are only available in brand name form and may not be readily available in hospital formularies. However, in the short term, they can potentially be therapeutically exchanged in the hospital with carbamazepine (or oxcarbazepine) and levetiracetam, respectively.

Rufinamide (Banzel) is an anticonvulsant medication approved as an adjunctive therapy for treatment of Lennox-Gastaut syndrome in individuals age 4 years or older. Perampanel (Fycompa) is a novel antiepileptic agent which acts as an AMPA receptor antagonist. Felbamate is approved for monotherapy for focal and generalized epilepsy and is a very effective treatment, but it is now only rarely prescribed in medically refractory epilepsy because of a significant risk of aplastic anemia and hepatic failure. None of these agents has convenient analogous treatments. If making adjustments to newer antiepileptic agents, or if a patient is using multiple antiepileptic agents that may interact with other medical therapies, neurological consultation is recommended.

Coordination with a neurologist is especially helpful when a patient is placed on multiple new antiepileptic agents during hospitalization. Generally, if a patient is on three or more antiepileptic agents at a time, it is because earlier agents were considered ineffective or less effective and were continued out of fear of precipitating additional seizures. The risk of polypharmacy effects are high in these patients, and it often can be useful to work with a neurologist to simplify the regimen and taper gradually down to the one or two most effective antiepileptic agents.

Certain sedative and anesthetic medications such as midazolam, propofol, ketamine, and pentobarbital are used in the intensive care setting to manage medically refractory status epilepticus and can be considered antiepileptic medications in their own right. However, their use (with the possible exception of ketamine) is limited to the ICU and is best done in coordination with a neurocritical care specialist.

Last, it is essential to effectively communicate with the outpatient physicians who will be managing a patient's antiepileptic care. This will help coordinate care, explain the rationale for the medication choices, and ensure ongoing prescribing of medications.

HELPFUL RESOURCES

Epilepsy Foundation Website: www.epilepsy.com/medications

REFERENCES

1. Marson A, Jacoby A, Johnson A, et al. Immediate versus deferred antiepileptic drug treatment for early epilepsy and single seizures: a randomised controlled trial. *Lancet.* 2005;365(9476):2007–2013.
2. Kim LG, Johnson TL, Marson AG, et al. Prediction of risk of seizure recurrence after a single seizure and early epilepsy: further results from the MESS trial. *Lancet Neurol.* 2006;5:317.
3. Berg, AT. Risk of recurrence after an unprovoked seizure. *Epilepsia.* 2008;49(Supp 1):13–18. doi: 10.1111/j.1528-1167.2008.01444.x
4. Yerram S, Katyal N, Premkumar K, Nattanmai P, Newey CR. Seizure prophylaxis in the neuroscience intensive care unit. *J Intens Care.* 2018;6:17. doi: 10.1186/s40560-018-0288-6.
5. Connolly ES Jr, Rabinstein AA, Carhuapoma JR, et al.; American Heart Association Stroke Council, Council on Cardiovascular Radiology and Intervention, Council on Cardiovascular Nursing, Council on Cardiovascular Surgery and Anesthesia, Council on Clinical Cardiology. Guidelines for the management of aneurysmal subarachnoid hemorrhage: a guideline for healthcare professionals from the American Heart Association/American Stroke Association. *Stroke.* 2012 Jun;43(6):1711–1737. Epub 2012 May 3.
6. Tolbert D, Cloyd J, Biton V, et al. Bioequivalence of oral and intravenous carbamazepine formulations in adult patients with epilepsy. *Epilepsia.* 2015;56(6):915–923.
7. Spina E. Carbamazepine. Chemistry, biotransformation, and pharmacokinetics. In Levy RH, Mattson RH, Meldrum BS, et al., eds., *Antiepileptic Drugs.* 5th ed. Philadelphia, PA: Lippincott Williams & Wilkins;2002: 236–246.
8. Patsalos PN, Berry DJ, Bourgeois BF, et al. Antiepileptic drugs: best practice guidelines for therapeutic drug monitoring: a position paper by the Subcommission on Therapeutic Drug Monitoring, ILAE Commission on Therapeutic Strategies. *Epilepsia.* 2008;49(7):1239–1276.
9. Ferrell PB, McLeod HL. Carbamazepine, HLA-B*1502 and risk of Stevens-Johnson syndrome and toxic epidermal necrolysis: US FDA recommendations. *Pharmacogenomics.* 2008;9(10):1543–1546.
10. Pack AM. The association between antiepileptic drugs and bone disease. *Epilepsy Curr.* 2003;3(3):91–95.
11. Hernández-Díaz S., Smith CR, Shean A, et al. Comparative safety of antiepileptic drugs during pregnancy. *Neurology.* May 2012;78(21):1692–1699. doi: 10.1212/WNL.0b013e3182574f39.

12. Guerreiro CAM, Guerreiro MM, Mintzer S. *Carbamazepine, Oxcarbazepine, and Eslicarbazepine*. 6th ed. Philadelphia, PA: Wolters Kluwer; 2015: 615–625.

13. Kellinghaus C. Lacosamide as treatment for partial epilepsy: mechanisms of action, pharmacology, effects, and safety. *Ther Clin Risk Manag*. 5(2009):757–766.

14. Kanner AM, Frey M. Adding valproate to lamotrigine: a study of their pharmacokinetic interaction. *Neurology* 2000;55:588–591

15. Glauser T, Shinnar S, Gloss D, et al. Evidence-based guideline: treatment of convulsive status epilepticus in children and adults: report of the Guideline Committee of the American Epilepsy Society. *Epilepsy Curr*. 2016;16(1):48–61.

16. Olsen RW. Drug interactions at the GABA receptor-ionophore complex. *Annu Rev Pharmacol Toxicol*. 1982;22:245–277.

17. Gallagher BB, Freer LS. Barbituric acid derivatives. In Frey H-H, Janz D, eds. *Antiepileptic Drugs*. New York: Springer-Verlag, 1985:421–447.

18. Tobler, A., Hösli, R., Mühlebach, S. et al. Free phenytoin assessment in patients: measured versus calculated blood serum levels. *Int J Clin Pharm*. 2016;38:303–309. https://doi.org/10.1007/s11096-015-0241-x.

19. Dager W, Inciardi J, Howe T. Estimating phenytoin concentration by the Sheiner-Tozer method in adults with pronounced hypoalbuminemia. Ann Pharmacother. 1995;2:667–670

20. Manno EM. Status Epilepticus: Current Treatment Strategies. *The Neurohospitalist*. 2011;1(1):23–31. doi:10.1177/1941875210383176.

21. Winter ME. *Basic Clinical Pharmacokinetics*, 5th ed. Philadelphia, PA: Lippincott Williams & Wilkins; 2010.

22. Conway JM, Morita DA, Glauser TA. *Phenytoin and Fosphenytoin*. 6th ed. Philadelphia, PA: Wolters Kluwer; 2015: 691–704.

23. Hernandez-Diaz S., Huybrechts KF, Desai RJ, et al. Topiramate use early in pregnancy and the risk of oral clefts. *Neurology*. 2018 Jan;90(4):e342–e351. doi: 10.1212/WNL.0000000000004857.

24. Rosenfeld WE. *Topiramate*. 6th ed. Philadelphia, PA: Wolters Kluwer; 2015: 712–725.

25. Tsanaclis LM, Allen J, Perucca E, Routledge PA, Richens A. Effect of valproate on free plasma phenytoin concentrations. *Br J Clin Pharmacol*. 1984 Jul;18(1):17–20.

26. Karas BJ, Wilder BJ, Hammond EJ, Bauman AW. Treatment of valproate tremors. *Neurology*. 1983 Oct 1;33(10):1380–1382.

27. Meador KJ, Baker GA, Browning N, et al.; NEAD Study Group. Fetal antiepileptic drug exposure and cognitive outcomes at age 6 years (NEAD study): a prospective observational study. *Lancet Neurol*. 2013 Mar;12(3):244–252.

28. Kerkhof M, Dielemans JC, van Breemen MS, Zwinkels H, Walchenbach R, Taphoorn MJ, Vecht CJ. Effect of valproic acid on seizure control and on survival in patients with glioblastoma multiforme. *Neuro Oncol*. 2013 Jul;15(7):961–967.

29. Lu VM, Texakalidis P, McDonald KL, Mekary RA, Smith TR. The survival effect of valproic acid in glioblastoma and its current trend: a systematic review and meta-analysis. *Clin Neurol Neurosurg*. 2018 Sep 15;174:149–155.

30. Welty, TE. *Zonisamide*. 6th ed. Philadelphia, PA: Wolters Kluwer; 2015: 615–625.

31. Gaston TE, Bebin EM, Cutter GR, Liu Y, Szaflarski JP. Interactions between cannabidiol and commonly used antiepileptic drugs. *Epilepsia*. 2017 Sept;58(9);1586–1592.

32. Sills GJ. The mechanisms of action of gabapentin and pregabalin. *Curr Opin Pharmacol*. 2006 Feb;6(1):108–113.

33. Bockbrader HN, Wesche D, Miller R, Chapel S, Janiczek N, Burger P. A comparison of the pharmacokinetics and pharmacodynamics of pregabalin and gabapentin. *Clin Pharmacokinet*. 2010;49 (10):661–669.

6 Acute Spinal Cord Injury

Geoffrey Stricsek, Omaditya Khanna, Alexandra Emes, and James Harrop

INTRODUCTION

Spinal cord injury (SCI) is a devastating event that can carry high rates of morbidity and mortality. The most common causes of mortality are respiratory and cardiac-related illnesses, accounting for 28% and 23% of deaths, respectively.[1,2] In the United States, the average age at time of injury was 43 years old in 2018, up from 28.7 years old in the 1970s, primarily attributed to an aging population.[3] The overall incidence of SCI has been relatively stable since the early 1990s; however, the incidence in patients younger than age 45 has been decreasing while the incidence in those over age 45 has been increasing.[4] Currently, the most common etiology of SCI is motor vehicle collision, accounting for 38% of injuries, followed by falls, which are responsible in 32% of cases.[3] Cervical injuries are more common than thoracolumbar injuries[3] and complete injuries are more common in the young.[5] Nearly 80% of SCIs occur in men.[3]

INITIAL MANAGEMENT

Care of the acute SCI patient begins prior to their arrival at the hospital and consists of the initial evaluation of the patient, resuscitation, immobilization, retrieval or extrication, and transport.[6,7] Since the 1970s, there has been a decrease in the number of patients who present to the emergency department with complete SCI, largely attributed to the standardization of EMS practices.[8,9] Once at the hospital, the initial evaluation of the spinal cord injured patient follows the Advanced Trauma Life Support (ATLS) ABCDE framework (Airway, Breathing, Circulation, Disability, Exposure). This provides a standardized pathway for identifying injuries and establishing treatment priorities to guide resuscitation efforts.

Once a patient's pulmonary and cardiac function has been found to be stable, a thorough neurological assessment can be performed. Speech, comprehension, level of arousal, and cranial nerves are examined to evaluate for intracranial injury. Next, strength is tested in all muscle groups in the bilateral upper and lower extremities while dermatomal sensation to light touch and pinprick is assessed in the extremities as well as the trunk. This thorough motor and sensory exam can help guide the clinician in choosing advanced imaging while also providing the necessary information

Table 6.1 American Spinal Injury Association (ASIA) grading system

ASIA grade	Type of injury	Description of injury
A	Complete	No motor or sensory function below the level of injury including S4-5
B	Incomplete	Preserved sensory but not motor function below the level of injury
C	Incomplete	Motor and sensory function preserved below the level of injury; >50% of muscle groups have strength <3 (out of 5)
D	Incomplete	Motor and sensory function preserved below the level of injury; >50% of muscle groups have strength ≥3 (out of 5)
E	Normal	Normal motor/sensory function

Adapted from Reference 72.

to assign an American Spinal Injury Association (ASIA) grade to the patient, thereby standardizing communication among treating physicians (Table 6.1).

Once the neurological exam is completed, the evaluation proceeds to advanced imaging. This often begins with CT imaging to assess for bony fractures and spinal alignment. MRI can supplement findings seen on CT imaging by identifying soft tissue and ligamentous injury, intrinsic SCI, and epidural hematoma.

MANAGEMENT

Care for patients with SCI is dictated by their neurological status and the structural morphology of their injury. Patients with any neurological injury and/or an unstable spinal fracture are often admitted to the ICU. The first goal in a patient with SCI is prevention of secondary injury which is implemented with attention to spinal stabilization and blood pressure management. Stabilization, in the form of a rigid cervical collar, halo placement, traction, and/or flat bed rest can reduce the risk of further spinal cord trauma in the setting of an unstable fracture. The goal of blood pressure management is to maintain perfusion to the spinal cord in the setting of extrinsic compression and intrinsic capillary compromise from spinal cord edema; higher mean arterial pressures (MAPs) have been correlated with improved outcomes in the setting of SCI.[10] Intravenous steroid administration in the setting of acute SCI has been extensively researched; however, the most recent guidelines from the American Association of Neurological Surgeons/ Congress of Neurological Surgeons (AANS/CNS) do not support its use in the setting of SCI.[11]

Once the patient has been stabilized and the nature of the injury has been characterized, a decision must be made regarding operative versus nonoperative management. Multiple decision-making guidelines have been published for operative versus nonoperative care of the neurologically intact patient with an injury to the spinal column. For any patient with neurological injury, early surgery (within 24 hours of injury) has been shown to improve neurological outcomes[12,13]; there is some recent literature that suggests that ultra-early surgery (within 12 hours of injury) may be even more beneficial.[12] Surgical management of the neurologically impaired SCI patient has specific goals that need to be accomplished to maximize a patient's chance for recovery.

1. *Decompression of the neural elements.* This can take different forms depending on the location of the injury. Often, decompression of the neural elements entails a laminectomy in order to relieve pressure on the spinal cord within the canal, but it also addresses dorsal pathology. If there is significant ventral spinal cord compression, alternative techniques may need to be utilized. A discussion of the nuances of making this choice is beyond the scope of this chapter, but is dependent on many factors including level, extent, and location of compression; medical fitness; and surrounding anatomic structures.
2. *Stabilization.* As discussed earlier, an important element in the care of the SCI patient involves prevention of secondary injury. Repeated spinal cord trauma can occur if unstable fracture segments are not stabilized. If rigid external orthoses are unable to provide definitive stabilization, internal fixation is required. As mentioned earlier in the context of neural decompression, the specific approach to stabilization depends on the nature of the underlying injury as well as its location along the spinal column. Stabilization can take the form of anterior, posterior, or combined fusion procedures. It can utilize screws, rods, plates, and cages. Unique risks and benefits exist for each approach, but, regardless of the technique, the aim is to prevent continued motion across the injured spinal segment.
3. *Arthrodesis.* Arthrodesis, or fusion, can be an important element when internal fixation is required. In the acute setting, stabilization will prevent or limit further injury to the spinal cord, but there is a finite repeated stress limit for implanted rods, screws, and plates. Over the long term, the goal is to have the patient grow his or her own bone across an unstable segment as their intrinsic bony fusion mass will be stronger than any implant.
4. *Restoration of alignment.* This may not be a goal in every procedure. If a patient is found to have significant subluxation of one vertebral body on another, it may be necessary to reduce that slip in order to achieve decompression of the neural elements. Additionally, if someone has a significant deformity that could limit rehabilitation potential, consideration should be given to correction (one potential example is the patient with significant thoracolumbar kyphosis that prevents them from comfortably sitting in a wheelchair).

OCCIPITAL-CERVICAL JUNCTION

Spinal injury at the occipital-cervical (OC) junction can be the result of ligamentous disruption, fracture of the occipital condyles, or both. Atlanto-occipital dislocation, or abnormal separation of the skull from the C1 vertebral body (the atlas) is classified into three types: anterior dislocation of the occiput relative to the atlas (type I), distraction or longitudinal dislocation (type II), and posterior dislocation of the occiput relative to the atlas (type III). Multiple techniques exist to quantify the degree of dislocation, including the ratio of the basion-axial interval to the basion-dental interval; the atlanto-occipital interval (distance between the occipital condyles and the superior articular surface of C1); and the Powers' ratio. Management initially consists of rigid halo immobilization, but the presence of radiographic evidence of atlanto-occipital dislocation should prompt internal fixation with occipito-cervical fusion.[14]

Occipital condyle fractures (OCFs) are uncommon, seen in less than 1% of trauma patients.[15] Suspicion should be high in the patient with lower cranial nerve palsies (e.g., hypoglossal); diagnosis is confirmed with CT imaging. Anderson and Montesano developed a classification in 1988 consisting of three types: type I, comminuted fracture; type II, extension of a basilar skull fracture; and type III, avulsion of condylar fragment. Type III was the only fracture morphology they believed had the potential to be unstable.[16] In the absence of neurological deficit, most patients with types I and II fractures can be treated with rigid external immobilization such as a cervical collar while patients with bilateral OCFs, OCF associated with atlantoaxial instability, or type III OCF with instability should be managed with halo immobilization.[17,18]

C1–C2 COMPLEX

There are multiple types of injury that can impact the C1–C2 complex. The first cervical vertebral body, the atlas, can have fracture of a single arch, the lateral mass(es), or multiple fracture points through the anterior and posterior arches of C1. Neurological deficit resulting from C1 injury is uncommon due to the wide canal diameter and the fact that fracture fragments tend to be displaced outward due to the axial loading mechanism of injury. Management of C1 fractures is predicated not on the bony pathology but based on ligamentous stability. Stability of the OC junction was outlined earlier; stability of the transverse ligament, responsible for the securing the articulation between the C2 dens and the anterior ring of C1, also needs to be assessed. Historically, this was evaluated using the Rule of Spence, where the cumulative overhang of the C1 lateral masses on C2 is quantified, and, if 7 mm or higher, there is presumed disruption of the transverse ligament.[18] More frequently, the Rule of Spence is combined with MR imaging to assess ligamentous injury. If there is suspicion for ligamentous instability, management options include halo immobilization and cervical fusion, with decision-making based on the extent of injury, patient age, and medical comorbidities.

The second cervical vertebral body is the axis. Fractures can occur through the dens, through the pars, or through the vertebral body and/or the posterior ring. There are three types of dens fractures: type I is through the tip of the dens, is rare, and, while not inherently unstable, is an indicator of a high-energy accident and should raise suspicion for ligamentous instability at the atlanto-occipital junction. Type II fractures are through the base of the dens and are often unstable. Type III fractures involve the body of the axis and are relatively stable fractures that can be managed with a cervical collar. Neurologically intact patients with type II dens fractures that have minimal displacement of the dens can be managed in a cervical collar with flexion-extension x-rays of the cervical spine in 6–8 weeks to assess for healing. Patients with displaced type II dens fractures or patients with nonunion after external immobilization should undergo a fusion procedure for definitive stabilization.

Bilateral fracture through the pars interarticularis of the axis is known as a "hangman's fracture." Often the result of hyperextension and an axial load on the cervical spine, they are classified using the Levine system,[19] a modification of Effendi's[20] original publication. These systems quantify the angulation between C2 and C3 as well as any subluxation between the two vertebral bodies. Surgical management is recommended for patients with bilateral pars fractures with associated C2–C3 disc and/or C2–C3 facet capsule disruption as these are unstable and can lead to neurological deterioration.

SUBAXIAL CERVICAL SPINE

In the cervical spine, the Subaxial Injury Classification (SLIC) scale was initially developed to standardize the description of subaxial cervical spine injuries.[21] The SLIC Scale utilizes three elements: fracture morphology, disco-ligamentous complex, and neurological status to arrive at a score out of a total possible score of 10 (Figure 6.1). Generally, scores less than 4 can be treated nonoperatively, scores of 5 or higher should be managed surgically, and a score of 4 may be managed either operatively or nonoperatively based on physician judgment and patient specifics.[22] A newer injury classification schema has also been published: the AOSpine subaxial cervical spine injury classification (Figure 6.2).[23] This system categorizes injury based on injury morphology, facet injury, neurological status, and any other case-specific modifiers. Morphology types include compression (type A), tension band injury (type B), and translation injury (type C). Facet injuries are broken down into nondisplaced facet fracture (F1), facet fracture with potential instability (F2), floating lateral mass (F3), and subluxation or perched/dislocated (F4). Neurological injury consists of intact (N0), transient deficit (N1), radiculopathy (N2), incomplete SCI (N3), and complete SCI (N4). Other modifiers include posterior ligamentous complex injury (M1), critical disc herniation (M2), hyperostosis or DISH (M3), and vertebral artery injury (M4). Surgical management is recommended for A3 and A4 fractures (incomplete and complete burst fractures) due to the risk of kyphotic deformity and instability, respectively.[24] Fusion-based stabilization is also recommended for B2 (posterior tension band injury involving bone and ligamentous structures), B3 (anterior tension band injury), and all type C injuries (translation).[24] Facet injuries of the F2, F3, and F4 varieties are typically associated with type B and C injuries and thus require surgical stabilization.[24]

	Points
Morphology	
No abnormality	0
Compression	1
Burst	+1 = 2
Distraction (*e.g.*, facet perch, hyperextension)	3
Rotation/translation (e.g., facet dislocation, unstable teardrop or advanced staged flexion compression injury)	4
Disco-ligamentous complex (DLC)	
Intact	0
Indeterminate (e.g., isolated interspinous widening, MRI signal change only)	1
Disrupted (e.g., widening of disc space, facet perch or dislocation)	2
Neurological status	
Intact	0
Root injury	1
Complete cord injury	2
Incomplete cord injury	3
Continuous cord compression in setting of neuro deficit (Neuro Modifier)	+1

FIGURE 6.1 Subaxial Injury Classification (SLIC) scoring.
From Vaccaro et al.[21]

THORACOLUMBAR SPINE

Fractures in the thoracic and lumbar spine are more common than in the cervical spine. The majority of thoracolumbar spine fractures occur in the transition zone between the lower thoracic and upper lumbar spine (between T11 and L2), accounting for approximately 20% of all spine fractures. This region is particularly susceptible to injury owing to the fact that it is a junction between the fixed, kyphotic thoracic spine and the more mobile lordotic lumbar spine, causing concentration of stress forces upon the ventral thoracolumbar vertebral column. The majority of thoracolumbar fractures are caused by high-energy mechanisms, which can result in concomitant injuries to other nearby organ and soft tissues; advanced imaging including CT of the abdomen and pelvis should be considered in these situations.

There are several systems in place to evaluate thoracolumbar fracture: the Denis three-column concept, the AOSpine thoracolumbar classification, and the Thoracolumbar Injury Classification and Severity Score (TLICS). Denis, in 1984, proposed a three-column classification scheme to describe the thoracolumbar spine, where any injury involving all three columns was deemed to be unstable and requiring surgical intervention.[25] In 2005, the Spine Trauma Study Group proposed a novel grading criteria for evaluation of thoracolumbar fractures: the TLICS. Injuries are defined according to insult morphology (compression, 1 point; burst, 2

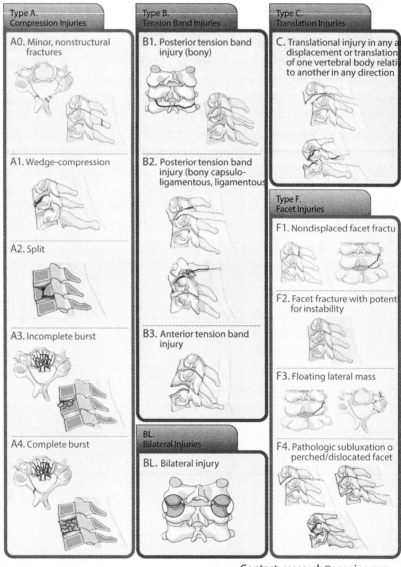

FIGURE 6.2 AO Spine subaxial cervical injury classification.
From AOSpine Subaxial Classification System.[73]

points; translational/rotational, 3 points; distraction, 4 points), patient's neurologic status (intact, 0 points; nerve root injury, 2 points; cord or conus medullaris incomplete injury, 2 points; cord or conus medullaris complete injury, 3 points; cauda equina syndrome, 3 points), and integrity of the posterior ligamentous complex (intact, 0 points; injury suspected/indeterminate, 2 points; injured, 3 points). Under the TLICS classification scheme, a summation of point values from the preceding categories of 3 or less can be treated with nonoperative management, scores of 4 may be treated either operatively or nonoperatively, and a cumulative score of 5 or above usually warrants surgical decompression and stabilization.[26,27] The AOSpine thoracolumbar classification system is similar to the cervical system and places injuries into three categories: type A, compression fractures; type B, anterior or posterior tension band injury without translation; and type C, dislocation or displacement in any plane (Figure 6.3).[28] Modifiers were incorporated for case-specific modifiers

AOSpine Thoracolumbar Classification System

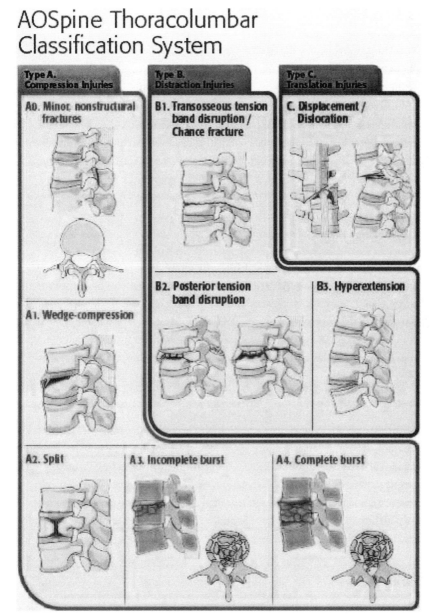

Type A. Compression Injuries	Type B. Distraction Injuries	Type C. Translation Injuries
A0. Minor nonstructural fractures	B1. Transosseous tension band disruption / Chance fracture	C. Displacement / Dislocation
A1. Wedge-compression	B2. Posterior tension band disruption	B3. Hyperextension
A2. Split	A3. Incomplete burst	A4. Complete burst

FIGURE 6.3 A0 Spine thoracolumbar classification.
From AOSPine Thoracolumbar Classification System.[74]

(using the letter M) and categorization of neurological status: N0, neurologically intact; N1, transient neurological symptoms which have resolved; N2, radiculopathy; N3, incomplete SCI or cauda equina syndrome; N4, complete SCI.[28]

Management of the patient with a thoracolumbar injury is predicated on neurological status and structural morphology of the injury. Any patient who presents with a neurological deficit and is medically stable should undergo surgery for stabilization of the fracture and decompression of the neural elements; the specific surgical approach will be influenced by the nature of the injury.

Management of the neurologically intact patient is more nuanced. Grossly unstable injuries such as the type B3 hyperextension and type C displacement/dislocation fracture should always be managed surgically. A poll of AOSpine surgeons worldwide demonstrated the variability in management of thoracolumbar injuries, but has provided some guidance for initial management.[29] Neurologically intact patients with split (A2) or incomplete burst fractures (A3) should be managed nonoperatively as a first-line strategy; the presence of neurological deficit in either would necessitate surgical intervention.[29] Although somewhat controversial, the recommendation based on the consensus opinion was that complete burst fractures (A4) should be managed surgically; other surgical fractures included single-level fractures involving all three columns with posterior tension band disruption (Chance fracture; B1) and incomplete burst fractures with posterior tension band disruption (B2).[29]

COMPLICATIONS
Intracranial Injury

Any traumatic mechanism sufficient to create a traumatic SCI has the potential to cause an intracranial injury. Approximately 5–23% of SCI patients have associated intracranial pathology, including subdural or extradural hematoma, intraparenchymal contusion, or diffuse axonal injury.[30–32] Patients with intracranial pathology are significantly more likely to experience pulmonary complications as well,[33] and these pulmonary complications are responsible for more than one-quarter of SCI deaths.[2,34]

Vascular Injury

The risk of vascular injury in patients with cervical spine injury is 15–30%.[35–37] Situations where vascular imaging with CT or MR angiography may be warranted include subaxial cervical spine subluxation, any fracture extending through a transverse foramen, craniocervical dislocation, or penetrating mechanism of injury as these are associated with increased risk of vertebral and carotid artery damage.[38,39] Early identification of vessel damage and initiation of appropriate therapy can reduce the risk of stroke.[40]

Dural Injuries

Dural injuries are commonly associated with traumatic SCI and are seen in 9–36% of thoracolumbar injuries and 9–13% of cervical injuries.[41–44] Traumatic dural injuries are more common in burst, flexion distraction, and fracture dislocation injuries and also are more likely to be associated with neurological injury.[44–47] The rate of complication associated with traumatic dural injuries is low $(0–2\%)$[43,44] but includes poor wound healing/wound breakdown, pseudomeningocele formation with associated headaches, and meningitis.

Medical Complications

Patients with SCI have an elevated risk of developing medical complications as a result of their injury: the more severe the injury, the higher the risk of medical complication.[30,32]

Pulmonary Complications

Pulmonary complications are the leading cause of mortality[2,34] and significantly increase lengths of hospital stay.[48] Specific complications can include acute lung injury, acute respiratory distress syndrome, respiratory failure, pulmonary embolus, pleural effusion, lobar collapse, mucus plug, pneumonia, aspiration, pneumothorax, and hemothorax.[32] Approximately 10–60% of patients with SCI will have some form of pulmonary complication,[32,49] but pneumonia is the most deadly.[50] Patients with complete SCIs are significantly more prone to pulmonary complications and have an increased risk with a more rostral level of injury: patients with a complete cervical SCI have a 60–70% risk of pneumonia compared with a 20–30% risk with incomplete SCI.[48,50] Early tracheostomy placement (within 7 days) can reduce the risk of ventilator-associated pneumonia and aspiration.[51] It also reduces the duration of mechanical ventilation and ICU stay, and decreases the rate of orotracheal intubation-associated complications such tracheal granuloma formation and stenosis.[52]

Hematologic Complications

Hematologic complications encountered in SCI include deep venous thrombus (DVT), anemia, thrombocytopenia, and coagulopathy.[32] DVT is the most common, but its incidence has fallen over the years and currently is cited at approximately 3–4%.[4,53] This reduction is most likely due to aggressive use of mechanical and chemoprophylactic agents. Interestingly, location of the SCI may play a role in risk for VTE as thoracic SCI patients have been found to have a higher rate for VTE than either cervical or lumbar patients (6% vs. 3%).[53] The biggest concern with any patient found with a DVT is the subsequent risk of pulmonary embolism (PE). While the rate of SCI-associated PE is approximately 1.5%,[4] all SCI patients should be managed with a combination of mechanical and pharmacologic prophylaxis beginning within 72 hours of injury and continuing for at least 3 months.[54] Research has demonstrated that there exists a synergistic effect when both techniques are used concurrently.[55] An inferior vena cava filter (IVCF) is not recommended as a first-line agent given the risk profile and absence of mortality benefit,[56] but it can be considered if a patient has failed first-line therapy or there is a contraindication to anticoagulation therapy.[54]

Cardiac Complications

The severity of cardiac dysfunction following SCI is correlated with the anatomic level and degree of SCI.[57,58] Patients with injuries in the cervical or upper thoracic spine to the level of T6 have the highest risk of cardiovascular dysfunction from impairment or loss of sympathetic vascular control, which subsequently allows unopposed parasympathetic input from the vagus nerve.[59] Cardiac complications are also more common in patients with more severe neurological injury (ASIA A and B) and are the second leading cause of death after pulmonary complications.[2,60,61] Common cardiac complications following SCI include arrhythmia, bradycardia, cardiac arrest, myocardial infarction, shock (defined as systolic blood pressure <80 mm Hg), congestive heart failure, and cardiogenic pulmonary edema.[32] In the acute setting, traumatic SCI requiring emergency surgery is associated with an increased risk of perioperative myocardial infarction (MI).[62] Loss of central sympathetic regulation of peripheral vascular tone can cause orthostatic hypotension, lower resting blood pressure, and, in severe cases, neurogenic shock when combined with persistent bradycardia.[63]

Gastrointestinal Complications

Similar to SCI-associated cardiac complications, many GI complications are thought to be the result of unopposed parasympathetic activity. Increased gastric and pancreatic secretions increase the risk of GI hemorrhage and pancreatitis, while autonomic imbalance and impaired gut motility increase the risk of ileus.[64] Delayed transit of gastric contents through the GI system has been found to increase the risk of aspiration in patients with cervical spine immobilization who are receiving nutrition via tube feeds.[65] SCI patients have also been found to have impaired glucose tolerance and insulin resistance attributed to skeletal muscle atrophy and decreased physical activity.[66,67]

Renal Complications

The risk of urinary tract infection is greater than 10% and is one of the most common complications associated with SCI.[68] While it remains controversial, sterile intermittent catheterization has been associated with a lower rate of urological complications compared with chronic indwelling catheters.[69] Improved outcomes have been demonstrated with a longer course (14 days instead of 3) of antibiotics for the treatment of acute urinary tract infections, but prophylactic antibiotic use is not supported for all SCI patients.[70,71]

CONCLUSION

Care of the SCI patient can be a complex process involving multiple care providers beginning prior to arrival in the hospital. Providing patients with the best chances for recovery relies on limiting the risk of secondary injury, appropriate diagnosis and management of the spinal pathology, and anticipation and treatment of secondary medical issues which arise in the setting of SCI.

REFERENCES

1. Weaver F, Smith B, Evans C, et al. Outcomes of outpatient visits for acute respiratory illness in veterans with spinal cord injuries and disorders. *Am J Phys Med Rehabil.* 85(9):718–726.

2. DeVivo M, Krause J, Lammertse D. Recent trends in mortality and causes of death among persons with spinal cord injury. *Arch Phys Med Rehabil.* 1999;80:1411–1419.

3. National Spinal Cord Injury Statistical Center. Facts and Figures at a Glance. Birmingham: University of Alabama at Birmingham; 2018.

4. Jain N, Ayers G, Peterson E, et al. Traumatic spinal cord injury in the United States, 1993–2012. *JAMA.* 2015;313(22):2236–2243.

5. Nobunaga A, Go B, Karunas R. Recent demographic and injury trends in people served by the Model Spinal Cord Injury Care Systems. *Arch Phys Med Rehabil.* 80:1372–1382.

6. Waters R, Meyer P, Adkins R, Felton D. Emergency, acute, and surgical management of spine trauma. *Arch Phys Med Rehabil.* 1999;80:1383–1390.

7. Soderstrom C, Brumback R. Early care of the patient with cervical spine injury. *Orthop Clin North Am.* 1986;17:3–13.

8. Green B, Eismont F, O'Heir J. Spinal cord injury: a systems approach: prevention, emergency medical services, and emergency room management. *Crit Care Clin.* 1987;3:471–493.

9. Dyson-Hudson T, Stein A. Acute management of traumatic cervical spinal cord injuries. *Mt Sinai J Med.* 1999;66:170–178.

10. Dhall S, Dailey A, Anderson P, et al. Congress of Neurological Surgeons systematic review and evidence-based guidelines on the evaluation and treatment of patients with thoracolumbar spine trauma: hemodynamic management. *Neurosurgery.* 2018;0(0):1–3.

11. Hurlbert R, Hadley M, Walters B, et al. Pharmacological therapy for acute spinal cord injury. *Neurosurgery.* 2013;72:93–105.

12. Burke J, Yue J, Ngwenya L, et al. Ultra-early (<12 hours) surgery correlates with higher rate of American Spinal Injury Association Impairment Scale conversion after cervical spinal cord injury. *Neurosurgery.* 2018;0:1–5.

13. Fehlings M, Vaccaro A, WIlson J, et al. Early versus delayed decompression for traumatic cervical spinal cord injury: results of the Surgical Timing in Acute Spinal Cord Injury Study (STASCIS). *PLoS ONE.* 2012;7(2):1–8.

14. Horn E, Feiz-Erfan I, Lekovic G. Survivors of occipitoatlantal dislocation injuries: imaging and clinical correlates. *J Neurosurg Spine.* 2007;6(2):113–120.

15. Maserati M, Stephens B, Zohny Z, et al. Occipital condyle fractures: clinical decision rule and surgical management. *J Neurosurg Spine.* 2009;11(4):388–395.

16. Anderson P, Montesano P. Morphology and treatment of occipital condyle fractures. *Spine.* 1988;13(7):731–736.

17. Theodore N, Aarabi B, Dhall S, et al. Occipital condyle fractures. *Neurosurgery.* 2013;72:106–113.

18. Greenberg M, ed. *Handbook of Neurosurgery.* 7th ed. New York: Thieme; 2010.

19. Levine A, Edwards C. The management of traumatic spondylolisthesis of the axis. *J Bone Jt Surg.* 1985;67A:217–226.

20. Effendi B, Roy D, Cornish B. Fractures of the ring of the axis: a classification based on the analysis of 131 cases. *J Bone Jt Surg.* 1985;63B:319–327.

21. Vaccaro A, Hulbert R, Patel A, et al. The subaxial cervical spine injury classification system: a novel approach to recognize the importance of morphology, neurology, and integrity of the disco-ligamentous complex. *Spine Phila Pa 1976.* 2007;32(21):2365–2374.

22. Joaquim A, Patel A, Vaccaro A. Cervical injuries scored accord to the Subaxial Injury Classification system: an analysis of the literature. *J Craniovertebr Junction Spine.* 2014;5(2):65–70.

23. Vaccaro A, Koerner J, Radcliff K, et al. AOSpine subaxial cervical spine injury classification system. *Eur Spine J.* 2016;25:2173–2184.

24. Schleicher P, Kobbe P, Kandziora F, et al. Treatment of injuries to the subaxial cervical spine: recommendations of the spine section of the German Society for Orthopaedics and Trauma (DGOU). *Glob Spine J.* 2018;8(25):255–335.

25. Denis F. The three column spine and its significance in the classification of acute thoracolumbar spinal injuries. *Spine.* 1983;8:817–831.

26. Vaccaro A, Lehman RJ, Hurlbert R, et al. A new classification of thoracolumbar injuries: the importance of injury morphology, the integrity of the posterior ligamentous complex, and neurologic status. *Spine Phila Pa 1976.* 2005;30(20):2325–2333.

27. Vaccaro A, Zeiller S, Hulbert R, et al. The thoracolumbar injury severity score: a proposed treatment algorithm. *J Spinal Disord Tech.* 2005;18(3):209–215.

28. Vaccaro A, Oner C, Kepler C, et al. AOSpine thoracolumbar spine injury classification system: fracture description, neurological status, and key modifiers. *Spine.* 2013;38:2028–2037.

29. Vaccaro A, Schroeder G, Kepler C, et al. The surgical algorithm for the AOSpine thoracolumbar spine injury classification system. *Eur Spine J.* 2016;25:1087–1094.

30. Silva Santos E, Santos Filho W, Possatti L, Azeredo Bittencourt L, Franca Fontoura E, Botelho R. Clinical complications in patients with severe cervical spine trauma: a ten year prospective study. *Arq Neuropsiquiatr.* 2012;70(7):524–528.

31. Chikuda H, Ohya J, Horiguchi H, et al. Ischemic stroke after cervical spine injury: analysis of 11,005 patients using the Japanese Diagnosis Procedure Combination database. *Spine J.* 2014;14:2275–2280.

32. Grossman R, Frankowski R, Burau K, et al. Incidence and severity of acute complications after spinal cord injury. *J Neurosurg Spine.* 2012;Suppl 17:119–128.

33. Fletcher D, Taddonio R, Byrne D, et al. Incidence of acute care complications in vertebral column fracture patients with and without spinal cord injury. *Spine Phila Pa 1976.* 1995;20(10):1136–1146.

34. Weaver F, Smith B, Evans C. Outcomes of outpatient visits for acute respiratory illness in veterans with spinal cord injuries and disorders. *Am J Phys Med Rehabil.* 2006;85:718–726.

35. Mueller C, Peters I, Podlogar M, et al. Vertebral artery injuries following cervical spine trauma: a prospective observational study. *Eur Spine J.* 2011;20(12):2202–2209.

36. Munera F, Cohn S, Rivas L. Penetrating injuries of the neck: use of helical computed tomographic angiography. *J Trauma.* 58:413–418.

37. Asensio J, Valenziano C, Falcone R, Grosh J. Management of penetrating neck injuries: the controversy surrounding zone II injuries. *Surg Clin North Am.* 1991;71:267–296.

38. Cothren C, Moore E, Biffl W, Ciesla D, Ray CJ, Johnson J. Cervical spine fracture patterns predictive in blunt cervical vascular injury. *J Trauma.* 2003;55:811–813.

39. Vilela M, Kim L, Bellabarba C, Bransford R. Blunt cerebrovascular injuries in association with craniocervical distraction injuries: a retrospective review of consecutive cases. *Spine J.* 2015;15:499–505.

40. Eastman A, Muraliraj V, Sperry J, Minei J. CTA-based screening reduces time to diagnosis and stroke rate in blunt cervical vascular injury. *J Trauma*. 2009;67:551–556.

41. Aydinli U, Karaeminogullari O, Tiskaya K, Ozturk C. Dural tears in lumbar burst fractures with greenstick lamina fractures. *Spine*. 26:E410–E415.

42. Silvestro C, Francaviglia N, Bragazzi R, Piatelli G, Viale G. On the predictive value of radiological signs for the presence of dural lacerations related to fractures of the lower thoracic or lumbar spine. *J Spinal Disord*. 1991;4:49–53.

43. Lee S, Chung C, Jahng T, Kim C. Dural tear and resultant cerebrospinal fluid leak after cervical spinal trauma. *Eur Spine J*. 2014;(23):1772–1776.

44. Luszczyk M, Blaisdell G, Wiater B, et al. Traumatic dural tears: what do we know and are they a problem? *Spine J*. 2014;14:49–56.

45. Miller C, Dewey R, Hunt W. Impaction fracture of the lumbar vertebra with dural tear. *J Neurosurg*. 1980;53:765–771.

46. Cammisa FJ, Eismont F, Green B. Dural laceration occurring with burst fractures and associated laminar fractures. *J Bone Jt Surg*. 1989;71:1044–1052.

47. Pickett J, Blumenkopf B. Dural lacerations and thoracolumbar fractures. *J Spinal Disord*. 1989;2:99–103.

48. Aarabi B, Harrop J, Tator C, et al. Predictors of pulmonary complications in blunt traumatic spinal cord injury. *J Neurosurg Spine*. 2012;Suppl 17:38–45.

49. Street J, Lenehan B, DiPaola C, et al. Morbidity and mortality of major adult spinal surgery. A prospective cohort analysis of 942 consecutive patients. *Spine J*. 2012;12:22–34.

50. Berney S, Bragge P, Granger C, Opdam H, Denehy L. The acute respiratory management of cervical spinal cord injury in the first 6 weeks after injury: a systemic review. *Spinal Cord*. 2011;49(1):17–29.

51. Jaeger J, Littlewood K, Durbin C. The role of tracheostomy in weaning from mechanical ventilation. *Respir Care*. 2002;47(4):469–480.

52. Romero J, Vari A, Gambarrutta C, Oliviero A. Tracheostomy timing in traumatic spinal cord injury. *Eur Spine J*. 2009;18(10):1452–1457.

53. Maung A, Schuster K, Kaplan L, Maerz L, Davis K. Risk of venous thromboembolism after spinal cord injury: not all levels are the same. *J Trauma*. 2011;71:1241–1245.

54. Dhall S, Hadley M, Aarabi B, et al. Deep venous thrombosis and thromboembolism in patients with cervical spinal cord injuries. *Neurosurgery*. 2013;72:244–254.

55. Merli G, Crabbe S, Doyle L, Ditunno J, Herbision G. Mechanical plus pharmacological prophylaxis for deep vein thrombosis in acute spinal cord injury. *Paraplegia*. 30(8):558–562.

56. Khansarinia S, Dennis J, Veldenz H, Butcher J, Hartland L. Prophylactic Greenfield filter placement in selected high-risk trauma patients. *J Vasc Surg*. 1995;22(3):231–235.

57. Furlan J, Fehlings M, Shannon P. Descending vasomotor pathways in humans: correlation between axonal preservation and cardiovascular dysfunction after spinal cord injury. *J Neurotrauma*. 2003;20:1351–1363.

58. Krassioukov A, Furlan J, Fehlings M. Autonomic dysreflexia in acute spinal cord injury: an under-recognized clinical entity. *J Neurotrauma*. 2003;20:707–716.

59. Garstang S, Miller-Smith S. Autonomic nervous system dysfunction after spinal cord injury. *Phys Med Rehabil Clin N Am*. 2007;18:275–296.

60. Popa C, Popa F, Grigorean V. Vascular dysfunctions following spinal cord injury. *J Med Life*. 2010;3:275–285.

61. Krassioukov A, Claydon V. The clinical problems in cardiovascular control following spinal cord injury: an overview. *Prog Brain Res*. 2006;152:223–229.

62. Wang T, Martin J, Loriaux D, et al. Risk assessment and characterization of 30-Day perioperative myocardial infarction following spine surgery: a retrospective analysis of 1346 consecutive adult patients. *Spine Phila Pa 1976.* 41(5):438–444.

63. Atkinson P, Atkinson J. Spinal shock. *Mayo Clin Proc.* 1996;71:384–389.

64. Albert T, Levine M, Balderston R, Cotler J. Gastrointestinal complications in spinal cord injury. *Spine Phila Pa 1976.* 16(Suppl 10):S522–S525.

65. Dvorak M, Noonan V, Belanger L. Early versus late enteral feeding in patients with acute cervical spinal cord injury: a pilot study. *Spine Phila Pa 1976.* 2004;29(9):E175–E180.

66. Jia X, Kowalski R, Sciubba D, Geocadin R. Critical care of traumatic spinal cord injury. *J Intensive Care Med.* 2013;28(1):12–23.

67. Raymond J, Harmer A, Temesi J, van Kemenade C. Glucose tolerance and physical activity level in people with spinal cord injury. *Spinal Cord.* 2010;48(8):591–596.

68. Dimar J, Fisher C, Vaccaro A, et al. Predictors of complications after spinal stabilization of thoracolumbar spine injuries. *J Trauma.* 2010;69:1497–1500.

69. Weld K, Dmochowski R. Effect of bladder management on urological complications in spinal cord injured patients. *J Urol.* 2000;163(3):768–772.

70. Dow G, Rao P, Harding G. A prospective, randomized trial of 3 or 14 days of ciprofloxacin treatment for acute urinary tract infection in patients with spinal cord injury. *Clin Infect Dis.* 2004;39(5):658–664.

71. Morton S, Shekelle P, Adams J. Antimicrobial prophylaxis for urinary tract infection in persons with spinal cord dysfunction. *Arch Phys Med Rehabil.* 2002;83(1):129–138.

72. McDonald J, Sadowsky C. Spinal-cord injury. *Lancet.* 2002;359:417–425.

73. AOSpine Classification Systems. Subaxial cervical. https://aospine.aofoundation.org/en/clinical-library-and-tools/aospine-injury-classification-system. Accessed December 30, 2018.

74. AOSpine Classification Systems. Thoracolumbar. https://aospine.aofoundation.org/en/clinical-library-and-tools/aospine-injury-classification-system. Accessed December 30, 2018.

7 Management of Bleeding Disorders in the Neurosurgical Patient

Vedavyas Gannamani and Sanaa Rizk

INTRODUCTION

Postoperative complications negatively impact both patient-centered outcomes and the quality indices of hospitals, thus affecting costs of care.[1,2] Postoperative bleeding (POB) and venous thromboembolism (VTE) are two frequently reported complications that affect surgery-related quality metrics like length of stay, 30-day readmission, and overall mortality. This emphasizes the need for identification and mitigation of risk factors associated with these preventable postoperative complications to improve patient care.[3–8]

Post operatively, neurosurgery patients are carefully monitored for bleeding complications due to their potential to result in dire situations, including death.[9,10] Due to the compact neuroanatomical space and flow-sensitive nervous tissue, a relatively small amount of bleeding at surgical site can be detrimental. Bleeding is one of the commonly reported postoperative complications, with an overall incidence of around 1%, although rates vary based on study population.[9,11,12] Prompt recognition and treatment of POB in these patients has been shown to minimize mortality and morbidity.[13,14] Risk reduction begins with identification of those conditions known to increase the chances of bleeding and correction of them preoperatively.[9,10,13,14]

Multiple studies were published describing risk factors that are associated with increased incidence of perioperative bleeding in neurosurgical patients. Commonly implicated factors include a patient's underlying disorders like hemophilia, older age, and preoperative use of anticoagulants.[10,15,16] Surgery-specific factors include degree of intraoperative blood loss, site of surgery, and condition requiring procedure.[9,15,17] Preoperative medical consultation provides an opportunity to recognize such risk factors and optimize the patient before undergoing surgery. Knowledge about these risk factors will also better prepare internists involved in the medical management of neurosurgical patients perioperatively.

Neurological patients are inherently at high risk of postoperative VTE events due to prolonged immobilization and the postoperative thrombogenic state.[5,6,18]

The risk is higher in patients undergoing brain surgery compared to spinal surgery, and additional patient-related factors have been implicated.[18–21] Reported incidence of VTE was 3.2–3.5% in brain surgery patients and 1.1–2.0% in spine surgery patients, but higher incidence was noted in other studies.[18–20,22,23] Patients with a history of VTE or underlying thrombophilia and those using anticoagulant or antiplatelet agents preoperatively pose a unique challenge for perioperative management of bleeding and VTE prevention. Prolonged interruptions in treatment of these conditions or medications will put patients at higher risk of cardiovascular and VTE events postoperatively.[24] Studies have shown the benefits of early initiation of VTE prophylaxis after neurosurgery, though the fear of POB inhibits aggressive use of appropriate medications.[25,26] Timing to safely initiate anticoagulant medications, especially at therapeutic doses, has not been established.

In this chapter, we outline the general principles of perioperative management of bleeding disorders and discuss interventions to reduce risk of bleeding in patients admitted for elective or emergent neurological surgeries. Management of patients primarily admitted for intracranial hemorrhage (subdural hematoma, subarachnoid hemorrhage) or trauma will be discussed separately. In addition, we review the current practice guidelines on perioperative adjustment of anticoagulant or antiplatelet agents in patients undergoing neurosurgery.

PREOPERATIVE EVALUATION

The objective of preoperative evaluation is to establish the risk factors associated with increased POB. These can be broadly divided into surgery-specific risk factors and patient-specific risk factors.

Surgery-Specific Risk Factors

Site and condition requiring surgery were consistently reported in majority studies as determinants of higher POB rates.[9,10] The incidence of POB was overall higher in patients undergoing brain than spine surgeries.[9,11] Prolonged duration of surgery and significant intraoperative blood loss were independently associated with increased POB events.[16,17,27,28]

Among brain surgeries, meningioma resection and craniotomy had higher POB compared to other procedures.[9,10,15,29] In patients undergoing craniotomy, incidence of POB differed depending on whether it was done as decompressive craniectomy, for trauma, or for epidural hematoma evacuation.[9,10] Chronic subdural hematoma was also reported as a risk factor for development of POB.[15,16] Aneurysm repair had lower incidence, while shunt placement had the lowest POB rates.[9] Technical aspects related to surgery, such as length and area of craniotomy and rapid drainage of cerebrospinal fluid, were also reported to be associated with higher POB.[27] Other described risk factors include emergency operation, surgery involving posterior fossa, and intrinsic supratentorial tumors.[10,15]

In patients undergoing spine surgeries, cervical and thoracic procedures had relatively higher incidences of bleeding than did lumbar surgeries.[9,30,31] Multilevel procedures were consistently reported to have been associated with higher POB.[13,28,30,32,33] Among lumbar spine surgeries, postoperative hematoma was noted to have developed after removal of suction drains.[31]

Patient-Specific Risk Factors

History of bleeding diathesis and use of antiplatelet/anticoagulant medications preoperatively remain the biggest risk factors for development of POB in neurosurgery.[10,15,16,28–30,33] The management of these conditions perioperatively will be discussed later in detail. Advanced age and hypertension are other risk factors commonly associated with increased POB.[16,29,32–34] Other reported risk factors include a higher level of comorbidities, pregnancy, alcohol consumption, Rh-positive blood type, and low serum calcium level.[13,30,33,35]

PLATELET DISORDERS

Platelet disorders affecting hemostasis can be those related to function (qualitative defect) and/or number (quantitative defect) and are classified as either congenital (usually rare) or acquired (more common). Due to the high risk of bleeding inherent to neurosurgical interventions, tests of hemostasis, including platelet count, are routinely checked preoperatively. Lower platelet count was shown to be associated with higher rates of postoperative hematoma as well as with higher rates of mortality in retrospective studies conducted on patients undergoing craniotomy.[29,36,37] Interestingly, a study conducted using the NSQIP database involving adult neurosurgical patients showed that preoperative platelet count has low sensitivity and specificity to predict hemostasis-related outcomes. The study also found patient history to be more sensitive than tests of hemostasis in predicting the outcomes.[38] It is, however, cost-effective and recommended to check platelet counts preoperatively in those with a known history of bleeding diathesis or taking antiplatelet or anticoagulant medications.[38,39]

There is a paucity of research evidence on the threshold of platelet count for patients undergoing neurosurgery. Studies also identified additional factors like chronicity of thrombocytopenia, response to transfusion, and swift drop in platelets perioperatively to have an impact on perioperative bleeding and outcomes.[36,40] Based on expert opinion, it is generally recommended to maintain a platelet count greater than 100,000/μL preoperatively for patients undergoing elective neurosurgery.[41–43] But in patients with chronic thrombocytopenia and underlying disorders like liver cirrhosis, immune thrombocytopenia (ITP), and chronic bone marrow suppression, a goal above 100,000/μL may not be achievable.[42,44,45] In conditions like liver disease or disseminated intravascular coagulation (DIC), thrombocytopenia can be complicated by other coagulation disorders and/or platelet function abnormalities. Additional therapies including intravenous desmopressin, immunoglobulins (IVIG), glucocorticoids, thrombopoietin receptor analogs (TPO-RA), and tranexamic acid may be used in certain situations instead of or in conjunction with platelet transfusions.[42,46] Hence, preoperative management of thrombocytopenia should be individualized, taking into account the underlying cause of thrombocytopenia, chronicity of the condition, presence of other coagulopathies, and urgency of the procedure.

Coagulopathy in liver disease patients is multifactorial, resulting from platelet dysfunction, thrombocytopenia, and coagulopathy. Due to splenic sequestration, the response to platelet transfusion is rarely as expected, and counts should be maintained close to patient's baseline, if it is not possible to keep levels above 100,000/μL.[47,48] TPO-RAs can be used but have to be administered 1–2 weeks prior to surgery.[42,49] Fresh frozen plasma (FFP) and cryoprecipitate to correct other coagulopathies are not usually recommended in cirrhosis patients, except in the setting of a bleed. In patients with ITP scheduled for elective neurosurgery, administration of a glucocorticoid course approximately 1–2 weeks prior to surgery and/or IVIG (if more rapid response needed) can raise the platelet count preoperatively.[44,46] Platelet transfusion or IVIG will be needed for urgent or emergent surgeries.[44,46] Platelet transfusion is relatively contraindicated in patients with consumptive disorders like thrombotic thrombocytopenic purpura (TTP) and heparin-induced thrombocytopenia (HIT) unless for an active bleed or for severe thrombocytopenia with a high risk of perioperative bleeding.[42,50,51]

There are no clear guidelines on transfusion of platelets in patients receiving antiplatelet agents preoperatively to correct the acquired platelet defect. Usually discontinuation of medication is sufficient, while transfusion of platelets is reserved for situations where urgent procedures are required and the patient did not have enough time to hold the medication or when severe/critical bleeding is anticipated.[42,52,53] Platelet function defects due to uremia can be treated with conjugated estrogen or desmopressin.[54] Correction of anemia also improves platelet function in renal failure patients.[42] For congenital platelet function disorders, there is a large disparity in bleeding manifestations, and the treatment approach should be individualized. Platelet transfusion (HLA-matched in Glanzmann thrombasthenia) is usually used to treat active bleeding or to prepare for a procedure, but it carries the risk of alloimmunization.[42] An alternative to platelet transfusion is desmopressin (DDAVP) in some patients with secretory defects. Antifibrinolytics are usually efficient in cases of mucosal bleed or menorrhagia but would not be of great benefits for neurosurgical procedures. Recombinant factor VIIa (rVIIa) is an option for refractory thrombocytopenia and alloimmunization.[55]

In patients with newly diagnosed thrombocytopenia during preoperative evaluation and with counts of less than 100,000/μL, elective surgery should be delayed until the diagnosis is established for better preoperative management of the condition. A hematology consultation will be required in such situations. However, in an emergency, delaying surgery is not recommended to evaluate the cause of low platelet counts. The surgical team may proceed with the required intervention with perioperative transfusion of platelets except in cases where it is contraindicated.[42] Hematology can be consulted to help with intraoperative and postoperative management.

The utility of platelet function testing—including platelet function analyzer (PFA)-100 and platelet aggregometry, as well as point-of-care tests (e.g., VerifyNow, thromboelastography [TEG] and rotational elastometry [ROTEM])—in the nontraumatic and elective neurosurgery setting has not been established.[56,57] However, referring to a hematologist to do the workup ahead of time for accurate diagnosis and appropriate perioperative planning is important for better outcome.

Threshold platelets counts have been proposed for different types of procedures. For diagnostic lumbar puncture, platelet counts of greater than 40,000/μL and for epidural or spinal anesthesia counts of greater than 80,000/μL are recommended.[42,45] Lower counts may be acceptable in certain situation like stable thrombocytopenia or hematological malignancy, and decisions must be made on a case-by-case basis.[45,58]

VON WILLEBRAND DISEASE

Von Willebrand disease (VWD) is the most common inherited bleeding disorder and is associated with abnormalities of both platelet function and coagulation cascade.[59] Acquired VWD is also noted with certain disease conditions.[59,60] Untreated patients present with skin and mucosal bleeding; however, symptoms vary based on the severity and type of VWD. Routine tests of hemostasis may show thrombocytopenia, normal prothrombin time (PT), abnormal activated partial thromboplastin time (aPTT; type 2N VWD with low plasma factor VIII concentrations), and prolonged bleeding time (BT).[61,62] VWD is diagnosed based on the patient's history with supporting laboratory tests that include plasma VWF antigen (VWF:Ag), plasma VWF activity (ristocetin cofactor activity, VWF:RCo), and factor VIII activity.[61,62] The VWF multimers distribution is also used to differentiate subtypes.

It is highly recommended to perform major bleeding risk procedures like neurosurgery in institutions with adequate laboratory and blood bank support and with the involvement of an experienced hematologist.[61,63] Preoperative evaluation comprises reviewing the type of VWD, severity of the disease, prior bleeding episodes and treatments, and documented response to desmopressin and VWF concentrate.[64] The main goal of perioperative management in VWD is to increase or replace VWF to achieve hemostasis by administering DDAVP (to enhance release of endogenous stores of VWF into the circulation) or by administering VWF-containing concentrates derived from human plasma. Outpatient testing for DDAVP response should be undertaken to determine DDAVP responders. If adequate hemostasis is not achieved, platelet transfusion can be considered, especially in type 3 VWD. Antifibrinolytics are used as adjuncts in surgeries involving mucosal incisions. In patients with acquired VWD, identification and treatment of the underlying cause should be attempted if possible. Various therapies including desmopressin, VWF concentrate, and recombinant factor VII are usually used in conjunction to minimize bleeding.[60,62]

In general, the treatment target is a VWF:RCo ratio of greater than 100 IU/dL preoperatively and a nadir of greater than 50 IU/dL up to 7–10 days postoperatively.[61,62,64] Similar levels should be targeted for factor VIII levels. Use of

VWF concentrate with low or no factor VIII is recommended over desmopressin in all types of VWD disease in major surgeries (like neurosurgery).[64] To reduce the risk of thromboembolism, VWF:RCo should be maintained below 200 IU/dL and factor VIII below 250 IU/dL. Levels are monitored every 12–24 hours to maintain in the desired range.[61,62,64]

COAGULATION FACTOR DEFICIENCIES

Patients with coagulation factor deficiencies need great attention when undergoing surgeries, especially those associated with high risk of bleeding, such as neurosurgical interventions. A hematologist or specialist with expertise in managing these disorders should be involved early to develop a perioperative management plan.[65,66] Coagulation factor deficiencies are either congenital or acquired later in life, with the latter being more frequently encountered. In a previously undiagnosed individual, certain clues such as a history of large ecchymosis or bleeding into joints or deep tissues should raise suspicion for bleeding disorders. A family history of bleeding disorders in an undiagnosed male patient may prompt testing for hemophilia. Immediate female relatives of hemophilia patients should be checked for factor levels when an intervention is planned.[67] Based on the specific coagulation factor deficiency, the tests of hemostasis—namely PT, PTT, or both—can be abnormal.

Hemophilia A (factor VIII deficiency) and hemophilia B (factor IX deficiency) are common inherited bleeding disorders (X-linked), and we will discuss their perioperative management here.[68] Hemophilia is categorized as mild, moderate, or severe depending on the factor level. Usually patients manifest prolonged PTT on screening tests. The next step in testing is PTT mixing studies to assess the presence or absence of an inhibitor. If PTT corrects on mixing, then a factor deficiency is present. Another key element during the preoperative assessment of hemophilia patients is determining the disease severity based on baseline factor activity level expressed as a percentage of normal or in international units (IU)/mL.[66,69] In cases where PTT does not correct on mixing studies, the clinician must rule out the presence of an inhibitor (either an auto- or allo-antibody against factor). If an inhibitor detected, a Bethesda assay of inhibitor must be performed, especially in those with severe disease.[70]

Required level of factor activity, dosage, and duration of coverage are determined based on patient, surgery, and bleeding risk. The recommended factor level for major procedures like neurosurgery is 80–100% in hemophilia A and hemophilia B patients.[66] The required dose of target factor to achieve the desired activity levels is calculated based on the patient's weight, baseline factor level, volume of distribution of factor, and presence of inhibitor. The calculated dose is usually given as a bolus preoperatively, and a peak level is checked prior to surgery to assess if the target level has been reached. If the target level is not reached, an additional bolus with half the initial dose can be given. Subsequent doses of clotting factor are based on activity levels that are checked at one half-life of the infused product (8–12 hours for factor VIII concentrate product and 18–24 hours for factor IX concentrate product).[66] Extended intervals of testing may be used for infused products with longer half-lives.[71]

Subsequent doses are also determined by the required factor activity level in the postoperative period. It is recommended to keep this level higher than 50%, assuming no complications occur. The duration of coverage with factor concentrate products varies with type of surgery; for neurosurgery it would be 10–14 days. In a situation with limited access to factor concentrate products, transfer to a well-equipped hospital with access to replacement factors and expert hematological consultation is preferred. If not possible, then targeting a lower percentage of activity levels pre- and postoperatively is suggested.[66]

In patients who were using emicizumab preoperatively, a bovine substrate-based chromogenic factor VIII assay, instead of routine factor assays should be used for monitoring.[72] Patients with inhibitors pose specific challenges preoperatively with factor supplementations, and an experienced hematologist should be on board. Bypassing agents are often used in these situations, especially for high inhibitor levels; these include activated prothrombin complex concentrate (aPCC or FEIBA) or recombinant human factor VIIa (Novoseven). Tests of activity will be of no use when bypass agents are used, and dosing is based on clinical response.[73]

Other inherited coagulation factor deficiencies are rare.[74,75] Replacement of deficient factor is the mainstay of perioperative management of these disorders. Based on availability, factor levels, and plasma half-lives, treatment modalities to consider include recombinant factor or factor concentrates, cryoprecipitate, or FFP.[74–76] Among patients with disorders of fibrinogen (congenital or acquired), a target level between 150 and 200 mg/dL should be achieved perioperatively until adequate hemostasis is obtained using plasma products or fibrinogen concentrates.[77,78] Management of acquired factor deficiencies secondary to inhibitors is specific to the affected factor and generally involves the use of plasma products and immunosuppression to eliminate inhibitor.[79]

MEDICATIONS AFFECTING HOMEOSTASIS

Drugs affecting hemostasis can be those affecting platelet function or clotting factors. Use of these medications preoperatively is a well-recognized risk factor associated with perioperative bleeding.[80,81] Patients typically take these medications for primary or secondary prevention of stroke and coronary artery disease or as treatment for VTE. Based on the drug being used, nonsteroidal anti-inflammatory medications (NSAIDs), should be stopped within at least five elimination half-lives before surgery.[82] Certain herbal medications and supplements are now increasingly recognized to cause coagulation abnormalities.[83,84] Over-the-counter supplements like garlic, ginkgo, and ginseng can affect coagulation and should be stopped preoperatively.[83] The evidence of fish oil in increasing bleeding events is under investigation.[85,86]

During preoperative consultation all prescription and over-the-counter medications should be reviewed to identify those that can potentially affect hemostasis. In a general sense, holding medications affecting hemostasis will reduce perioperative bleeding complications and related outcomes but may also increase the risk of perioperative vascular complications depending on the indication for their use. Hence perioperative management of these medications must weigh the benefits versus the risks associated with holding them. These medications differ widely in their mechanisms of action, pharmacodynamics, and pharmacokinetics and thus require specific, drug-based approaches.

Aspirin

Aspirin acts by irreversibly inhibiting cyclooxygenase-1 and -2 and thus affecting platelet aggregation and clot formation. The effects of aspirin on platelets lasts for remainder for their life span (i.e., 7–10 days). Common indications of use include primary or secondary prevention of stroke or coronary artery disease and in patients with stent placement (coronary artery or peripheral arteries). In patients using aspirin as monotherapy, it is recommended to stop aspirin at least 7 days prior to neurosurgery. In those undergoing carotid endarterectomy (CEA) and for patients on dual antiplatelet therapy (DAPT), aspirin should be continued.[87,88]

P2Y12 Receptor Blocking Agents

P2Y12 receptor blocking agents include clopidogrel, prasugrel, and ticagrelor, which are generally used in patients with previous cerebrovascular accidents or as part of DAPT in patients with recent coronary or peripheral vascular stenting. Nonemergent procedures should be delayed when possible until the patient completes the recommended duration of DAPT, which is 6 months for bare metal and newer drug-eluting stenting.[88–90] If delaying surgery is not possible for longer periods or until completion of DAPT, the minimum recommended duration is 3 months.[88] When discontinued, interruption of treatment should be kept to the minimum possible. Suggested stop dates for P2Y12 receptor blockers preoperatively are 5 days (clopidogrel), 7 days (prasugrel), and 3–5 days (ticagrelor).[88,91] These patients will be continued on aspirin. In urgent or emergent situations, the risks and benefits of DAPT must be reviewed in discussion with the patient, cardiologist, and surgeon before arriving at a decision. No formal management guidelines are formulated for patients using antiplatelet therapy for cerebrovascular disease or peripheral stenting.[92]

Anticoagulant Medications

The steps in the preoperative evaluation of patients taking anticoagulant medications are (1) determine the indication for use and the risk of thrombosis if anticoagulation is interrupted, (2) evaluate the need for bridging therapy, and (3) decide on the appropriate timing of discontinuation of anticoagulants. Based on indication for use, time of recent stroke or VTE, underlying thrombophilia, CHADS2 score, and other patient characteristics, the American College of Chest Physicians guidelines stratified perioperative risk of thromboembolism into high, medium, and low categories.[82]

As neurosurgical interventions are considered at high risk for bleeding, it is generally recommended to stop anticoagulant medications prior to surgery.[93,94] However, situations with increased thrombotic risk will require bridging therapy preoperatively.[82] In patients with recent VTE, stroke, or transient ischemic attack (TIA) (i.e., < 3 months), the risk of thrombosis is high but transient, and, if possible, surgery should be delayed beyond the 3-month period.[82] Short-acting medications like heparin products—unfractionated heparin (UFH) or low-molecular-weight (LMW) heparin—are used for bridging, while direct thrombin and factor Xa inhibitors are not recommended. LMWH should be stopped 24 hours before surgery, while UFH can be stopped 4–6 hours before the procedure.[82] Oral anticoagulant medications must be stopped at the appropriate preoperative time.[82,93–95] Patient-related factors like age and renal function also must to be taken into consideration when determining the time to discontinue anticoagulants.[93] Coagulation tests (PT, INR, and PTT) can be checked the day before or the morning of the day of surgery.

A valuable instrument for preoperative assessment is obtaining a patient history detailing medical problems, prior surgical history, current medication use, and family history.[38,39] Patients should be asked about a history of platelet disorders, clotting factor deficiencies, or thrombophilia, and, if diagnosed with a specific disease, the time of diagnosis, severity of disease, and current therapy or medication use must be elicited.[39]

Information pertaining to conditions that are associated with bleeding disorders, such as chronic liver disease and cirrhosis, end-stage renal disease, connective tissue disorders, antiphospholipid antibody syndrome, and vitamin K deficiency, will also be valuable.

In patients with no known history of bleeding or clotting disorders, questions about severity of bleeding following past injuries, tooth extractions, or prior surgical procedures; history of ecchymosis, bruises, or hematoma formation; epistaxis; menorrhagia; and history of hepatitis or alcohol use might provide clues to undiagnosed conditions. The complete list of medications a patient is taking, including prescription drugs, over-the-counter medications, and herbal supplements must be reviewed. A positive family history of bleeding and clotting disorders may point to an undiagnosed condition depending on the modes of inheritance. Use of instruments like the HAS-BLED score gives the clinician a better understanding of the general risk of bleeding in a patient.[96]

In patients with a history of thrombophilia or VTE, data pertaining to the timeline of diagnosis, current anticoagulant medications, recurrences of VTE, and inferior vena cava filter placement will be of help for appropriate perioperative management of these conditions.

In addition to underlying medical conditions, other patient-related factors were also identified in various studies as described above. Surgery-specific factors are also well-recognized to have an impact on perioperative bleeding risks and VTE events, and they have to be given equal importance during preoperative assessment. Both these categories of risk factors were reviewed in detail above in the chapter. Tests of hemostasis—namely platelet count, PT, INR, and aPTT—are generally not recommended unless the patient's history points toward an underlying bleeding diathesis.[38,97,98] Specific tests like platelet function assays (P2Y12 activity), VWF activity, and clotting factor assays should be ordered on individual basis.[56]

The following list is a general outline of the preoperative assessment of bleeding risks (also see Figure 7.1):

1. Obtain history pertaining to platelet and clotting factor disorders.
2. Obtain history of liver or renal disease, connective tissue disorder, vasculitis, conditions predisposing to vitamin K deficiency, alcoholism.
3. Obtain any history of thrombophilia, VTE, recurrences, IVC filter placement.
4. Review medications including prescription and over-the-counter medicines and herbal supplements.
5. Review surgery-specific factors.
6. Obtain necessary preoperative laboratory tests.

INTRAOPERATIVE CARE

The role of an internist in the intraoperative management of any surgical patient is minimal; however, relevant recommendations must be laid out preoperatively for management of bleeding in the operating room. Based on the underlying coagulopathy, use of platelets, blood products like FFP or factor replacement have to be considered. Intraoperative blood loss can be associated with hemodynamic instability and, in such situations, red blood cell (RBC) transfusion is appropriate.

POSTOPERATIVE CARE

The aim of postoperative care is to monitor patients for medical or surgery-related complications while they recover to discharge from hospital. Certain neurological procedures may be performed as same-day surgeries, but most patients are admitted to the hospital postoperatively.[99,100] Those with underlying bleeding diathesis or with interruptions to their antiplatelet or anticoagulant medications usually require hospitalization following surgery. The postoperative level of care is determined by the surgeon based on intraoperative complications, the patient's known risk factors, and the type of surgery.[101–103] Patients undergoing brain biopsies, shunt procedures, diagnostic angiograms, and most spine surgeries can be transferred to telemonitored units postoperatively, whereas procedures like tumor resections, skull base surgeries, cranioplasty, and multilevel spine surgery are associated with a high risk of bleeding and usually need an ICU level of care.[101] Intraoperative blood loss is a risk factor for POB and complications, and it warrants a closer monitoring of those patients.

Postoperative hematoma is reported to commonly occur within the first 6 hours postoperatively in both brain and spine surgery patients. The majority of POB complications are reported within first 24 hours after surgery.[15,31] Delayed hematoma (>24 hours postsurgery) formation can occur in spine patients especially after removal of suction drains.[31] As opposed to most surgeries, clinically significant bleeding requiring repeat surgery or evacuation in neurosurgery patients occurs at

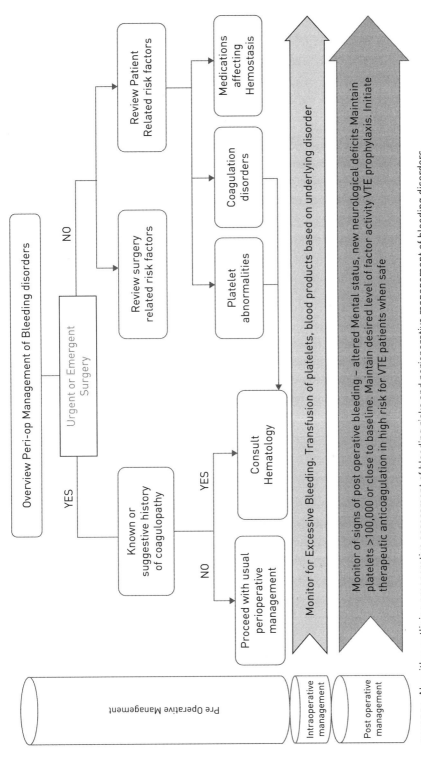

FIGURE 7.1 Algorithm outlining preoperative assessment of bleeding risks and perioperative management of bleeding disorders.

relatively smaller amounts of bleed. Changes in mental status, new or worsening of baseline neurological deficits, intractable back pain, and urine retention or incontinence should prompt evaluation for POB. Neurological deficits precede more systemic signs and symptoms, and hypotension in postoperative period most likely reflects significant intraoperative blood loss.

Radiologist should be aware of normal postoperative findings in neurosurgery patients and be able to differentiate expected findings from abnormal findings.[104] Prompt recognition of POB and treatment improves mortality and other outcomes.[13,14] In patients with underlying bleeding diathesis with suspected POB, laboratory evaluation should occur in conjunction with needed surgical intervention. Correction of incomplete local hemostasis when present is usually sufficient even in patients with bleeding diathesis. Blood transfusion is indicated only in appropriate patients based on the clinical situation.[105–108]

Patients can develop thrombocytopenia after surgery without an established diagnosis preoperatively. Thrombocytopenia was reported in cardiovascular procedures and certain orthopedic interventions, but studies are lacking on its incidence in neurosurgery patients.[109–111] Platelet count may be reduced as a physiologic response to tissue injury through various mechanisms including complement activation, release of cytokines, and VWF causing platelet activation and consumption. Other etiologies to consider for low platelets in the immediate postoperative period include pseudo-thrombocytopenia, hemodilution, massive transfusion, and type 1 HIT.[109] Thrombocytopenia that persists or develops 4–5 days after surgery may have a more serious cause; sepsis, HIT type 2, thrombotic microangiopathy, and drug-induced immune thrombocytopenia should be considered,[109,112] and the hematology team should be on board.

For patients with a known history of thrombocytopenia, treatment options are based on the underlying diagnosis, as mentioned earlier in the preoperative section. Use of desmopressin is associated with tachyphylaxis and with fluid retention and hyponatremia. Platelet transfusion is indicated in clinically significant bleeding. In patients with VWD and clotting factor deficiencies, monitoring of levels should be continued postoperatively and target levels maintained for up to 14 days. Those who received factor replacement are at risk of inhibitor development and hence screening should occur after a few weeks.[66]

VTE prophylaxis is crucial in the postoperative period, and the use of a multimodal approach through mechanical and pharmacologic therapies has been effective in reducing VTE events. Use of subcutaneous UFH or LMWH, although it carries the risk of POB, is relatively safe and effective especially in high-risk patients.[25,26,113–116] Age of more than 60 years, comorbidity burden, dependent functional status, prior history of VTE, corticosteroid use, and postoperative sepsis, urinary tract infection, and pneumonia are frequently noted predictors of VTE.[18–24] Surgery-related risks commonly identified include emergent surgery, duration of surgery longer than 4 hours, craniotomy for brain tumors, multilevel and fusion spine surgeries, and higher intraoperative blood loss.[18,20,21,23,24,117] Time to initiate anticoagulation (prophylactic and therapeutic) has not been standardized, and there is wide variation in current practices.[118,119] Available studies on safety have reported the use of prophylactic heparin based on type of surgery from postoperative day 1 (spine) or later (day 4 for intracranial bleed).[26,117,120,121] Routine screening ultrasound for VTE in neurosurgery patients is not cost-effective.[122,123] The decision to initiate therapeutic anticoagulation is more challenging and available literature is mostly from trauma patients. A multidisciplinary team approach to start therapeutic anticoagulation by taking into account the type of surgery, risk of bleeding and VTE, indication for anticoagulation, and perioperative complications is recommended.

CONCLUSION

Neurosurgical interventions are generally considered high risk for bleeding procedures. Preoperative evaluation gives an opportunity not only to address cardiopulmonary risk assessment but also to review factors associated with bleeding.

REFERENCES

1. Healy MA, Mullard AJ, Campbell DA, Dimick JB. Hospital and payer costs associated with surgical complications. *JAMA Surg.* 2016;151(9):823–830. doi: 10.1001/jamasurg.2016.0773.
2. Tevis SE, Kennedy GD. Postoperative complications and implications on patient-centered outcomes. *J Surg Res.* 2013;181(1):106–113. doi: 10.1016/j.jss.2013.01.032.
3. Wong JM, Panchmatia JR, Ziewacz JE, et al. Patterns in neurosurgical adverse events: intracranial neoplasm surgery. *Neurosurg Focus.* 2012;33(5):E16. doi: 10.3171/2012.7.FOCUS12183.
4. Rolston JD, Han SJ, Lau CY, Berger MS, Parsa AT. Frequency and predictors of complications in neurological surgery: national trends from 2006 to 2011. *J Neurosurg.* March 2014:736–745. doi: 10.3171/2013.10.JNS122419.
5. Bekelis K, Desai A, Bakhoum SF, Missios S. A predictive model of complications after spine surgery: the National Surgical Quality Improvement Program (NSQIP) 2005–2010. *Spine J.* 2014;14(7):1247–1255. doi: 10.1016/j.spinee.2013.08.009.
6. Karhade AV, Vasudeva VS, Dasenbrock HH, et al. Thirty-day readmission and reoperation after surgery for spinal tumors: a National Surgical Quality Improvement Program analysis. *Neurosurg Focus.* 2016;41(2):E5. doi: 10.3171/2016.5.FOCUS16168.
7. Basques BA, Fu MC, Buerba RA, Bohl DD, Golinvaux NS, Grauer JN. Using the ACS-NSQIP to identify factors affecting hospital length of stay after elective posterior lumbar fusion. *Spine (Phila Pa 1976).* 2014;39(6):497–502. doi: 10.1097/BRS.0000000000000184.
8. Gruskay JA, Fu M, Bohl DD, Webb ML, Grauer JN. Factors affecting length of stay after elective posterior lumbar spine surgery: a multivariate analysis. *Spine J.* 2015;15(6):1188–1195. doi: 10.1016/j.spinee.2013.10.022.
9. Lillemäe K, Järviö JA, Silvasti-Lundell MK, Antinheimo JJ-P, Hernesniemi JA, Niemi TT. Incidence of postoperative hematomas requiring surgical treatment in neurosurgery: a retrospective observational study. *World Neurosurg.* 2017;108:491–497. doi: 10.1016/j.wneu.2017.09.007.
10. Palmer JD, Sparrow OC, Iannotti F. Postoperative hematoma: a 5-year survey and identification of avoidable risk factors. *Neurosurgery.* 1994;35(6):1061–1064; discussion 1064–1065. http://www.ncbi.nlm.nih.gov/pubmed/7885549. Accessed November 30, 2018.

11. Glotzbecker MP, Bono CM, Wood KB, Harris MB. Postoperative spinal epidural hematoma: a systematic review. *Spine (Phila Pa 1976)*. 2010;35(10):E413–E420. doi: 10.1097/BRS.0b013e3181d9bb77.

12. Cramer DE, Maher PC, Pettigrew DB, Kuntz C. Major neurologic deficit immediately after adult spinal surgery: incidence and etiology over 10 years at a single training institution. *J Spinal Disord Tech*. 2009;22(8):565–570. doi: 10.1097/BSD.0b013e318193452a.

13. Amiri AR, Fouyas IP, Cro S, Casey ATH. Postoperative spinal epidural hematoma (SEH): incidence, risk factors, onset, and management. *Spine J*. 2013;13(2):134–140. doi: 10.1016/j.spinee.2012.10.028.

14. Kao F-C, Tsai T-T, Chen L-H, et al. Symptomatic epidural hematoma after lumbar decompression surgery. *Eur Spine J*. 2015;24(2):348–357. doi: 10.1007/s00586-014-3297-8.

15. Nittby HR, Maltese A, Ståhl N. Early postoperative haematomas in neurosurgery. *Acta Neurochir (Wien)*. 2016;158(5):837–846. doi: 10.1007/s00701-016-2778-4.

16. Seifman MA, Lewis PM, Rosenfeld J V, Hwang PYK. Postoperative intracranial haemorrhage: a review. *Neurosurg Rev*. 2011;34(4):393–407. doi: 10.1007/s10143-010-0304-3.

17. Liu J-M, Deng H-L, Zhou Y, et al. Incidence and risk factors for symptomatic spinal epidural haematoma following lumbar spinal surgery. *Int Orthop*. 2017;41(11):2297–2302. doi: 10.1007/s00264-017-3619-7.

18. Cote D, Dubois H, Karhade A, Smith T. Venous thromboembolism in patients undergoing craniotomy for brain tumors: a U.S. nationwide analysis. *Semin Thromb Hemost*. 2016;42(08):870–876. doi: 10.1055/s-0036-1592306.

19. Wang T, Yang S-D, Huang W-Z, Liu F-Y, Wang H, Ding W-Y. Factors predicting venous thromboembolism after spine surgery. *Medicine (Baltimore)*. 2016;95(52):e5776. doi: 10.1097/MD.0000000000005776.

20. Piper K, Algattas H, DeAndrea-Lazarus IA, et al. Risk factors associated with venous thromboembolism in patients undergoing spine surgery. *J Neurosurg Spine*. 2017;26(1):90–96. doi: 10.3171/2016.6.SPINE1656.

21. Kimmell KT, Jahromi BS. Clinical factors associated with venous thromboembolism risk in patients undergoing craniotomy. *J Neurosurg*. 2015;122(5):1004–1011. doi: 10.3171/2014.10.JNS14632.

22. Algattas H, Kimmell KT, Vates GE, Jahromi BS. Analysis of venous thromboembolism risk in patients undergoing craniotomy. *World Neurosurg*. 2015;84(5):1372–1379. doi: 10.1016/j.wneu.2015.06.033.

23. Yoshioka K, Murakami H, Demura S, Kato S, Tsuchiya H. Prevalence and risk factors for development of venous thromboembolism after degenerative spinal surgery. *Spine (Phila Pa 1976)*. 2015;40(5):E301–E306. doi: 10.1097/BRS.0000000000000727.

24. Smith TR, Nanney AD, Lall RR, et al. Development of venous thromboembolism (VTE) in patients undergoing surgery for brain tumors: results from a single center over a 10-year period. *J Clin Neurosci*. 2015;22(3):519–525. doi: 10.1016/j.jocn.2014.10.003.

25. Collen JF, Jackson JL, Shorr AF, Moores LK. Prevention of venous thromboembolism in neurosurgery: a metaanalysis. *Chest*. 2008;134(2):237–249. doi: 10.1378/chest.08-0023.

26. Cox JB, Weaver KJ, Neal DW, Jacob RP, Hoh DJ. Decreased incidence of venous thromboembolism after spine surgery with early multimodal prophylaxis. *J Neurosurg Spine*. 2014;21(4):677–684. doi: 10.3171/2014.6.SPINE13447.

27. Kim SH, Lee JH, Joo W, et al. Analysis of the risk factors for development of postoperative extradural hematoma after intracranial surgery. *Br J Neurosurg*. 2015;29(2):243–248. doi: 10.3109/02688697.2014.967749.

28. Kou J, Fischgrund J, Biddinger A, Herkowitz H. Risk factors for spinal epidural hematoma after spinal surgery. *Spine (Phila Pa 1976)*. 2002;27(15):1670–1673. http://www.ncbi.nlm.nih.gov/pubmed/12163731. Accessed December 2, 2018.

29. Gerlach R, Raabe A, Scharrer I, Meixensberger J, Seifert V. Postoperative hematoma after surgery for intracranial meningiomas: causes, avoidable risk factors and clinical outcome. *Neurol Res*. 2004;26(1):61–66. doi: 10.1179/016164104773026543.

30. Domenicucci M, Mancarella C, Santoro G, et al. Spinal epidural hematomas: personal experience and literature review of more than 1000 cases. *J Neurosurg Spine*. 2017;27(2):198–208. doi: 10.3171/2016.12.SPINE15475.

31. Aono H, Ohwada T, Hosono N, et al. Incidence of postoperative symptomatic epidural hematoma in spinal decompression surgery. *J Neurosurg Spine*. 2011;15(2):202–205. doi: 10.3171/2011.3.SPINE10716.

32. Sokolowski MJ, Garvey TA, Perl J, et al. Prospective study of postoperative lumbar epidural hematoma: incidence and risk factors. *Spine (Phila Pa 1976)*. 2008;33(1):108–113. doi: 10.1097/BRS.0b013e31815e39af.

33. Awad JN, Kebaish KM, Donigan J, Cohen DB, Kostuik JP. Analysis of the risk factors for the development of postoperative spinal epidural haematoma. *J Bone Joint Surg Br*. 2005;87(9):1248–1252. doi: 10.1302/0301-620X.87B9.16518.

34. Zrinzo L, Foltynie T, Limousin P, Hariz MI. Reducing hemorrhagic complications in functional neurosurgery: a large case series and systematic literature review. *J Neurosurg*. 2012;116(1):84–94. doi: 10.3171/2011.8.JNS101407.

35. Goldstein CL, Bains I, Hurlbert RJ. Symptomatic spinal epidural hematoma after posterior cervical surgery: incidence and risk factors. *Spine J*. 2015;15(6):1179–1187. doi: 10.1016/j.spinee.2013.11.043.

36. Chan KH, Mann KS, Chan TK. The significance of thrombocytopenia in the development of postoperative intracranial hematoma. *J Neurosurg*. 1989;71(1):38–41. doi: 10.3171/jns.1989.71.1.0038.

37. Dasenbrock HH, Devine CA, Liu KX, et al. Thrombocytopenia and craniotomy for tumor: a National Surgical Quality Improvement Program analysis. *Cancer*. 2016;122(11):1708–1717. doi: 10.1002/cncr.29984.

38. Seicean A, Schiltz NK, Seicean S, Alan N, Neuhauser D, Weil RJ. Use and utility of preoperative hemostatic screening and patient history in adult neurosurgical patients. *J Neurosurg*. 2012;116(5):1097–1105. doi: 10.3171/2012.1.JNS111760.

39. Chee YL, Crawford JC, Watson HG, Greaves M. Guidelines on the assessment of bleeding risk prior to surgery or invasive procedures. British Committee for Standards in Haematology. *Br J Haematol*. 2008;140(5):496–504. doi: 10.1111/j.1365-2141.2007.06968.x.

40. Abdelfatah M. Management of chronic subdural hematoma in patients with intractable thrombocytopenia. *Turk Neurosurg*. 2018;28(3):400–404. doi: 10.5137/1019-5149.JTN.18825-16.1.

41. Li D, Glor T, Jones GA. Thrombocytopenia and neurosurgery: a literature review. *World Neurosurg*. 2017;106:277–280. doi: 10.1016/j.wneu.2017.06.097.

42. Estcourt LJ, Birchall J, Allard S, et al. Guidelines for the use of platelet transfusions. *Br J Haematol*. 2017;176(3):365–394. doi: 10.1111/bjh.14423.

43. Hogshire LC, Patel MS, Rivera E, Carson JL. Evidence review: periprocedural use of blood products. *J Hosp Med*. 2013;8(11):647–652. doi: 10.1002/jhm.2089.

44. Cines DB, Bussel JB. How I treat idiopathic thrombocytopenic purpura (ITP). *Blood*. 2005;106(7):2244–2251. doi: 10.1182/blood-2004-12-4598.

45. Schiffer CA, Bohlke K, Delaney M, et al. Platelet transfusion for patients with cancer: American Society of Clinical Oncology clinical practice guideline update. *J Clin Oncol*. 2018;36(3):283–299. doi: 10.1200/JCO.2017.76.1734.

46. Neunert C, Lim W, Crowther M, Cohen A, Solberg L, Crowther MA. The American Society of Hematology 2011 evidence-based practice guideline for immune thrombocytopenia. *Blood.* 2011;117(16):4190–4207. doi: 10.1182/blood-2010-08-302984.

47. Afdhal N, McHutchison J, Brown R, et al. Thrombocytopenia associated with chronic liver disease. *J Hepatol.* 2008;48(6):1000–1007. doi: 10.1016/j.jhep.2008.03.009.

48. Abbas N, Makker J, Abbas H, Balar B. Perioperative care of patients with liver cirrhosis: a review. *Heal Serv Insights.* 2017;10:117863291769127. doi: 10.1177/1178632917691270.

49. Kim ES. Lusutrombopag: first global approval. *Drugs.* 2016;76(1):155–158. doi: 10.1007/s40265-015-0525-4.

50. Linkins L-A, Dans AL, Moores LK, et al. Treatment and prevention of heparin-induced thrombocytopenia. *Chest.* 2012;141(2):e495S–e530S. doi: 10.1378/chest.11-2303.

51. Swisher KK, Terrell DR, Vesely SK, Kremer Hovinga JA, Lämmle B, George JN. Clinical outcomes after platelet transfusions in patients with thrombotic thrombocytopenic purpura. *Transfusion.* 2009;49(5):873–887. doi: 10.1111/j.1537-2995.2008.02082.x.

52. Kaufman RM, Djulbegovic B, Gernsheimer T, et al. Platelet transfusion: a clinical practice guideline from the AABB. *Ann Intern Med.* 2015;162(3):205. doi: 10.7326/M14-1589.

53. Ghadimi K, Levy JH, Welsby IJ. Perioperative management of the bleeding patient. *Br J Anaesth.* 2016;117(Suppl 3):iii18–iii30. doi: 10.1093/bja/aew358.

54. Livio M, Mannucci PM, Viganò G, et al. Conjugated estrogens for the management of bleeding associated with renal failure. *N Engl J Med.* 1986;315(12):731–735. doi: 10.1056/NEJM198609183151204.

55. Alamelu J, Liesner R. Modern management of severe platelet function disorders. *Br J Haematol.* 2010;149(6):813–823. doi: 10.1111/j.1365-2141.2010.08191.x.

56. Rodgers GM. Evaluation of coagulation in the neurosurgery patient. *Neurosurg Clin N Am.* 2018;29(4):485–492. doi: 10.1016/j.nec.2018.06.001.

57. Beynon C, Wessels L, Unterberg A. Point-of-care testing in neurosurgery. *Semin Thromb Hemost.* 2017;43(04):416–422. doi: 10.1055/s-0037-1599159.

58. van Veen JJ, Nokes TJ, Makris M. The risk of spinal haematoma following neuraxial anaesthesia or lumbar puncture in thrombocytopenic individuals. *Br J Haematol.* 2010;148(1):15–25. doi: 10.1111/j.1365-2141.2009.07899.x.

59. Sadler JE, Mannucci PM, Berntorp E, et al. Impact, diagnosis and treatment of von Willebrand disease. *Thromb Haemost.* 2000;84(2):160–174. http://www.ncbi.nlm.nih.gov/pubmed/10959685. Accessed January 1, 2019.

60. Tiede A, Rand JH, Budde U, Ganser A, Federici AB. How I treat the acquired von Willebrand syndrome. *Blood.* 2011;117(25):6777–6785. doi: 10.1182/blood-2010-11-297580.

61. Laffan MA, Lester W, O'Donnell JS, et al. The diagnosis and management of von Willebrand disease: a United Kingdom Haemophilia Centre Doctors Organization guideline approved by the British Committee for Standards in Haematology. *Br J Haematol.* 2014;167(4):453–465. doi: 10.1111/bjh.13064.

62. Nichols WL, Hultin MB, James AH, et al. von Willebrand disease (VWD): evidence-based diagnosis and management guidelines, the National Heart, Lung, and Blood Institute (NHLBI) Expert Panel report (USA). *Haemophilia.* 2008;14(2):171–232. doi: 10.1111/j.1365-2516.2007.01643.x.

63. Zulfikar B, Koc B, Ak G, et al. Surgery in patients with von Willebrand disease. *Blood Coagul Fibrinolysis.* 2016;27(7):812–816. doi: 10.1097/MBC.0000000000000500.

64. Miesbach W, Berntorp E. Von Willebrand disease—the 'dos' and 'don'ts' in surgery. *Eur J Haematol.* 2017;98(2):121–127. doi: 10.1111/ejh.12809.

65. Escobar MA, Brewer A, Caviglia H, et al. Recommendations on multidisciplinary management of elective surgery in people with haemophilia. *Haemophilia.* 2018;24(5):693–702. doi: 10.1111/hae.13549.

66. Srivastava A, Brewer AK, Mauser-Bunschoten EP, et al. Guidelines for the management of hemophilia. *Haemophilia.* 2013;19(1):e1–47. doi: 10.1111/j.1365-2516.2012.02909.x.

67. Plug I, Mauser-Bunschoten EP, Bröcker-Vriends AHJT, et al. Bleeding in carriers of hemophilia. *Blood.* 2006;108(1):52–56. doi: 10.1182/blood-2005-09-3879.

68. Carcao MD. The diagnosis and management of congenital hemophilia. *Semin Thromb Hemost.* 2012;38(7):727–734. doi: 10.1055/s-0032-1326786.

69. Blanchette VS, Key NS, Ljung LR, et al. Definitions in hemophilia: communication from the SSC of the ISTH. *J Thromb Haemost.* 2014;12(11):1935–1939. doi: 10.1111/jth.12672.

70. Teitel JM, Carcao M, Lillicrap D, et al. Orthopaedic surgery in haemophilia patients with inhibitors: a practical guide to haemostatic, surgical and rehabilitative care. *Haemophilia.* 2009;15(1):227–239. doi: 10.1111/j.1365-2516.2008.01840.x.

71. Poon MC, Aledort LM, Anderle K, Kunschak M, Morfini M. Comparison of the recovery and half-life of a high-purity factor IX concentrate with those of a factor IX complex concentrate. Factor IX Study Group. *Transfusion.* 1995;35(4):319–323. http://www.ncbi.nlm.nih.gov/pubmed/7701550. Accessed January 1, 2019.

72. Adcock DM, Strandberg K, Shima M, Marlar RA. Advantages, disadvantages and optimization of one-stage and chromogenic factor activity assays in haemophilia A and B. *Int J Lab Hematol.* 2018;40(6):621–629. doi: 10.1111/ijlh.12877.

73. Kempton CL, White GC. How we treat a hemophilia A patient with a factor VIII inhibitor. *Blood.* 2009;113(1):11–17. doi: 10.1182/blood-2008-06-160432.

74. Peyvandi F, Duga S, Akhavan S, Mannucci PM. Rare coagulation deficiencies. *Haemophilia.* 2002;8(3):308–321. http://www.ncbi.nlm.nih.gov/pubmed/12010428. Accessed January 19, 2019.

75. Mannucci PM, Duga S, Peyvandi F. Recessively inherited coagulation disorders. *Blood.* 2004;104(5):1243–1252. doi: 10.1182/blood-2004-02-0595.

76. di Paola J, Nugent D, Young G. Current therapy for rare factor deficiencies. *Haemophilia.* 2001;7(s1):16–22. doi: 10.1046/j.1365-2516.2001.00100.x.

77. Casini A, de Moerloose P, Congenital Fibrinogen Disorders Group. Management of congenital quantitative fibrinogen disorders: a Delphi consensus. *Haemophilia.* 2016;22(6):898–905. doi: 10.1111/hae.13061.

78. Bornikova L, Peyvandi F, Allen G, Bernstein J, Manco-Johnson MJ. Fibrinogen replacement therapy for congenital fibrinogen deficiency. *J Thromb Haemost.* 2011;9(9):1687–1704. doi: 10.1111/j.1538-7836.2011.04424.x.

79. Hurwitz A, Massone R, Lopez BL. Acquired bleeding disorders. *Hematol Oncol Clin North Am.* 2017;31(6):1123–1145. doi: 10.1016/j.hoc.2017.08.012.

80. Dagi TF. The management of postoperative bleeding. *Surg Clin North Am.* 2005;85(6):1191–1213. doi: 10.1016/j.suc.2005.10.013.

81. Glotzbecker MP, Bono CM, Wood KB, Harris MB. Postoperative spinal epidural hematoma. *Spine (Phila Pa 1976).* 2010;35(10):E413–E420. doi: 10.1097/BRS.0b013e3181d9bb77.

82. Douketis JD, Spyropoulos AC, Spencer FA, et al. Perioperative management of antithrombotic therapy: Antithrombotic Therapy and Prevention of Thrombosis, 9th

ed.: American College of Chest Physicians Evidence-Based Clinical Practice Guidelines. *Chest.* 2012;141(2 Suppl):e326S–e350S. doi: 10.1378/chest.11-2298.

83. Ang-Lee MK, Moss J, Yuan CS. Herbal medicines and perioperative care. *JAMA.* 2001;286(2):208–216. http://www.ncbi.nlm.nih.gov/pubmed/11448284. Accessed November 29, 2018.

84. Rowe DJ, Baker AC. Perioperative risks and benefits of herbal supplements in aesthetic surgery. *Aesthetic Surg J.* 2009;29(2):150–157. doi: 10.1016/j.asj.2009.01.002.

85. Kepler CK, Huang RC, Meredith D, Kim J-H, Sharma AK. Omega-3 and fish oil supplements do not cause increased bleeding during spinal decompression surgery. *J Spinal Disord Tech.* 2012;25(3):129–132. doi: 10.1097/BSD.0b013e3182120227.

86. Meredith DS, Kepler CK, Hirsch B, et al. The effect of omega-3 fatty-acid supplements on perioperative bleeding following posterior spinal arthrodesis. *Eur Spine J.* 2012;21(12):2659–2663. doi: 10.1007/s00586-012-2365-1.

87. Graham MM, Sessler DI, Parlow JL, et al. Aspirin in patients with previous percutaneous coronary intervention undergoing noncardiac surgery. *Ann Intern Med.* 2018;168(4):237–244. doi: 10.7326/M17-2341.

88. Valgimigli M, Bueno H, Byrne RA, et al. 2017 ESC focused update on dual antiplatelet therapy in coronary artery disease developed in collaboration with EACTS: the Task Force for dual antiplatelet therapy in coronary artery disease of the European Society of Cardiology (ESC) and of the European Association for Cardio-Thoracic Surgery (EACTS). *Eur Heart J.* 2018;39(3):213–260. doi: 10.1093/eurheartj/ehx419.

89. Colombo A, Chieffo A, Frasheri A, et al. Second-generation drug-eluting stent implantation followed by 6- versus 12-month dual antiplatelet therapy. *J Am Coll Cardiol.* 2014;64(20):2086–2097. doi: 10.1016/j.jacc.2014.09.008.

90. Schulz-Schupke S, Byrne RA, ten Berg JM, et al. ISAR-SAFE: a randomized, double-blind, placebo-controlled trial of 6 vs. 12 months of clopidogrel therapy after drug-eluting stenting. *Eur Heart J.* 2015;36(20):1252–1263. doi: 10.1093/eurheartj/ehu523.

91. Dweck MR, Cruden NL. Noncardiac surgery in patients with coronary artery stents. *Arch Intern Med.* 2012;172(14). doi: 10.1001/archinternmed.2012.3025.

92. Childers CP, Mak S, Miake-Lye IM, et al. *Management of Antiplatelet Therapy Among Patients on Antiplatelet Therapy for Cerebrovascular or Peripheral Vascular Diseases Undergoing Elective Non-Cardiac Surgery.* Department of Veterans Affairs (US); 2017. http://www.ncbi.nlm.nih.gov/pubmed/29608260. Accessed January 19, 2019.

93. Spyropoulos AC, Al-Badri A, Sherwood MW, Douketis JD. Periprocedural management of patients receiving a vitamin K antagonist or a direct oral anticoagulant requiring an elective procedure or surgery. *J Thromb Haemost.* 2016;14(5):875–885. doi: 10.1111/jth.13305.

94. van Veen JJ, Makris M. Management of peri-operative anti-thrombotic therapy. *Anaesthesia.* 2015;70:58–e23. doi: 10.1111/anae.12900.

95. Healey JS, Eikelboom J, Douketis J, et al. Periprocedural bleeding and thromboembolic events with dabigatran compared with warfarin. *Circulation.* 2012;126(3):343–348. doi: 10.1161/CIRCULATIONAHA.111.090464.

96. Lip GYH. Implications of the CHA(2)DS(2)-VASc and HAS-BLED Scores for thromboprophylaxis in atrial fibrillation. *Am J Med.* 2011;124(2):111–114. doi: 10.1016/j.amjmed.2010.05.007.

97. Levy JH, Szlam F, Wolberg AS, Winkler A. Clinical use of the activated partial thromboplastin time and prothrombin time for screening. *Clin Lab Med.* 2014;34(3):453–477. doi: 10.1016/j.cll.2014.06.005.

98. Schramm B, Leslie K, Myles PS, Hogan CJ. Coagulation studies in preoperative neuro-surgical patients. *Anaesth Intensive Care.* 2001;29(4):388–392. http://www.ncbi.nlm.nih.gov/pubmed/11512650. Accessed December 31, 2018.

99. Turel MK, Bernstein M. Outpatient neurosurgery. *Expert Rev Neurother.* 2016;16(4):425–436. doi: 10.1586/14737175.2016.1158104.

100. Purzner T, Purzner J, Massicotte EM, Bernstein M. Outpatient brain tumor surgery and spinal decompression: a prospective study of 1003 patients. *Neurosurgery.* 2011;69(1):119–127. doi: 10.1227/NEU.0b013e318215a270.

101. Hanak BW, Walcott BP, Nahed B V., et al. Postoperative intensive care unit requirements after elective craniotomy. *World Neurosurg.* 2014;81(1):165–172. doi: 10.1016/j.wneu.2012.11.068.

102. Kay HF, Chotai S, Wick JB, Stonko DP, McGirt MJ, Devin CJ. Preoperative and surgical factors associated with postoperative intensive care unit admission following operative treatment for degenerative lumbar spine disease. *Eur Spine J.* 2016;25(3):843–849. doi: 10.1007/s00586-015-4175-8.

103. Memtsoudis SG, Stundner O, Sun X, et al. Critical care in patients undergoing lumbar spine fusion. *J Intensive Care Med.* 2014;29(5):275–284. doi: 10.1177/0885066613491924.

104. Chughtai KA, Nemer OP, Kessler AT, Bhatt AA. Postoperative complications of craniotomy and craniectomy. *Emerg Radiol.* September 2018. doi: 10.1007/s10140-018-1647-2.

105. Simon GI, Craswell A, Thom O, Fung YL. Outcomes of restrictive versus liberal transfusion strategies in older adults from nine randomised controlled trials: a systematic review and meta-analysis. *Lancet Haematol.* 2017;4(10):e465–e474. doi: 10.1016/S2352-3026(17)30141-2.

106. Docherty AB, O'Donnell R, Brunskill S, et al. Effect of restrictive versus liberal transfusion strategies on outcomes in patients with cardiovascular disease in a non-cardiac surgery setting: systematic review and meta-analysis. *BMJ.* 2016;352:i1351. doi: 10.1136/bmj.i1351.

107. Gruskay JA, Fu M, Bohl DD, Webb ML, Grauer JN. Factors affecting length of stay after elective posterior lumbar spine surgery: a multivariate analysis. *Spine J.* 2015;15(6):1188–1195. doi: 10.1016/j.spinee.2013.10.022.

108. Basques BA, Fu MC, Buerba RA, Bohl DD, Golinvaux NS, Grauer JN. Using the ACS-NSQIP to identify factors affecting hospital length of stay after elective posterior lumbar fusion. *Spine (Phila Pa 1976).* 2014;39(6):497–502. doi: 10.1097/BRS.0000000000000184.

109. Ali N, Auerbach HE. New-onset acute thrombocytopenia in hospitalized patients: pathophysiology and diagnostic approach. *J community Hosp Intern Med Perspect.* 2017;7(3):157–167. doi: 10.1080/20009666.2017.1335156.

110. Chang JC. Review: postoperative thrombocytopenia: with etiologic, diagnostic, and therapeutic consideration. *Am J Med Sci.* 1996;311(2):96–105. http://www.ncbi.nlm.nih.gov/pubmed/8615383. Accessed January 14, 2019.

111. Zacharia G, Walczyszyn BA, Lee D, Stoffels G, Spaccavento C, Levine RL. Characteristics of the postsurgical decrease in platelet counts in orthopedic patients. *Blood.* 2016;128(22). http://www.bloodjournal.org/content/128/22/2554?sso-checked=true. Accessed January 14, 2019.

112. Naqvi TA, Baumann MA, Chang JC. Postoperative thrombotic thrombocytopenic purpura: a review. *Int J Clin Pract.* 2004;58(2):169–172. doi: 10.1111/j.1368-5031.2004.0080.x.

113. Algattas H, Damania D, DeAndrea-Lazarus I, et al. Systematic review of safety and cost-effectiveness of venous thromboembolism prophylaxis strategies in patients undergoing craniotomy for brain tumor. *Neurosurgery.* 2018;82(2):142–154. doi: 10.1093/neuros/nyx156.

114. Alshehri N, Cote DJ, Hulou MM, et al. Venous thromboembolism prophylaxis in brain tumor patients undergoing craniotomy: a meta-analysis. *J Neurooncol.* 2016;130(3):561–570. doi: 10.1007/s11060-016-2259-x.

115. Hamilton MG, Yee WH, Hull RD, Ghali WA. Venous thromboembolism prophylaxis in patients undergoing cranial neurosurgery: a systematic review and meta-analysis. *Neurosurgery.* 2011;68(3):571–581. doi: 10.1227/NEU.0b013e3182093145.

116. Sharpe JP, Gobbell WC, Carter AM, et al. Impact of venous thromboembolism che-moprophylaxis on postoperative hemorrhage following operative stabilization of spine fractures. *J Trauma Acute Care Surg.* 2017;83(6):1108–1113. doi: 10.1097/TA.0000000000001640.

117. Dhillon ES, Khanna R, Cloney M, et al. Timing and risks of chemoprophylaxis after spinal surgery: a single-center experience with 6869 consecutive patients. *J Neurosurg Spine.* 2017;27(6):681–693. doi: 10.3171/2017.3.SPINE161076.

118. Scales DC, Riva-Cambrin J, Le TL, et al. Prophylaxis against venous thromboem-bolism in neurointensive care patients: survey of Canadian practice. *J Crit Care.* 2009;24(2):176–184. doi: 10.1016/j.jcrc.2009.03.010.

119. Glotzbecker MP, Bono CM, Harris MB, Brick G, Heary RF, Wood KB. Surgeon practices regarding postoperative thromboembolic prophylaxis after high-risk spinal surgery. *Spine (Phila Pa 1976).* 2008;33(26):2915–2921. doi: 10.1097/BRS.0b013e318190702a.

120. Agarwal N, Zenonos GA, Agarwal P, et al. Risk-to-benefit ratio of venous thrombo-embolism prophylaxis for neurosurgical procedures at a quaternary referral center. *Neurosurgery.* 2019;84(2):355–361. doi: 10.1093/neuros/nyy035.

121. Strom RG, Frempong-Boadu AK. Low-molecular-weight heparin prophylaxis 24 to 36 hours after degenerative spine surgery. *Spine (Phila Pa 1976).* 2013;38(23):E1498–E1502. doi: 10.1097/BRS.0b013e3182a4408d.

122. Needleman L, Cronan JJ, Lilly MP, et al. Ultrasound for lower extremity deep venous thrombosis. *Circulation.* 2018;137(14):1505–1515. doi: 10.1161/CIRCULATIONAHA.117.030687.

123. Samuel S, Patel N, McGuire MF, Salazar M, Nguyen T. Analysis of venous thromboem-bolism in neurosurgical patients undergoing standard versus routine ultrasonography. *J Thromb Thrombolysis.* November 2018. doi: 10.1007/s11239-018-1761-8.

8 Fever in the Neurosurgical Patient

Rakhshanda Akram, Crystal Benjamin,
Linda Mwamuka, and Katherine A. Belden

INTRODUCTION

Postoperative fever falls under the broad category of nosocomial (healthcare-associated) fever of unknown origin, defined as a temperature greater than 38.3°C (or greater than 100.9°F) for more than 3 days not present or incubating before surgery.[1]

Many studies have highlighted that early postoperative fever is more frequently associated with a physiologic response to surgically induced tissue injury releasing pyrogenic cytokines and interleukins.[2-5] However, there are well-recognized pathologic, infectious, and noninfectious etiologies of postoperative fever frequently attributable to risk factors encountered in the healthcare environment that can lead to increased morbidity, mortality, and healthcare cost. Therefore, it is important to differentiate physiologic from pathologic postoperative fever to reduce unnecessary testing and treatment and to institute timely therapy, when indicated, for treatable causes of fever to decrease overall morbidity and mortality.

The American College of Surgeons National Surgical Quality Improvement Program showed the rate of postoperative neurosurgical infection to be 5.3% from 2006 to 2014.[6] In neurosurgical patients, fever is a presenting symptom in 22% of patients with postoperative infections.[7] In this chapter, we aim to address the pathophysiology of fever and present a thorough initial evaluation and management plan for postoperative fever, followed by a detailed description of nosocomial infections specific to the neurosurgical patient population.

FEVER IN THE CONTEXT OF NEUROSURGICAL PATIENTS

While fever is an important manifestation of the body's immune response to infectious insults, it is of significance in neurosurgical patients because of its deleterious effects on an already injured brain. Elevated temperature (>37.9°C) within the first 7 days after stroke was shown to be an independent predictor of poor outcome during the first month and was also associated with a higher mortality rate in the first 10 days after a stroke.[8] The exact mechanism of hyperthermia-induced brain injury is unclear. However, hyperthermia has been demonstrated to increase the release of excitatory neurotransmitters and oxygen free radicals, to cause more extensive blood–brain barrier breakdown, to impair recovery of energy metabolism via increased enzymatic inhibition of protein kinases, and to worsen cytoskeletal proteolysis.[9] Hypothermia to 34°C, on the other hand, has been shown to control intracranial hypertension.[10] Therefore, management of fever in this patient population is vital to improve patient outcomes and decrease the cost of medical care.

Preoperative Fever

Fever present prior to neurosurgery is important to recognize. While neurosurgical patients may have noninfectious fever related to their underlying condition, it is important to assess patients with fever for the possibility of an infectious etiology. In cases where emergent or urgent surgery is indicated for the stability of the patient, delaying surgery in order to evaluate for infection is not always feasible. However, in febrile patients undergoing nonurgent or elective procedures, it is often appropriate to delay the procedure in order to evaluate for a source of fever. A complete history and physical examination should be performed, with careful consideration given to any new symptoms, sick contacts, or relevant exposures. Further workup including blood, urine, or sputum cultures; testing for respiratory viruses; testing for *Clostridium difficile* enterocolitis; and chest radiography or additional imaging may be indicated. If an active infection is identified, this should be resolved prior to proceeding with elective surgery.

Postoperative Fever
Pathophysiology

Cytokines, including interleukins and interferons, are key players in mediating the body's inflammatory response to surgical tissue injury. Activated macrophages and monocytes in the damaged tissues release interleukin-1 (IL-1) and tumor necrosis factor-alpha (TNF-α) which stimulate the production of IL-6. IL-6 is responsible for the acute phase response characterized by fever, granulocytosis, and hepatic production of acute-phase proteins such as C-reactive protein (CRP), fibrinogen, and alpha-2 macro globulin.[7]

The degree of tissue trauma determines the levels of cytokine production, which tends to peak 24 hours postoperatively and remain elevated for about 2–3 days afterward. Less invasive procedures are associated with less tissue trauma and thus fewer episodes of postoperative fever. D-dimer may also remain elevated for weeks after surgery. More specifically, central nervous system (CNS) trauma in neurosurgical patients results in production of cytokines in the brain raising the hypothalamic set point. Experimental animal models have shown that the concentration of a cytokine required to cause fever is much lower when injected directly into the brain substance than with systemic injections.[11]

Systemic inflammatory response syndrome (SIRS) criteria were described more than two decades ago, and the signs meeting these criteria have been assumed to indicate a clinical response to inflammation.[12] Patients may be diagnosed with SIRS when two or more of the following criteria are met:

- Body temperature <36°C (96.8°F) or >38°C (100.4°F)
- Heart rate >90 bpm
- Respiratory rate >20 breaths/min; or an arterial pco_2 <32 mmHg (4.3 kPa)
- White blood cell count <4,000 cells/mm³ (4 × 10⁹ cells/L) or >12,000 cells/mm³ (12 × 10⁹ cells/L); or the presence of >10% bands

The presence of signs meeting two or more SIRS criteria is common but is not specific for infection.[13] Studies have shown no difference in the presence of SIRS criteria at the onset of fever in neurologic intensive care patients with central versus infectious fever.[14] SIRS had a cumulative incidence of 1.6% at a median of 3 days in the National Surgical Quality Improvement Program (NSQIP) study.[6] Up to 70% of neurologically injured patients develop fever, typically not as an isolated event but rather as a sustained response seen for as long as 2 weeks following injury.[9,15] Only some of these febrile episodes are attributable to an infectious process, with nosocomial pulmonary infections being the most common. Since fever and leukocytosis could reflect a physiologic response to surgical trauma in the first 48 hours after surgery, routine infectious workup or antibiotic treatment is not indicated in most cases.

In the event of an infectious process, cytokine release is stimulated by bacterial endotoxins and exotoxins. Self-limited postoperative fever from a similar mechanism may occur as a result of bacterial translocation from the colon due to preoperative ileus or hypotension in the absence of a true clinical infection.[16] In one-fifth to one-third of cases of fever in neurologically injured patients, fever remains unexplained even after extensive diagnostic workup.[17]

Timing of Postoperative Fever

The timing of fever onset after surgery is the most useful factor in determining the initial evaluation and management.[18] Based on the timing of onset, postoperative fever can be classified into four categories:

- *Immediate*: Onset of fever during or within hours after surgery
- *Acute*: Onset of fever within the first week of surgery
- *Subacute*: Onset of fever after the first week and up to 4 weeks after surgery
- *Delayed*: Onset of fever 1 month after surgery

Causes of postoperative fever based on time of onset are listed in Box 8.1.

Assessment of Postoperative Fever

Fever in a postoperative neurosurgical patient should be evaluated systematically, taking into account the timing of onset as well as various patient- and

Box 8.1 Causes of Postoperative Fever

Immediate Postoperative Fever (During and Within Hours After Surgery)

Drug fever (anesthetic agents/ medications used during surgery)

Febrile transfusion reaction

Preoperative Infections

SIRS

Malignant hyperthermia

Neuroleptic malignant syndrome

Fulminant skin/ soft tissue infection (Group A streptococcus and *Clostridium perfringens*)

Thyroid storm

Adrenal insufficiency

Alcohol withdrawal

Acute Postoperative Fever (First Postoperative Week)

Nosocomial pneumonia (hospital-acquired, ventilator-associated, and aspiration)

Urinary tract infection (usually with an indwelling urinary catheter)

Venous thromboembolism (DVT/ PE)

Thrombophlebitis

Myocardial infarction

Stroke

Acute pancreatitis

Acute gout

Acalculous cholecystitis

Skin and soft tissue infections (more likely subacute)

Nosocomial meningitis (more likely subacute)

Catheter (CSF drain) exit site infection (more likely subacute)

Central venous catheter associated blood stream infection (more likely subacute)

Atelectasis (not causal)

Subacute Postoperative Fever (>1 Week–4 Weeks Postoperatively)

Skin and soft tissue infections

Central venous catheter associated blood stream infection

Antibiotic-associated diarrhea (including *Clostridium difficile* colitis)

Nosocomial infections including nosocomial meningitis, pneumonia, and UTI

CSF drain infections, ventriculitis

Early shunt infections

Sinusitis

Febrile drug reactions (e.g., antimicrobials, H_2-blockers, heparin, etc.)

Thrombophlebitis

Venous thromboembolism (DVT/ PE)

Delayed Postoperative Fever (>1 Month Postoperatively)

Postoperative intracranial abscess (intracerebral and subdural)

Postoperative epidural abscess

Shunt infections

Cranial/spinal osteomyelitis

Transfusion-related viral infections (CMV, hepatitis viruses, HIV)

Transfusion-related parasitic infections (toxoplasmosis, babesiosis, *Plasmodium malariae* infection)

Skin and soft tissue infections from more indolent microorganisms (e.g., coagulase negative staphylococci)

Delayed cellulitis (in patients with postsurgical disrupted venous or lymphatic drainage)

Nosocomial infective endocarditis

procedure-specific risk factors. Most fevers within the first 48 hours of surgery either represent a response to surgery or a noninfectious etiology which should be investigated and managed based on the history and physical examination clues. Routine chest radiography, urinalysis, and blood and urine cultures are not recommended in febrile postoperative patients within the first 72 hours. A high level of suspicion should be maintained for deep venous thrombosis, superficial thrombophlebitis, and pulmonary embolism, especially in patients who are sedentary, have lower limb immobility, have a malignant neoplasm, or are taking an oral contraceptive.[19] Fever that begins on or after postprocedure day 5 is much more likely to represent a clinically significant infection, so appropriate diagnostics to look for an infectious source and use of empiric antibiotics are more useful.

A thorough history and physical examination is an integral component of initial evaluation of postoperative fever. It is important to review the preoperative presentation and hospital course and the operating room records for any intraoperative complications and postoperative course. Emergent surgeries are more likely to be associated with postoperative sepsis. It is important to recognize underlying chronic medical conditions such as diabetes mellitus, heart failure, chronic obstructive pulmonary disease (COPD) and the like as part of the evaluation of fever after surgery. Reviewing drug allergies and medications and blood products administered before, during, or after surgery may provide useful clues. Careful attention should be paid to the time of placement and location of various catheters, including intravascular lines, Foley catheters, nasogastric tubes, surgical site drains, and implanted devices and hardware. New-onset symptoms should be carefully reviewed with the patient. Nursing staff can provide useful information regarding new-onset diarrhea, skin break down, rash, and character and amount of respiratory secretions.

In addition to monitoring vital signs and particularly the association of changes in heart rate and blood pressure with hyperthermia, American College of Critical Care Medicine and Infectious Diseases Society of America (IDSA) guidelines from 2008 recommend daily examination of the surgical incision for erythema, purulence, or tenderness.[19] A thorough neurologic examination in a postoperative neurosurgical patient may have inherent limitations but is still one of the most useful tools to determine a CNS infection. However, absence of focal abnormalities in this patient population should not rule out the possibility of a CNS infection.[19] A thorough skin examination should be performed to look for a new rash, ecchymoses, catheter and drain insertion and exit sites, injection sites, and hematomas in addition to the routine abdominal, cardiac, and pulmonary examination.

If the initial patient evaluation suggests an infectious etiology, it is appropriate to initiate workup for an underlying infectious process. Complete blood count with differential is the first step, followed by routine chemistry, liver function tests, and a lactate level. Serum procalcitonin level can be used to discriminate bacterial infection as the cause of fever.[19] Three to four blood cultures should be obtained within the first 24 hours of the onset of fever and ideally before the initiation of antibiotic therapy.[19] Urinalysis and urine culture are indicated in patients at high risk for urinary tract infection (UTI). Although the absence of an infiltrate on a chest radiograph does not exclude the possibility of nosocomial pneumonia, it remains an important initial diagnostic tool in the workup of postoperative fever. Gram stain and culture of respiratory secretions (expectorated, induced, nasopharyngeal washings, deep tracheal suctioning, and bronchoscopic or nonbronchoscopic lavage) not only provide useful diagnostic information but can also be helpful for deescalation of antibiotics. New-onset diarrhea in a hospitalized patient is rarely due to enteric pathogens other than *Clostridium difficle*. Once the more common noninfectious etiologies of nosocomial diarrhea have been excluded, testing for *C. difficle* colitis is appropriate in patients with more than two loose, watery bowel movements in a day. Gram stain and cultures from superficial surgical site infections are likely to be contaminated and not routinely recommended. However, any expressed purulence obtained from levels within the incision consistent with a deep incisional or organ/space surgical site infection should be sent for Gram stain and culture.[19] Routine cultures of a removed intravenous catheter are not indicated unless there is a high pretest probability of catheter sepsis.[20]

While a noncontrast head CT is more helpful to rule out a noninfectious pathology such as new or worsening hemorrhage, mass lesion, or obstructive hydrocephalous, it may point toward a CNS focus of infection, such as an abscess, and is also helpful to rule out contraindications for LP, which is almost always indicated in postoperative neurosurgical patients with new fever. In febrile patients with an intracranial device, cerebrospinal fluid (CSF) should be obtained from the CSF reservoir as well as from the lumbar space when the CSF flow to the subarachnoid space is obstructed.[19] In addition to cell counts, differential, glucose, and protein evaluation, CSF should be tested for Gram stain and bacterial cultures. Other tests to be performed on CSF are usually dictated by the clinical situation and the patient's immune status. In patients with ventriculostomies, the removed catheter tip should be cultured.[19] A CT or MRI may be indicated in patients with spinal surgeries, depending upon the site of surgery.

Additional blood and radiographic studies may be indicated based on specific findings or for the evaluation of silent sources of infection when all other workup remains negative. In such situations, it is useful to look for clinical and/or radiographic evidence of sinusitis, otitis media, parotitis, ileus, cholecystitis, pancreatitis, sacral decubiti, and perineal or perianal abscess. Rarely, testing for transfusion-related infections such as cytomegalovirus (CMV), hepatitis B (HBV), hepatitis C (HCV), human immunodeficiency virus (HIV) and/or babesiosis may be indicated.

Noninfectious Postoperative Fever

It is important to recognize central fevers, dysautonomia, and drug fevers in neurosurgical patients to avoid inappropriate and potentially dangerous treatment with unnecessary antimicrobial therapy.

Central Fever Central fever related to loss of the physiological regulation of body temperature by the hypothalamus is often proposed as a possible cause for persistent fever in acute neurosurgical patients with no evidence of infection.[21] Direct damage to thermoregulatory centers in the preoptic nucleus of the hypothalamus and focal centers in the pons has been shown to cause an increase in CNS temperature.[22] Other studies have indicated that the presence of blood within the CSF, especially in intraventricular spaces[23] where blood may mechanically irritate hypothalamic thermoregulatory centers, may lead to fevers.

Several variables for central fever were identified by Hocker et al. in a retrospective study of 8,761 neurocritical patients.[24] Those included negative cultures; chest radiographs without infiltrates; onset of fever within 3 days of hospitalization especially in the setting of subarachnoid hemorrhage (SAH), intraventricular hemorrhage (IVH), or brain tumor; and greater fever burden persisting for a longer period. It is also important to differentiate central fever from other noninfectious causes of fever in patients with brain injury such as neuroleptic malignant syndrome, malignant hyperthermia, paroxysmal dysautonomia, and autonomic dysreflexia related to spinal cord injury.[25] With lack of definite criteria to diagnose central fever,[21] it is usually considered to be a diagnosis of exclusion.

Dysautonomia (Autonomic Storm) A complication of severe brain injury, regardless of etiology, is a syndrome of marked agitation, diaphoresis (as opposed to central fever), hyperthermia (temperature of at least 38.5°C), hypertension, tachycardia (pulse of at least 130 beats/min), and tachypnea (respiratory rate of at least 140 breaths/min) accompanied by hypertonia and extensor posturing; this constellation may persist for weeks to months, well beyond the acute care setting.[25] It was first identified as *brainstem attacks* in 1956 by Strich and has since taken various labels.[26] Treatment may include morphine, propranolol, bromocriptine, clonidine, or Thorazine. Benzodiazepines and haloperidol can be used acutely.[25]

Drug Fever Drug fever is characterized by a new fever coinciding with administration of a drug and disappearing after the discontinuation of the drug, when no other cause for the fever is evident after a careful physical examination and laboratory

Box 8.2 Medications Associated with Fever

- *Drug fever*: PCN, Vancomycin
- *Inflammatory response*: Rifampin, erythromycin, tetracycline
- *Hypersensitivity*: Captopril, hydralazine, labetalol
- *Pyrogen release*: Ranitidine
- *Endogenous pyrogen release*: Interferon

investigation.[27] The most common type of drug fever is due to a hypersensitivity reaction. The fever most commonly occurs after 7–10 days of drug administration, persists as long as the drug is continued, disappears soon after stopping the drug, and will rapidly reappear if the drug is restarted.[28] It is important to remember that the lag time between starting a new drug to onset of drug fever can be as long as several years. Presence of a drug rash may provide a valuable clue, but its absence does not rule out the diagnosis. Laboratory findings in a patient with drug fever may include leukocytosis with accompanying eosinophilia, but these findings occur in fewer than 20% of cases.[27] An elevated erythrocyte sedimentation rate (ESR) and CRP may be noted but are often nonspecific. Unexplained transaminitis and/or acute kidney injury (AKI) may also be seen. A positive urine eosinophil stain in such patients with pyuria may point toward accompanying interstitial nephritis. Discontinuation of the most probable offending drug first, followed sequentially by cessation of other drugs if fever persists, is usually the only way to confirm drug fever. In most, but not all cases, resolution of drug fever will occur within 72–96 hours of discontinuing the offending drug. Multiple medications are associated with postoperative drug fever (Box 8.2).

Infectious Postoperative Fever

Healthcare-associated infection (HAI) includes nosocomial infection that is described as infection, absent on hospital admission, which develops during the treatment course of a disparate condition.[29] The Center for Disease Control and Prevention (CDC) estimates that on any given day 1 in 31 hospitalized patients in the United States has at least one HAI.[30] The incidence in critically ill patients is highest and is associated with the use of invasive devices such as catheters and ventilators. In high-income countries up to 30% of patients in ICUs are affected by at least one HAI. In low- and middle-income countries rates can be two- to three-fold higher.[31] The impact is far-reaching with prolonged length of hospitalization, increased morbidity and mortality, and the increased use of antibiotics contributing to the emergence of multidrug-resistant organisms.[31,32]

Neurosurgical patients are especially vulnerable to HAI due to the increased incidence of altered mental status, risk for aspiration, concomitant trauma, and critical illness in this patient population. Furthermore, they are at risk for a subset of infections including procedure-related meningitis, ventriculitis, and hardware-related infections.[33] The 30-day rate of any postoperative infection after neurosurgery was 5.3% in a large, US multicenter analysis.[33] Fever is often, although not always, present in infections after neurosurgery.

Postoperative Meningitis Infectious and aseptic meningitis can complicate neurosurgical procedures that breach the blood–brain barrier. Bacterial meningitis is a life-threatening purulent infection of the subarachnoid space associated with an inflammatory reaction in the brain parenchyma and cerebral vasculature. The incidence of bacterial meningitis after both cranial and spinal surgery is low, with rates of 0.3–1.9% and 0.1–0.2% reported, respectively, although rates may be higher if combined with other infections such as ventriculitis.[34,35] Postoperative CSF drainage and perioperative steroid use are reported risk factors.

The predominant causative bacterial pathogens are *Staphylococcus aureus*, coagulase-negative staphylococci, gram-negatives including *Pseudomonas aeruginosa* and Enterobacteriaceae, and *Cutibacterium acnes* (formerly *Propionibacterium acnes*).[36,37] Multidrug-resistant gram negatives such as extended-spectrum beta-lactamase (ESBL) and carbapenemase (CRE)-producing *Klebsiella pneumoniae* and *Acinetobacter* spp., and gram positives including methicillin-resistant *S. aureus* (MRSA) and vancomycin-resistant enterococci (VRE) are of concern.[38] Meningitis and encephalitis due to herpes simplex virus (HSV) has been reported after neurosurgery.[39]

Evaluation for meningitis in the neurosurgical patient can be challenging as clinical manifestations are often nonspecific. A high index of suspicion for meningitis is essential as a delay in diagnosis can lead to adverse outcomes. Infectious and aseptic meningitis have similar presentations. Headache and nuchal rigidity can be seen in uninfected patients with meningeal irritation from hemolyzed blood. CSF parameters including protein and cell composition can be modified by the procedure itself or by infection, thus making interpretation of laboratory studies difficult.[40,41] The patient presenting with meningitis is typically febrile and lethargic, and there may be rapid deterioration of consciousness. Coma is a result of increased intracranial pressure.[42]

Diagnosis If there is concern for meningitis, an LP for CSF examination should be performed. In patients after lumbar spine surgery, CT guidance is advised. CSF abnormalities seen in bacterial meningitis include an increased opening pressure, decreased glucose concentration to less than 45 mg/dL, and an increased protein concentration. Elevated CSF lactate and CSF procalcitonin have correlated with bacterial infection in some studies.[35,42,43] Gram stain and bacterial culture should be obtained. Nucleic acid amplification testing (NAAT) can be performed on CSF to provide a more rapid pathogen identification and increased yield after antibiotic exposure and in atypical infections. Assays that test simultaneously for multiple pathogens or broad-range 16s rRNA polymerase chain reaction (PCR) are available. Neuroimaging with MRI or contrast-enhanced CT should be performed to exclude concomitant abscess, subdural and epidural empyema, surgical site infection, and hydrocephalus.[42,43]

Management Empiric antibiotics should be started immediately if meningitis is suspected after neurosurgery. Empiric antibiotic therapy for the neurosurgical patient includes a combination of vancomycin covering for staphylococci including MRSA, plus cefepime, ceftazidime, or meropenem covering for gram-negative bacilli. (Table 8.1). Awareness of local antibiotic resistance patterns is imperative. High local rates of carbapenem-resistant gram-negative organisms necessitates expanded empiric antibiotic coverage.

Therapy should be adjusted to target identified pathogens (Table 8.2), and duration is typically between 7 and 21 days, individualized based on pathogen identification and clinical response.[37] If cultures are negative, a shortened course of less than 7 days is appropriate.[40]

Ventriculitis/CSF Shunt and Drain Infections Management of hydrocephalus involves placement of an internalized or externalized CSF shunt. The proximal end of the shunt is most commonly placed in a cerebral ventricle and sometimes in an intracranial cyst or lumbar arachnoid space. The distal end can be internalized to drain CSF into the peritoneal cavity (ventriculoperitoneal [VP] shunt) or less commonly into a vascular space (ventriculoatrial [VA] shunt) or the pleural space (ventriculopleural shunt). Alternatively, when used temporarily, shunts can be externalized as tunneled ventriculostomy catheters or external ventricular drains (EVDs). The Ommaya reservoir is another externalized CSF drainage device used for the administration of antimicrobial or chemotherapeutic drugs.

CSF shunts and drains are prone to infections. VP shunt infections can be superficial, involving the skin and soft tissue adjacent to the shunt valve or reservoir, or can be deeper, involving the cerebral ventricles proximally or the peritoneum distally. Drain infections can be tunnel infections, catheter exit site infections, or ventriculitis. The case incidence of CSF shunt infection ranges from 5% to 41% in various series.[44] The operative incidence ranges from 2.8% to 14%, although most series have generally reported rates of less than 6%.[1] Factors associated with an increased risk of CSF shunt infection include premature birth (especially when associated with intraventricular hemorrhage), younger age, previous shunt infection, cause of hydrocephalus (more likely after purulent meningitis, hemorrhage, and myelomeningocele), longer duration of the shunt procedure, insertion of the catheter below the level of the T7 vertebral body in those with VA shunting, improper patient skin preparation, shaving of skin, and shunt revision (risk is especially high in those undergoing three or more revisions).[45,46]

The most frequent mechanism of shunt infection is shunt colonization at the time of surgery and is most relevant in the context of fever in a hospitalized neurosurgical patient due to its earlier onset. Other mechanisms responsible for delayed-onset infection include retrograde infection from the distal end of the shunt, hematogenous seeding, and infection through the skin after accessing the shunt or reservoir.[47] The incidence of infection in patients with EVDs ranges from 0% to 22%[d]. Factors associated with increased risk of these infections include intraventricular or subarachnoid hemorrhage, CSF leak, craniotomy or cranial fracture, ventriculostomy catheter irrigation, and duration of catheterization of more than 5 days.[47,48] Common pathogens are *S. aureus*, coagulase negative staphylococci, streptococci, *C. acnes* and

Table 8.1 Empiric antimicrobial therapy for neurosurgical infections.

Infection	First choice	Alternatives due to anaphylactic allergy	Duration; tailor ABX to cultures
Postoperative meningitis	Vancomycin plus an antipseudomonal beta-lactam (cefepime, ceftazidime, meropenem)	Linezolid or daptomycin for gram-positive coverage; Azactam or ciprofloxacin for gram-negative coverage	10–14 days, consider 21 days for gram-negative infection
Ventriculitis/CSF shunt infection	Vancomycin plus an antipseudomonal beta-lactam (cefepime, ceftazidime, meropenem)	Linezolid or daptomycin for gram-positive coverage; Azactam or ciprofloxacin for gram-negative coverage	10–14 days from the last positive CSF culture, consider 21 days for gram-negative infection
Surgical site infection	Vancomycin plus an antipseudomonal beta-lactam (cefepime, ceftazidime, meropenem)	Linezolid or daptomycin for gram-positive coverage; Azactam or ciprofloxacin for gram-negative coverage	Dependent on severity, extent of debridement and clinical response
Epidural abscess	Vancomycin plus an antipseudomonal beta-lactam (cefepime, ceftazidime, meropenem)	Linezolid or daptomycin for gram-positive coverage; Azactam or ciprofloxacin for gram-negative coverage	4–6 weeks
Vertebral osteomyelitis	In stable patients hold empiric antimicrobial therapy until a microbiologic diagnosis is established		6 weeks

(*continued*)

Table 8.1 Continued

Infection	First choice	Alternatives due to anaphylactic allergy	Duration; tailor ABX to cultures
Brain abscess, community acquired	Vancomycin plus ceftriaxone or cefotaxime plus metronidazole	Linezolid or daptomycin for gram-positive coverage; Azactam or ciprofloxacin for gram-negative coverage	6–8 weeks with careful clinical and imaging follow-up
Brain abscess, post-neurosurgery	Vancomycin plus an antipseudomonal beta-lactam (cefepime, ceftazidime, meropenem)	Linezolid or daptomycin for gram-positive coverage; Azactam or ciprofloxacin for gram-negative coverage	6–8 weeks with careful clinical and imaging follow-up
Brain abscess, HIV infection, concern for toxoplasmosis	Pyrimethamine plus sulfadiazine	Pyrimethamine plus clindamycin	6 weeks with careful clinical and imaging follow-up

gram-negative bacteria including *P. Aeruginosa*. Fungal infection, especially due to *Candida* species, as well as mycobacterial infections are reported.

Symptoms may be absent, nonspecific, or local based on site of involvement. Patients with shunt obstruction can present with headache, confusion, and vomiting. Symptoms and signs of peritonitis or pleuritis may represent infection of the distal end of the shunt. VA shunts can cause bacteremia and subsequent endocarditis. Soft tissue infection may be associated with the distal end infection of an EVD.

Diagnosis The Centers for Disease Control and Prevention's National Healthcare Safety Network (CDC/NHSN) definition of healthcare-associated ventriculitis or meningitis includes at least 1 of the following criteria (CDC/NHSN Surveillance Definitions; January 2015)[49]:

- Organism cultured from CSF
- At least two of the following symptoms with no other recognized cause in patients aged >1 year: fever >38°C or headache, meningeal signs, or cranial nerve signs, or at least two of the following symptoms with no other recognized cause

Microorganism	First choice	Alternatives for anaphylactic allergy or antimicrobial resistance
Staphylococci, oxacillin susceptible	Nafcillin or oxacillin 1.5–2 g IV q4–6h; consider adding rifampin 600 mg PO q24h if retained hardware	Vancomycin 15–20 mg/kg IV q12h or daptomycin 6–8 mg/kg IV q24h or linezolid 600 mg PO/IV q12h or trimethoprim-sulfamethoxazole 5 mg/kg IV/PO q8–12h; consider adding rifampin 600 mg PO q24h if retained hardware
Staphylococci, oxacillin resistant	Vancomycin 15–20 mg/kg IV q12h, consider alternative agent if MIC is ≥1, consider adding rifampin 600 mg PO q24h if retained hardware	Daptomycin 6–8 mg/kg IV q24h or linezolid 600 mg PO/IV q12h or trimethoprim-sulfamethoxazole 5 mg/kg IV/PO q8–12h, consider adding rifampin 600 mg PO q24h if retained hardware
Streptococci, confirm susceptibility testing for viridans streptococci	Penicillin G 18–24 million units IV q24h continuously or in 6 divided doses, or ceftriaxone 2g q12–24h	Vancomycin 15–20 mg/kg IV q12h
Enterococci, penicillin susceptible	Penicillin G 20–24 million units IV q24h continuously or in 6 divided doses, or ampicillin sodium 12g IV q24h continuously or in 6 divided doses	Vancomycin 15–20 mg/kg IV q12h or daptomycin 6–8 mg/kg IV q24h or linezolid 600 mg PO/IV q12h
Enterococci, penicillin resistant	Vancomycin 15–20 mg/kg IV q12h	Daptomycin 6–8 mg/kg IV q24h or linezolid 600 mg PO/IV q12h
Cutibacterium acnes	Penicillin G 20 million units IV q24h continuously or in 6 divided doses, or ceftriaxone 2g q12–24h	Vancomycin 15–20 mg/kg IV q12h or daptomycin 6–8 mg/kg IV q24h or clindamycin 600–900 mg IV q8h

(continued)

Table 8.2 Continued

Microorganism	First choice	Alternatives for anaphylactic allergy or antimicrobial resistance
Enterobacteriaceae, confirm susceptibility testing	Ceftriaxone 2g q12–24h or cefepime 2g IV q8h or ertapenem 1g IV q24h	Meropenem 1–2 g q8h or ciprofloxacin 400 mg IV q12h (or 500 mg PO q12h) or trimethoprim-sulfamethoxazole 5 mg/kg IV/PO q8–12h
Pseudomonas species, confirm susceptibility testing	Cefepime 2 g q8h, ceftazidime 2 g q8h or meropenem 1–2 g q8h	Azactam 2 g q8h or ciprofloxacin 400 mg IV q8h (or 750 mg PO q12h)
Acinetobacter species, confirm susceptibility testing	Meropenem 1–2 g IV q8h	Ciprofloxacin 400 mg IV q12h (or 500 mg PO q12h or ampicillin-sulbactam 3g/1.5g IV q6h or polymyxin B 1.5–2.5 mg/kg IV q24h in 2 divided doses
Candida species, confirm susceptibility testing	Liposomal amphotericin 5 mg/kg IV q24h	Fluconazole 400–800 mg IV/PO q24h, consider adding flucytosine 25 mg/kg q6h

in patients aged ≤1 year: fever >38°C or hypothermia <36°C, apnea, bradycardia, or irritability and at least one of the following:

- Increased white cells, elevated protein, and decreased glucose in CSF
- Organisms seen on Gram stain of CSF
- Organisms cultured from blood
- Positive nonculture diagnostic laboratory test from CSF, blood, or urine

When a shunt or EVD infection is suspected, direct aspiration of the CSF shunt is preferred over ventricular tap or LP. CSF should be sent for cell count and differential, protein and glucose concentrations, Gram stain, and culture. An elevated CSF lactate or procalcitonin may point toward a bacterial infection. It is reasonable to order CSF beta-D-glucan and galactomannan when a fungal infection is suspected. CSF NAAT can be helpful to identify a specific pathogen. Blood cultures should be obtained before initiation of antibiotics. MRI with diffusion weighting (DWI) is the most helpful imaging modality for evaluation of CSF shunts. Distal ends of shunts can be visualized with chest or abdominal imaging.

Management Removal of the infected device, parenteral antimicrobials and shunt replacement after the CSF is sterile are the mainstay of CSF shunt infection management. If removal of the infected device is not feasible, intraventricular antibiotics may be used.[47] Empiric coverage should include antibiotics against nosocomial gram-positive and gram-negative organisms (Table 8.1). Most frequently employed regimens include vancomycin with ceftazidime, cefepime, or meropenem. In patients with penicillin allergy, aztreonam or ciprofloxacin could be used. Targeted therapy is dictated by culture results (Table 8.2). Duration of treatment is 10–21 days depending on the severity of infection and the infecting organism. It may need to be extended to several weeks if cultures remain positive despite optimal antibiotic treatment. Although repeat CSF cultures during the treatment course are indicated to document sterility of CSF, daily CSF cultures are not recommended. The timing of a new shunt placement is variable depending on the CSF studies, culture results, and clinical response. Delays of 48 hours to 10 days or longer after externalization of the old device[47] may be implemented.

Surgical Site Infection Surgical site infection (SSI) is defined as an infection related to an operative procedure occurring at or near the surgical incision. SSI can involve the superficial incision, deep incision, or underlying organ space.[30,50] Most surgical site infections are caused by microbial contamination with endogenous flora at the surgical site. Other routes of infection include hematogenous seeding and traumatic wound inoculation. Typical pathogens causing SSI after neurosurgery include *S. aureus* including MRSA, coagulase-negative staphylococci, Enterobacteriaceae, and *C. acnes*.[51] Rates of SSI after neurosurgery vary widely with estimates of 0.7–16% reported.[32,33,51,52]

The clinical presentation of SSI after neurosurgery depends on the location of the surgical incision. Patients typically present within 2–4 weeks of surgery, although delayed presentations do occur. Typical findings include incisional erythema, swelling, tenderness, purulent discharge, and wound dehiscence. An abscess may form at the surgical site involving deep soft tissues with a healed incision. Systemic signs of infection such as fever and leukocytosis may be present.[53,54]

Risk factors for SSI after cranial surgery include the number of previous surgeries, prolonged operative duration, the presence of other infections, extended ICU stay, CSF leakage, CSF external drainage, and venous sinus entry.[51,53] Risk factors for SSI after spine surgery include prolonged operative time, a posterior approach, implanted foreign body, and multilevel fusion.[55] Patient-related risk factors for SSI include diabetes mellitus, obesity, smoking and *S. aureus* colonization.[51,55,56] Antibiotic prophylaxis has been shown to decrease the incidence of SSI after neurosurgery.[34]

SSI after neurosurgery can be related to the presence of a foreign body. Free craniotomy flaps are devascularized bones. Infection involving a bone flap often requires debridement, bone flap removal, treatment with targeted antibiotics, and delayed cranioplasty with acrylic, titanium, or other material for optimal outcome. In some cases, preservation of the bone flap is attempted after sterilization and is followed by systemic antibiotic therapy.[57] Spinal implants are used in spinal fusion procedures. Given the need for stabilization of the spine, removal of hardware in early-onset infections (<1 month from surgery) is not usually an option, and debridement with retention of hardware and extended antibiotic therapy is recommended. In late-onset spine infection after the spine has fused, implant removal followed by 4–6 weeks of targeted antibiotic therapy is recommended.[58]

Diagnosis A thorough examination of the surgical wound is imperative. Fever without a clear source after neurosurgery should always warrant consideration of SSI even if the incision appears intact. If not evident from physical examination of the incision, imaging with either CT scan or MRI should be obtained to evaluate for deep collection and/or osteomyelitis. Blood cultures should be obtained if the patient is febrile or appears systemically ill. Lack of response to antimicrobial therapy should raise suspicion for a deep infection.

Management Irrigation and debridement of infected or devitalized tissue should be pursued with procurement cultures including Gram stain to guide therapy. Removal of foreign bodies if deep infection is found is often necessary for cure. Empiric antimicrobial therapy for SSI after neurosurgery should include coverage for both gram-positive and gram-negative organisms.

Epidural Abscess An epidural abscess is a localized collection of purulent fluid between the dura mater and overlying skull (cranial epidural abscess) or vertebral column (spinal epidural abscess).[57]

Cranial Epidural Abscess Cranial epidural abscess may develop as a complication of sinusitis or otitis, following trauma, or after neurosurgery including craniotomy and transnasal or transmastoid procedures. Common causative pathogens include staphylococci, gram-negative organisms, and, if related to sinus disease, streptococci and anaerobes with polymicrobic infection. Presentation includes fever and headache with variation in time to presentation. Epidural abscess after neurosurgery can present with rapid progression. Findings of cranial epidural abscess include focal neurologic deficits, seizures, nausea, vomiting, altered mental status, and increased intracranial pressure with papilledema.[57]

Cranial epidural abscess can extend into the subdural space causing subdural empyema. Subdural empyema may also result from direct infection of the subdural space during a neurosurgical procedure (e.g., drainage of subdural hematoma). Both cranial epidural abscess and subdural empyema can be complicated by meningitis, cortical venous thrombosis, and brain abscess.[58]

Spinal Epidural Abscess Spinal epidural abscess is more common than cranial epidural abscess and is reported in 2.5–3.0 per 10,000 hospitalized patients, with the posterior spine more frequently involved.[57] The incidence has been increasing due to the spread of injection drug abuse (IVDA) and the increased use of therapeutic spinal interventions. Up to 75% of cases of spinal epidural abscess may be misdiagnosed on first presentation, and such delays in diagnosis can have a significant impact on morbidity and mortality.[59] Spinal epidural abscess is caused by hematogenous spread from a remote site of infection, such as skin infection, UTI, pneumonia, indwelling vascular access, or endocarditis in about half of cases.

Contiguous spread from osteomyelitis in an adjacent vertebral body, direct extension of infection from a decubitus ulcer or psoas muscle abscess, or direct infection of the epidural space from spine surgery are other routes of infection. Risk factors include transient bacteremia, diabetes mellitus, immunosuppressive therapy, HIV infection, alcoholism, and placement of a spine stimulator or catheter.

Spinal epidural abscess is most commonly due to *S. aureus* (60–90% of cases) with MRSA accounting for a significant number of infections. Coagulase-negative staphylococci, aerobic and anaerobic streptococci, and aerobic gram-negative bacilli are other pathogens. Spinal epidural abscess due to *Escherichia coli* is seen in patients with a history of UTI, and *Pseudomonas aeruginosa* is seen with IVDA. Coagulase-negative staphylococci are associated with spinal procedures such as placement of catheters for analgesia, steroid injections, and surgery.[60] Atypical infections including mycobacteria and fungi can also cause spinal epidural abscess.[59]

Spinal epidural abscesses may develop within hours to days or over weeks to months. Clinical presentation includes back pain with local tenderness, nerve root pain, radiculopathy, and paresthesia. Progression of infection can lead to neurologic deficits including spinal cord dysfunction with motor weakness, sensory loss, sphincter dysfunction (loss of bowel and bladder control), and paraplegia. Fever is present in 50–60% of patients, while the classic triad of back pain, fever, and neurologic deficits is seen in only a minority.[59,60]

Vertebral Osteomyelitis Vertebral osteomyelitis, also termed *spinal osteomyelitis* or *spondylodiskitis*, can be acute or chronic and accounts for 3–5% of all cases of osteomyelitis annually in the United States, with an estimated incidence of 4.8 cases per 100,000 population and increasing rates in the past few decades (similar to spinal epidural abscess). Hematogenous seeding of the adjacent disk space from a distant source is the primary route of infection, with direct inoculation from spine surgery or extension from a contiguous focus as additional sources.[61,62] Most patients presenting with vertebral osteomyelitis have an underlying medical condition or use intravenous drugs. *S. aureus* is the most common cause of pyogenic infection. Coagulase-negative staphylococci and *C. acnes* are found after spinal surgery especially with hardware retention and are associated with biofilm formation. Sustained bacteremia and endocarditis with *S. aureus* as well as with less virulent pathogens can predispose to vertebral osteomyelitis. *E. coli* and streptococci are associated with UTI and odontogenic sources, respectively. Atypical pathogens including *Brucella*, mycobacteria, and fungi can be seen in endemic regions or immunocompromised hosts. Vertebral osteomyelitis can be complicated by paravertebral, epidural, or psoas abscess in many cases.[61–63]

The clinical presentation of vertebral osteomyelitis is variable. Back pain correlating with the site of infection is the most common initial symptom. The lumbar spine is most frequently involved, followed by the thoracic and cervical spine locations, respectively. Fever is reported in 30–50% of cases. Neurologic impairment including sensory loss, radiculopathy, and weakness is reported in one-third of cases. A source of infection is identified in one-half of cases, with endocarditis reported in up to one-third.[61]

Diagnosis The diagnosis of vertebral osteomyelitis is often delayed as symptoms may be attributed to arthritis or muscular pain. Elevation of CRP and ESR are sensitive tests for diagnosis, while an increased leukocyte count or percentage of neutrophils is not. MRI is the imaging study of choice. An imaging-guided or intraoperative disc space aspiration or vertebral endplate sample should be obtained and sent for culture and pathologic diagnosis, and, if negative, a second biopsy should be considered prior to initiating antimicrobial therapy. Cultures for mycobacteria and fungi should be sent if epidemiologic or host risk factors or imaging findings are suggestive of atypical infection. Blood cultures should be obtained (reportedly positive in 30–78% of cases), and a positive blood culture for *S. aureus*, *S. lugdunensis*, or other suspected true pathogen in the preceding 3 months with comparable spine MRI changes precludes the need for disc space sampling.[61–63] Echocardiography is indicated in most cases of vertebral osteomyelitis to exclude endocarditis.

Management Empiric antimicrobial therapy should be withheld until a microbiologic diagnosis is confirmed except in cases of sepsis, shock, or worsening neurologic deficit. Once a diagnosis is established a 6-week course of targeted parental or highly bioavailable oral antibiotic therapy is recommended for the treatment of most cases of vertebral osteomyelitis (Table 8.2). Surgical intervention is indicated in patients with progressive neurologic deficits, deformity, or spinal instability. Persistent bloodstream infection or worsening pain in spite of appropriate antibiotic therapy would also warrant surgical intervention with or without stabilization. Inflammatory markers can be followed after 4 weeks of therapy in combination with clinical assessment to monitor progress. A poor clinical response to therapy merits repeat MRI and surgical evaluation.[63]

In cases of infection related to retained spinal implants, extended oral antibiotic suppression for 6–12 months or longer after the initial treatment course is often indicated. The optimal duration of suppression has not been established but suppression has been shown to decrease the risk of relapse, especially in early-onset infections (<1 month from fusion surgery). In delayed-onset infections, removal of hardware is associated with improved outcomes.[64]

Psoas Abscess Psoas abscess is most commonly the result of direct extension (secondary infection) from a bony site, including vertebral infection. *S. aureus* is the most common identified pathogen. Psoas abscess can also form after osteomyelitis of the ilium, septic arthritis of the sacroiliac joint, or after total hip arthroplasty. Extension from a gastrointestinal source, infected aortic aneurysm, or UTI are other routes of infection. Hematogenous seeding (primary infection) is more commonly seen in children and young adults and in those with risk factors for bacteremia and immune suppression. Primary infection is most often due to *S. aureus*, *E. coli*, and streptococci. Psoas abscess due to *Mycobacterium tuberculosis* is well described in endemic regions. Secondary infections are often polymicrobic and due to enteric organisms if from a gastrointestinal source.

Clinical presentation of psoas abscess includes fever, lower abdominal or back pain, or pain referred to hip or knee, and limping.[65] The "psoas sign," pain with extension of the hip, may be present. Psoas abscess can present as a fever of un-known origin.[66]

Diagnosis CT scan is the most sensitive imaging technique identifying phlegmon with diffuse enlargement of the psoas muscle, abscess with sharply circumscribed low-density fluid collection within muscle, and gas within muscle.

Management CT-guided catheter drainage or surgical drainage should be pursued, with cultures sent for pathogen identification. Empirical antibiotic therapy should be initiated based on the origin of infection and narrowed based in microbiologic findings (Table 8.2). The optimal duration of antibiotic therapy is not known. Typically, a 4- to 6-week course of therapy after drainage is appropriate, with longer courses implemented in cases of osteomyelitis. Relapse can occur in cases of incomplete drainage or inadequate antibiotic therapy.[66]

Brain Abscess Brain abscess is a life-threatening pyogenic infection of brain parenchyma that begins as cerebritis or unencapsulated inflammation and progresses to encapsulated necrotic infection. It arises from extension of a contiguous infection such as otitis, mastoiditis, sinusitis, or odontogenic infection; from hematogenous seeding from a distant source such as endocarditis, pneumonia, or abdominal or skin infection; or from head trauma or neurosurgical procedure. No primary site of infection can be identified in up to 40% of cases in some series.[67,68–71] Direct spread typically causes a single abscess, while hematogenous seeding usually causes multiple abscesses in the distribution of the middle cerebral artery. The incidence of brain abscess in developed countries is estimated to be 0.3–0.9 per 100,000 inhabitants per year with a risk of 0.2% after neurosurgery.[69]

The most common pathogens causing brain abscess are viridans streptococci, in particular the *S. milleri* group of oral streptococci, and *S. aureus*, with a wide variety of reported pathogens differing based on the primary site of infection, host immune status, and epidemiology. Polymicrobic infection including anaerobes is not uncommon, in particular with a head and neck source of infection. Gram-negative pathogens causing brain abscess include *Klebsiella pneumoniae, E. coli*, and *P. aeruginosa*. Fungal, mycobacterial, and parasitic infections are also described. Opportunistic infections seen in immune-suppressed patients include *Toxoplasma gondii, M. tuberculosis, Nocardia* spp., and *Aspergillus* spp. Neurocysticercosis due to *Taenia solium* is a common cause of brain abscess in patients from Central and South America. Brain abscess seen in the context of the neurosurgical patient is usually a result of direct inoculation after a neurosurgical procedure. The etiology is typically due to staphylococci, gram-negative bacilli, Enterobacteriaceae, or *P. aeruginosa*.[70,71]

Patients with brain abscess can present with headache, altered mental status, focal neurologic symptoms, nausea and vomiting, or generalized seizure. Fever is common, reported in up to 80% of patients. Neck stiffness occurs in patients with concomitant meningitis or intraventricular rupture. Papilledema may be seen with increased intracranial pressure. Because presentation can vary, a high index of suspicion for brain abscess is imperative for prompt diagnosis.[67–70] Patients with brain abscess may be admitted to the hospital without a clear diagnosis or with a misdiagnosis of presumed brain tumor. It is important to exclude underlying conditions that can predispose to brain abscess such as HIV infection, bacterial endocarditis, and intrapulmonary right-to-left shunting with pulmonary arteriovenous malformation.

Diagnosis Brain MRI is the imaging test of choice for diagnosis of brain abscess and is preferred over contrast-enhanced CT scan. Stereotactic needle aspiration provides specimens for Gram stain and culture, as well as therapeutic drainage of the abscess. Blood work may reveal a peripheral leukocytosis and elevated ESR. Blood cultures should be obtained and are positive in 15–50% of cases. CSF may show pleocytosis, elevated protein, and decreased glucose, but it may be normal. Brain herniation can occur in patients with brain abscess undergoing LP, therefore, LP should be reserved for those with limited mass effect where a pathogen cannot be identified through other methods.[67,68,71]

Management All patients with brain abscess should be started on empiric antibiotics (Table 8.1). While medical management alone is an option in patients without mass effect and abscess size of less than 2.5 cm, in most cases, surgical drainage is needed for cure. Stereotactic aspiration by CT guidance is usually pursued, while open excision is preferred in some cases. Cultures should be obtained and are noted to isolate a pathogen in up to 68% of cases. Molecular diagnostics will likely improve this yield in the near future.[69] Posterior fossa abscess can be complicated by obstructing hydrocephalus requiring CSF diversion.[68]

Brain abscess is treated with a 6- to 8-week course of targeted parenteral antibiotics (Table 8.2), followed by an additional 2- to 3-month course of oral antimicrobial therapy. Extended antibiotic courses may be required in immune-suppressed patients or for atypical infections. Imaging should be repeated at the completion of antibiotics or for any signs of clinical deterioration as recurrence is not uncommon, especially after aspiration.[69–71] Seizure prophylaxis should also be given during treatment and for at least 3 months after the resolution of brain abscess. Corticosteroids are not recommended in brain abscess unless severe edema with mass effect is present.[68]

Non-neurosurgical Nosocomial Infections

Nosocomial Pneumonia Nosocomial pneumonia encompasses both hospital-associated pneumonia (HAP) and ventilator-associated pneumonia (VAP). Together, they are among the most common HAIs, accounting for 22% of all HAIs in a multistate point-prevalence survey.[72] Incidence of VAP in the setting of traumatic brain injury is around 40%.[73] Early VAP (occurring within first 7 days of intubation) bears significant morbidity in patients with severe SAH.[74] Lepelletier et al. indicated in a study that achieving a rate of enteral feeding of 2,000 kcal/d or more before day 5 is a protective factor regarding the occurrence of early-onset VAP in head trauma patients.[73]

Pneumonia was defined in the 2005 IDSA guidelines as the presence of new lung infiltrate plus clinical evidence that the infiltrate is of an infectious origin, which includes the new onset of fever, purulent sputum, leukocytosis, and decline in oxygenation.[75] Nonetheless, the panel recognized that there is no gold standard for the diagnosis of HAP or VAP. HAP is defined as a pneumonia not incubating at the time of hospital admission and occurring 48 hours or more after admission but not associated with ventilation.[31] VAP is defined as a pneumonia occurring more than 48 hours after endotracheal intubation.[76] Ventilator-associated tracheobronchitis (VAT) may be an intermediate condition between lower respiratory tract colonization and VAP. It is a challenging clinical diagnosis, usually made in the absence of radiographic evidence of a new infiltrate or pneumonia. Management of VAT is virtually identical to the management of VAP.

Common pathogens include aerobic gram-negative bacilli (e.g., *E. coli*, *Klebsiella pneumoniae*, *Enterobacter* spp., *Pseudomonas aeruginosa*, *Acinetobacter* spp.) and gram-positive cocci (e.g., *S. aureus*, including MRSA, *Streptococcus* spp.). Host factors and hospital flora may also influence the patterns of pathogens seen. Although several risk factors have been identified for antimicrobial resistance in patients with HAP and VAP, only prior use of intravenous antibiotics in past 90 days has a significant association with both MRSA and multidrug-resistant *Pseudomonas* as well as all-cause multidrug-resistant HAP and VAP.[77,78]

No signs or symptoms, alone or in combination, have a high sensitivity or specificity for diagnosis.[79] The presence of a new or progressive radiographic infiltrate plus at least two of three clinical features (fever >38°C, leukocytosis or leukopenia, and purulent secretions) has a 69% sensitivity and 75% specificity for VAP.[79] Respiratory samples should ideally be obtained prior to initiation (or change in patients already on antibiotics) of antibiotics to improve the diagnostic yield. IDSA recommends noninvasive sampling (spontaneous expectoration, sputum induction, nasotracheal suctioning, and endotracheal aspiration in intubated patients) with semiquantitative cultures for microbiologic diagnosis.[76] Invasive sampling such as (nonbronchoscopic) mini bronchoalveolar lavage, (bronchoscopic) bronchoalveolar lavage, or protected specimen brush may occasionally be indicated in nonintubated patients and is the preferred sampling method for diagnosis of VAP based on 2017 guidelines issued by the European Respiratory Society (ERS)/European Society of Intensive Care Medicine (ESCIM)/European Society of Clinical Microbiology/Infectious Diseases (ESCMID)/Asociación Latinoamericana del Tórax (ALAT).[80] The use of biomarkers such as procalcitonin, soluble triggering receptor expressed on myeloid cells (sTREM-1), and CRP, as well as the use of a Clinical Pulmonary Infection Score is not encouraged by IDSA for making a diagnosis of HAP or VAP.[76] Blood cultures in patients with VAP are clearly useful if there is suspicion of another probable infectious condition, but the isolation of a microorganism in the blood does not confirm that microorganism as the pathogen causing VAP.[81]

IDSA recommends regular generation and dissemination of a local antibiogram addressing local distribution of pathogens, their associations with VAP, and their antimicrobial susceptibilities to direct empiric treatment regimens.[76] Empiric antimicrobials should provide coverage for *S. aureus, Pseudomonas aeruginosa*, and other gram-negative bacilli. Use of vancomycin or linezolid is encouraged if the prevalence of MRSA in an institution is unknown or is greater than 10–20%, or if the patient has other risk factors for multidrug-resistant infection.[76] Two antipseudomonal antibiotics from two different drug classes are recommended as part of the empiric regimen if the institutional prevalence of gram-negative isolates resistant to the agent being considered for monotherapy is greater than 10%, if local antimicrobial susceptibility rates are not available, or if patient has other risk factors for multidrug-resistant infection.[76] If patient is not high risk for MRSA, piperacillin-tazobactam, cefepime, levofloxacin, or meropenem can be used for empiric coverage. Aminoglycosides and colistin should be avoided if alternative agents are available.[76] Deescalation of empiric antibiotics to pathogen-specific antibiotics is highly encouraged. The recommended duration of antimicrobial therapy is 7 days unless otherwise indicated.[76]

Nosocomial Diarrhea Diarrhea is defined as at least 1 day with three or more unformed stools or a significant increase in stool frequency above baseline. Nosocomial diarrhea is an acute episode of diarrhea in a hospitalized patient that was not present on admission and arises after 3 or more days after hospitalization.[82] Given the inherent complicated nature of most neurosurgical diseases often requiring prolonged hospitalization, this patient population is at an increased risk of developing nosocomial diarrhea.

Physicians often consider *C. difficle* infection (CDI) as the primary cause of nosocomial diarrhea. However, only around 20% of cases are attributable to CDI.[82] Important noninfectious causes to consider are medications, enteral feeding, underlying illness, and alterations in the intestinal microbiome. Among noninfectious causes, toxin-producing strains of *Clostridium perfringens* and *Klebsiella oxytoca* can cause severe colitis.[83,84]

CDI rates have plateaued at historic highs in the United States since about 2010.[85] Healthcare facility-onset CDI remains a significant consideration in postoperative neurosurgical patients with new-onset fever and/or diarrhea. It is important to remember that postoperative patients may present with ileus, toxic megacolon, or leukocytosis without diarrhea as the manifestation of *C. difficile* disease.[19]

Testing algorithms differ markedly among institutions. A stool enzyme immunoassay for toxin A and B as part of a multistep algorithm (i.e., glutamate dehydrogenase [GDH] plus toxin; GDH plus toxin, arbitrated by NAAT; or NAAT plus toxin) rather than a NAAT alone is considered to be the best performing method for detecting patients at increased risk for clinically significant CDI.[85] Cultures for *C. difficle*, although technically demanding, time-consuming, and nonspecific for distinguishing asymptomatic carriage, may be useful in the setting of nosocomial outbreaks when isolates are needed for strain typing.[86] The NAP 1 strain has been epidemic in many hospitals in the United States, Canada, and Europe; it is associated with serious complications (toxic megacolon, leukemoid reactions, sepsis, and death) and is often refractory to standard therapy.[19] IDSA recommends against repeat testing (within 7 days) during the same episode of diarrhea and testing stool from asymptomatic patients.[85]

Treatment for CDI based on 2018 IDSA guidelines is summarized here.[87]

Clinical Definition	Supportive Clinical Data	Recommended Treatment
Initial episode, nonsevere	Leukocytosis with a white blood cell count of ≤15,000 cells/mL and a serum creatinine level <1.5 mg/dL	VAN 125 mg given 4 times daily for 10 days, OR FDX 200 mg given twice daily for 10 days Alternate if above agents are unavailable: metronidazole, 500 mg 3 times per day by mouth for 10 days
Initial episode, severe	Leukocytosis with a white blood cell count of ≥15,000 cells/mL or a serum creatinine level >1.5 mg/dL	VAN, 125 mg 4 times per day by mouth for 10 days, OR FDX 200 mg given twice daily for 10 days
Initial episode, fulminant	Hypotension or shock, ileus, megacolon	VAN, 500 mg 4 times per day by mouth or by nasogastric tube. If ileus, consider adding rectal instillation of VAN. Intravenously administered metronidazole (500 mg every 8 hours) should be administered together with oral or rectal VAN, particularly if ileus is present.
First recurrence		VAN 125 mg given 4 times daily for 10 days if metronidazole was used for the initial episode, OR Use a prolonged tapered and pulsed VAN regimen if a standard regimen was used for the initial episode (e.g., 125 mg 4 times per day for 10–14 days, 2 times per day for a week, once per day for a week, and then every 2 or 3 days for 2–8 weeks), OR FDX 200 mg given twice daily for 10 days if VAN was used for the initial episode

Clinical Definition	Supportive Clinical Data	Recommended Treatment
Second or subsequent recurrence		VAN in a tapered and pulsed regimen, OR VAN, 125 mg 4 times per day by mouth for 10 days followed by rifaximin 400 mg 3 times daily for 20 days, OR FDX 200 mg given twice daily for 10 days, OR Fecal microbiota transplantation

Catheter-Associated Urinary Tract Infections Many neurosurgical conditions (e.g., neurogenic bladder, cauda equina syndrome, opiate-induced urinary retention) are associated with an impairment of urinary bladder function. This subset of patients frequently requires urinary bladder catheterization thus increasing the risk of bacteriuria which can be clinically benign or may result in serious infections. It is therefore important to understand the difference between asymptomatic and symptomatic catheter-associated bacteriuria.

IDSA defines symptomatic bacteriuria as culture growth of 10^3 colony-forming units (cfu)/mL or more of uropathogenic bacteria in the presence of symptoms or signs compatible with UTI without other identifiable source in a patient with indwelling urethral, indwelling suprapubic, or intermittent catheterization. Compatible symptoms include fever, suprapubic or costovertebral angle tenderness, and otherwise unexplained systemic symptoms such as altered mental status, hypotension, or evidence of a systemic inflammatory response syndrome. Culture growth of 10^5 cfu/mL or more of uropathogenic bacteria in the absence of symptoms compatible with UTI in a patient with indwelling urethral, indwelling suprapubic, or intermittent catheterization is defined as asymptomatic bacteriuria.[88]

Bacteriuria related to short-term catheters ($\leq$30 days) is usually monomicrobial.[89] Common pathogens are *E. coli, Klebsiella* spp., *Serratia* spp., *Citrobacter* spp., *P. aeruginosa,* gram-positive cocci such as coagulase-negative staphylococci and enterococci, and *Candida* spp. Long-term catheterization (>30 days) is often associated with polymicrobial infections. In addition to the pathogens just mentioned, *Proteus mirabilis, Proteus stuartii,* and *Morganella morganii* are commonly seen in polymicrobial infections.

Symptoms of catheter-associated UTI (CAUTI) are often variable and not always referred to the urinary tract.[89] Fever, new-onset delirium, flank or suprapubic discomfort, costovertebral angle tenderness, and catheter obstruction are nonspecific but common findings. Patients with spinal cord injury may experience increased spasticity and autonomic dysreflexia. Patients whose catheter was removed within the past 48 hours may report dysuria or urinary urgency and frequency.

It is advisable to replace the catheter before collecting a urine sample for culture. A mid-stream urine sample is the preferred sample in patients with condom catheters to prevent contamination with skin flora.[90] Absence of pyuria helps to rule out a diagnosis of UTI, but its presence does not support the diagnosis. In general, bacteriuria (as defined by IDSA) in a catheterized patient who has signs and symptoms consistent with UTI or systemic infection that are otherwise unexplained is diagnostic for CAUTI.[88] A UTI diagnosed in a patient who had a catheter removed within the past 48 hours is also considered a CAUTI. Given the lack of specificity of signs and symptoms, a fair degree of clinical judgment and individualization is required for the diagnosis of CAUTI.

The presence of clinical findings suggesting an ascending or systemic infection along with supportive laboratory data (blood and urine cultures) with or without imaging studies (renal ultrasound and CT scan of abdomen and pelvis) provide useful information to guide the selection of empiric antimicrobial regimen. Choice of empiric antibiotics is also influenced by risk factors for antibiotic resistance which include healthcare exposure, community prevalence of antimicrobial resistance, use of antimicrobial therapy, and patient's past urine culture data if available. Standard-spectrum empiric antibiotics for UTI in patients with no risk factors for antimicrobial resistance include ceftriaxone, piperacillin-tazobactam, and fluoroquinolones such as ciprofloxacin or levofloxacin. In patients with hemodynamic instability and multidrug-resistant/ESBL risk factors, carbapenems may be used for empiric coverage. In patients with suspected or documented urinary tract obstruction or urine Gram stain showing gram-positive cocci, addition of MRSA coverage is reasonable. Antimicrobial regimen should be tailored to the pathogenic organism once the culture speciation and sensitivity data are available. Optimal duration of therapy varies anywhere from 7 to 14 days depending on clinical response, infecting organism, and the antimicrobial agent used.

The use of indwelling catheters should be minimized whenever possible. In patients requiring long-term catheterization, use of intermittent catheterization decreases the rate of bacteriuria.[91] When intermittent catheterization is not a possibility, an indwelling catheter should be replaced at the initiation of antimicrobial therapy due to poor biofilm penetration of most antimicrobials.

Nosocomial Sinusitis It is not uncommon for neurosurgical patients to require mechanical ventilation. Sinus drainage can be obstructed by nasotracheal or nasogastric tubes, leading to collection of uninfected fluid within the sinuses. Nosocomial sinusitis results from infection of these fluid collections. Although the prevalence of nosocomial sinusitis is low in comparison with other nosocomial infections, it is still worthwhile to consider in the differential diagnoses of nosocomial fever as it is often an occult infection with serious consequences. Complications include bacteremia, VAP, orbital infection, meningitis, mastoiditis, cerebral abscess, or thrombosis of the sinus cavernosus. While the incidence of sinus opacification is common, prevalence of sinusitis secondary to transnasal intubation of the airway is estimated to be 33% after 7 days of intubation.[19] Maxillofacial trauma is another clear risk factor.

Nosocomial sinus infections are often polymicrobial. Apart from nasopharyngeal flora, gram-negative bacilli (particularly *P. aeruginosa*), gram-positive cocci (typically *S. aureus* and coagulase-negative staphylococci), anaerobes (such as *Prevotella* and *Fusobacterium*), and fungi are important key players.[92]

Major and minor diagnostic criteria used for the diagnosis of acute sinusitis in the outpatient setting are of little help in intubated patients. Only 25% of proved cases of sinusitis had purulent nasal discharge.[92] CT scan is more sensitive than plain radiographs.[93] Sinus ultrasonography can also detect sinus opacification. Culture of sinus fluid obtained by minimally invasive sinus puncture or endoscopy is the gold standard for diagnosis. A common threshold used to declare a quantitative culture positive is 10^3 cfu/mL. Tissue biopsy may be needed to rule to invasive fungal sinusitis in patients with specific risk factors. Secretions collected from the nares or oral cavity are unreliable.

Systemic empiric antimicrobial coverage for nosocomial sinusitis is essentially similar to that of VAP, followed by deescalation as guided by pathogen identification and sensitivity from the sinus fluid cultures. It is interesting to note that patients may develop nosocomial sinusitis despite being on systemic antimicrobials targeting the pathogenic organisms. Lower sinus mucosal concentrations of systemic antimicrobials and formation of biofilms are some of the proposed mechanisms.[94] Therefore, supportive measures such as semi-recumbent positioning, removal of nasotracheal and nasogastric tubes, topical decongestants and antimicrobials, and occasionally intranasal glucocorticoids play an important role in the management of this infection. Sinus drainage is indicated in patients who fail to improve on antimicrobial therapy.

Superficial Thrombophlebitis Suppurative thrombophlebitis is an inflammation of the vein wall caused by the presence of microorganisms and is frequently associated with thrombosis and bacteremia.[1] Nosocomial superficial thrombophlebitis occurs secondary to an indwelling intravenous catheter. The risk goes up with prolonged duration of cannulation ($\geq$5 days) and increased frequency of catheter manipulations.[95] The most common causative organism is *S. aureus*. Streptococci and *Enterobacteriaceae* are other important pathogens.

Fever and local findings such as warmth, erythema, tenderness, swelling, lymphangitis, palpable cord, or purulent drainage at the site of the involved vessel are the most common clinical manifestations. Complications include bacteremia and septic pulmonary emboli, which may be the presenting features. Imaging by ultrasound or, less commonly, CT can aid the diagnosis.[96] The microbiologic diagnosis can be made based on culture of blood or purulent material expressed from the site.

Treatment includes removing the catheter, prompt administration of intravenous antibiotics, and a consideration for surgery and anticoagulation. Empiric antibiotic therapy should include an agent with anti-staphylococcal activity such as vancomycin and an agent with activity against *Enterobacteriaceae* such as ceftriaxone followed by targeted antibiotics based on culture and sensitivity data when available. Two weeks of intravenous antibiotics is generally considered to be an optimum duration of therapy.[97] Shorter durations of intravenous antibiotics (at least >7 days) followed by oral antibiotics have also shown promising results.[96] Phlebitis in the absence of an evidence of infection does not require antimicrobial therapy. There are no controlled studies or guidelines regarding anticoagulation in these settings, and a decision for anticoagulation is made on a case-by-case basis when there is evidence of significant extension of thrombus or ongoing sepsis despite antibiotic treatment. Surgical incision and drainage or vein excision may be warranted if there is persistent or recurrent bacteremia despite antimicrobial therapy.

Central Line–Associated Bloodstream Infections Central line–associated blood stream infection (CLABSI) should be suspected in patients with central venous catheters with evidence of bloodstream infection in the absence of another source. Fever is a common but nonspecific presenting symptom. Local inflammatory signs and symptoms and purulence at the site of insertion may be less common but more specific. Clinical improvement within 24 hours of catheter removal is also suggestive of CLABSI. Frequently encountered pathogens include coagulase-negative staphylococci, *S. aureus*, enterococci, *Enterobacteriaceae*, and *Candida* spp. (especially in patients on parenteral nutrition).

Ideally, two sets of peripheral blood cultures (20 mL blood/set) drawn from separate sites should be obtained. When this is not feasible, one set may be drawn from a catheter hub and the other set obtained through a peripheral venipuncture.[98] There is no role for routine catheter cultures at the time of catheter removal.

A positive catheter tip culture or a positive blood culture drawn from a catheter with negative peripheral blood cultures and no clinical evidence of infection do not require systemic antimicrobial therapy. When indicated, empiric therapy is guided by clinical circumstances and severity of infection. In general, an anti-staphylococcal agent is always indicated with additional coverage for gram negatives (including *P. aeruginosa*) and *Candida* as needed. Targeted therapy for uncomplicated CLABSI is continued for 7–14 days once the blood cultures are sterile. Removal of a central venous catheter is particularly important for *S. aureus*, *P. aeruginosa*, and *Candida* species. A new catheter can be placed once the blood cultures are negative for 48–72 hours.

Acalculous Cholecystitis Acalculous cholecystitis is typically a disease of hospitalized and critically ill patients. Pathogenesis is complex and involves gallbladder stasis and ischemia leading to a local inflammatory response in gallbladder wall. Once acalculous cholecystitis is established, secondary infection with enteric pathogens including *E. coli*, *Enterococcus faecalis*, *Klebsiella* spp., *Pseudomonas* spp., *Proteus* spp., and *Bacteroides fragilis* and related species is common.[99] Severe cases may be complicated by gallbladder perforation. Major trauma, diabetes mellitus, end-stage renal disease, heart failure, and AIDS are important comorbid conditions associated with an increased risk of acalculous cholecystitis. Mechanical ventilation, total parenteral nutrition, immunosuppression, and nonbiliary surgery also increase the risk of this inadvertent complication of critical illness.

Appearance of unexplained fever in critically ill patients may be the only sign of acalculous cholecystitis. Jaundice and right upper quadrant tenderness on physical examination may provide additional clues. Leukocytosis and abnormal liver function tests with an elevated alkaline phosphatase and direct hyperbilirubinemia should raise the suspicion of acalculous cholecystitis in critically ill and postoperative patients with new jaundice and fever. Abdominal ultrasonography is the initial imaging modality in suspected cases followed by contrast-enhanced CT, if needed. A hepatobiliary iminodiacetic acid (HIDA) scan is useful in stable patients with unclear diagnosis despite an abdominal ultrasound and CT scan. Imaging studies alone cannot make a diagnosis of acalculous cholecystitis and should be interpreted in the context of clinical settings.

Broad-spectrum antibiotics (piperacillin-tazobactam or meropenem alone or combination therapy with ceftazidime or cefepime plus metronidazole plus ampicillin or vancomycin) should be started after blood cultures are obtained. Percutaneous or endoscopic gallbladder drainage is indicated for source control in patients who are poor surgical candidates.

REFERENCES

1. Wright WF, Mackowiak PA. Fever of unknown origin. In Bennett JE, Dolin R, Blaser MJ, eds. *Mandell, Douglas, and Bannett's Principles and Practice of Infectious Diseases.* Philadelphia, PA: Elsevier Saunders; 2015: 722.

2. Netea MG, Kullberg BJ, Van der Meer JW. Circulating cytokines as mediators of fever. *Clin Infect Dis.* 2000;31 Suppl 5:S178.

3. Blatteis CM, Sehic E, Li S. Pyrogen sensing and signaling: old views and new concepts. *Clin Infect Dis.* 2000;31 Suppl 5:S168.

4. Saper CB, Breder CD. The neurologic basis of fever. *N Engl J Med.* 1994;330:1880.

5. Mitchell JD, Grocott HP, Phillips-Bute B, et al. Cytokine secretion after cardiac surgery and its relationship to postoperative fever. *Cytokine.* 2007;39:37.

6. Karhade AV, Cote DJ, Larsen AMG, Smith TR. Neurosurgical infection rates and risk factors: a National Surgical Quality Improvement Program analysis of 132,000 patients, 2006–2014. *World Neurosurg.* 2015;97:205–212.

7. Cevasco M, Ashley S, Cooper Z. Physiologic response to surgery. In MecKean SC, Ross JJ, Dressler DD, Brotman DJ, Ginsberg JS, eds. *Principles and Practice of Hospital Medicine.* New York: McGraw Hill; 2012: 291.

8. Azzimondi G, Bassein L, Nonino F, Fiorani L, Vignatelli L, Re G, D'Alessandro R. Fever in acute stroke worsens prognosis: a prospective study. *Stroke.* 1995;26:2040–2043.

9. Kilpatrick MM, Lowry DW, Firlik AD, et al. Hyperthermia in the neurosurgical intensive care unit. *Neurosurgery.* 2000;47:850–855;discussion 855–856.

10. Shiozaki T, Sugimoto H, Taneda M, Yoshida H, Iwai A, Yoshioka T, Sugimoto T. Effect of mild hypothermia on uncontrollable intracranial hypertension after severe head injury. *J Neurosurg.*1993;79:363–368.

11. Dinarello CA, Porat R. Fever. In Kasper DL, Hauser SL, Jameson JL, Fauci AS, Longo DC, Coscalzo J, eds. *Harrison's Principles of Internal Medicine.* New York: McGraw Hill; 2015: 123.

12. Kaukonen K-M, Bailey M, Pilcher D, Cooper DJ, Bellomo R. Systemic inflammatory response syndrome criteria in defining severe sepsis. *N Engl J Med.* 2015;372:1629–1638.

13. Sprung CL, Sakr Y, Vincent JL, et al. An evaluation of systemic inflammatory response syndrome signs in the Sepsis Occurrence in Acutely Ill patients (SOAP) study. *Intensive Care Med.* 2006;32:421–427.

14. Hocker SE, Tian L, Li G, Steckelberg JM, Mandrekar JN, Rabinstein AA. Indicators of central fever in the neurologic intensive care unit. *JAMA Neurol.* 2013;70: 1499–1504.

15. Diringer MN, Reaven NL, Funk SE, et al. Elevated body temperature independently contributes to increased length of stay in neurologic intensive care unit patients [see comment] [published correction appears in *Crit Care Med.* 2004;32:2170]. *Crit Care Med.* 2004;32:1489–1495.

16. Albrecht RF II, Wass CT, Lanier WL. Occurrence of potentially detrimental temperature alterations in hospitalized patients at risk for brain injury. *Mayo Clin Proc.* 1998;73:629–635.

17. Kane TD, Alexander JW, Johannigman JA. The detection of microbial DNA in the blood: a sensitive method for diagnosing bacteremia and/or bacterial translocation in surgical patients. *Ann Surg.* 1998;227:1.

18. Garibaldi RA, Brodine S, Matsumiya S, Coloman M. Evidence for the noninfectious etiology of early postoperative fever. *Infect Control.* 1985;6:273.

19. O'Grady NP, Barie PS, Bartlett JG, Bleck T, Carroll K, et al. Guidelines for evaluation of new fever in critically ill adult patients: 2008 update from the American College of Critical Care Medicine and the Infectious Diseases Society of America. *Crit Care Med.* 2008;36 (1330–1349).

20. Mermeel LA, Farr BM, Sherertz RJ, et al. Guidelines for the management of intravascular catheter-related infections. *Clin Infect Dis.* 2001;32:1249–1272.

21. Rabinstein AA, Sandhu K. Noninfectious fever in the neurological intensive care unit: incidence, causes and predictors. *J Neurol Neurosurg Psychiatry.* 2007;78:1278–1280.

22. Badjatia N. Hyperthermia and fever control in brain injury. *Crit Care Med.* 2009;37[Suppl.]:S250–S257.

23. Commichau C, Scarmeas N, Mayer SA. Risk factors for fever in the neurologic intensive care unit. *Neurology.* 2003;60:837–841.

24. Hocker SE, Tian L, Li G, Steckelberg JM, Mandrekar JN, Rabinstein AA. Indicators of central fever in the neurologic intensive care unit. *JAMA Neurol.* 2013;70:1499–1504.

25. Blackman JA, Patrick PD, Buck ML, Rust RS. Paroxysmal autonomic instability with dystonia after brain injury. *Arch Neurol.* 2004;61:321–328.

26. Strich SJ. Diffuse degeneration of the cerebral white matter in severe dementia. *J Neurol Neurosurg Psychiatry.* 1956;19:163–185.

27. Mackowiak PA, LeMaistre CF. Drug fever: a critical appraisal of conventional concepts. An analysis of 51 episodes in two Dallas hospitals and 97 episodes reported in the English literature. *Ann Intern Med.* 1987;106:728.

28. Tabor PA. Drug-induced fever. *Drug Intell Clin Pharm.* 1986;20:413.

29. Cardoso T, Almeida M, Friedman ND, et al. Classification of healthcare-associated infection: a systematic review 10 years after the first proposal. *BMC Med.* 2014. doi: 10.1186/1741-7015-12-40.

30. CDC. CDC/NHSN surveillance definitions for specific types of infections. *Surveill Defin.* 2016. doi: 10.1016/j.ajic.2008.03.002.

31. World Health Organization (WHO). Report on the burden of endemic health care–associated infection worldwide. 2011. http://whqlibdoc.who.int/publications/2011/9789241501507_eng.pdf. Accessed 12/24/18.

32. Rosenthal VD, Bijie H, Maki DG, et al. International Nosocomial Infection Control Consortium (INICC) report, data summary of 36 countries, for 2004–2009. *Am J Infect Control.* 2012. doi: 10.1016/j.ajic.2011.05.020.

33. Karhade AV, Cote DJ, Larsen AMG, Smith TR. Neurosurgical infection rates and risk factors: a National Surgical Quality Improvement Program analysis of 132,000 patients, 2006–2014. *World Neurosurg.* 2017. doi: 10.1016/j.wneu.2016.09.056.

34. McClelland S, Hall WA. Postoperative central nervous system infection: incidence and associated factors in 2111 neurosurgical procedures. *Clin Infect Dis.* 2007. doi: 10.1086/518580.

35. Lin TY, Chen WJ, Hsieh MK, et al. Postoperative meningitis after spinal surgery: a review of 21 cases from 20,178 patients. *BMC Infect Dis.* 2014. doi: 10.1186/1471-2334-14-220.

36. Tunkel AR, Hartman BJ, Kaplan SL, et al. Practice guidelines for the management of bacterial meningitis. *Clin Infect Dis.* 2004. doi: 10.1086/425368.

37. Roos KL. Bacterial infections of the central nervous system. *Contin Lifelong Learn Neurol.* 2015. doi: 10.1212/CON.0000000000000242.

38. Kourbeti IS, Vakis AF, Ziakas P, et al. Infections in patients undergoing craniotomy: risk factors associated with post-craniotomy meningitis. *J Neurosurg.* 2015. doi: 10.3171/2014.8.JNS132557.

39. Aldea S, Joly LM, Roujeau T, Oswald AM, Devaux B. Postoperative herpes simplex virus encephalitis after neurosurgery: case report and review of the literature. *Clin Infect Dis.* 2003. doi: 10.1086/368090.

40. Zarrouk V, Vassor I, Bert F, et al. Evaluation of the management of postoperative aseptic meningitis. *Clin Infect Dis.* 2007. doi: 10.1086/518169.

41. Brown, J. de Louvois, R. Bayston, P EM. The management of neurosurgical patients with postoperative bacterial or aseptic meningitis or external ventricular drain-associated ventriculitis. Infection in Neurosurgery Working Party of the British Society for Antimicrobial Chemotherapy. *Br J Neurosurg.* 2000. doi: 10.1080/02688690042834.

42. Hussein K, Bitterman R, Shofty B, Paul M, Neuberger A. Management of post-neurosurgical meningitis: narrative review. *Clin Microbiol Infect.* 2017. doi: 10.1016/j.cmi.2017.05.013.

43. Tunkel AR, Hasbun R, Bhimraj A, et al. 2017 Infectious Diseases Society of America's clinical practice guidelines for healthcare-associated ventriculitis and meningitis. *Clin Infect Dis.* 2017. doi: 10.1093/cid/cix152.

44. Kaufman BA. Infections of cerebrospinal fluid shunts. In Scheld WM, Whitley RJ, Durack DT, eds. *Infections of the Central Nervous System.* 2nd ed. Philadelphia, PA: Lippincott-Raven; 1997: 555–577.

45. van de Beek D, Drake JM, Tunkel JR. Nosocomial bacterial meningitis. *N Engl J Med.* 2010;362:146–154.

46. Simon TD, Butler J, Whitlock KB, et al. Risk factors for first cerebrospinal fluid shunt infection: findings from a multi-center prospective cohort study. *J Pediatr.* 2014;164:1462–1468.e2.

47. Tunnel AR, Hasbun R, Bhimraj A, et al. 2017 Infectious Diseases Society of America's clinical practice guidelines for healthcare-associated ventriculitis and meningitis. *Clin Infect Dis.* 2017;64:e34–e65.

48. Lozier AP, Sciacca RR, Romagnoli MF, Connolly ES Jr. Ventriculostomy related infections: a critical review of the literature. *Neurosurgery.* 2002;51:170–181.

49. CDC/NHSN Surveillance definitions for specific types of infection. January 2015.

50. Centers for Disease Control and Prevention. Surgical site infection event. *Procedure Assoc Modul.* 2015. doi: E07-10-1046 [pii]\r10.1091/mbc.E07-10-1046.

51. Cassir N, De La Rosa S, Melot A, et al. Risk factors for surgical site infections after neurosurgery: a focus on the postoperative period. *Am J Infect Control.* 2015. doi: 10.1016/j.ajic.2015.07.005.

52. Smith JS, Shaffrey CI, Sansur CA, et al. Rates of infection after spine surgery based on 108,419 procedures: a report from the Scoliosis Research Society morbidity and mortality committee. *Spine (Phila Pa 1976)*. 2011. doi: 10.1097/BRS.0b013e3181eadd41.

53. Sneh-Arbib O, Shiferstein A, Dagan N, et al. Surgical site infections following craniotomy focusing on possible postoperative acquisition of infection: prospective cohort study. *Eur J Clin Microbiol Infect Dis*. 2013. doi: 10.1007/s10096-013-1904-y.

54. Nichols RL, Florman S. Clinical presentations of soft-tissue infections and surgical site infections. *Clin Infect Dis*. 2001. doi: 10.1086/321862.

55. Meng F, Cao J, Meng X. Risk factors for surgical site infections following spinal surgery. *J Clin Neurosci*. 2015. doi: 10.1016/j.jocn.2015.03.065.

56. Akins PT, Belko J, Banerjee A, et al. Perioperative management of neurosurgical patients with methicillin-resistant *Staphylococcus aureus*. *J Neurosurg*. 2010. doi: 10.3171/2009.5.JNS081589.

57. Yadla S, Campbell PG, Chitale R, Maltenfort MG, Jabbour P, Sharan AD. Effect of early surgery, material, and method of flap preservation on cranioplasty infections: a systematic review. *Neurosurgery*. 2011. doi: 10.1227/NEU.0b013e31820a5470.

58. Kowalski TJ, Berbari EF, Huddleston PM, Steckelberg JM, Mandrekar JN, Osmon DR. The management and outcome of spinal implant infections: contemporary retrospective cohort study. *Clin Infect Dis*. 2007. doi: 10.1086/512194.

59. Pradilla G, Ardila GP, Hsu W, Rigamonti D. Epidural abscesses of the CNS. *Lancet Neurol*. 2009. doi: 10.1016/S1474-4422(09)70044-4.

60. Agrawal A, Timothy J, Pandit L, Shetty L, Shetty JP. A review of subdural empyema and its management. *Infect Dis Clin Pract*. 2007. doi: 10.1097/01.idc.0000269905.67284.c7.

61. Darouiche MD RO. Current concepts: spinal epidural abscess. *N Engl J Med*. 2006.

62. Berbari EF, Kanj SS, Kowalski TJ, et al. 2015 Infectious Diseases Society of America (IDSA) clinical practice guidelines for the diagnosis and treatment of native vertebral osteomyelitis in adults. *Clin Infect Dis*. 2015;61(6):e26–e46. doi: 10.1093/cid/civ482.

63. Bond A, Manian FA. Spinal epidural abscess: a review with special emphasis on earlier diagnosis. *Biomed Res Int*. 2016. doi: 10.1155/2016/1614328.

64. Zimmerli W. Clinical practice. Vertebral osteomyelitis. *N Engl J Med*. 2010. doi: 10.1056/NEJMcp0910753.

65. Graeber A, Cecava ND. Osteomyelitis, *Vertebral*.;2018. doi: 30335289.

66. Shields D, Robinson P, Crowley TP. Iliopsoas abscess: a review and update on the literature. *Int J Surg*. 2012. doi: 10.1016/j.ijsu.2012.08.016.

67. López VN, Ramos JM, Meseguer V, et al. Microbiology and outcome of iliopsoas abscess in 124 patients. *Medicine (Baltimore)*. 2009. doi: 10.1097/MD.0b013e31819d2748.

68. Brouwer MC, Coutinho JM, Van De Beek D. Clinical characteristics and outcome of brain abscess: systematic review and meta-analysis. *Neurology*. 2014. doi: 10.1212/WNL.0000000000000172.

69. Patel K, Clifford DB. Bacterial brain abscess. *Neurohospitalist*. 2014. doi: 10.1177/1941874414540684.

70. Sonneville R, Ruimy R, Benzonana N, et al. An update on bacterial brain abscess in immunocompetent patients. *Clin Microbiol Infect*. 2017. doi: 10.1016/j.cmi.2017.05.004.

71. Brouwer MC, Tunkel AR, McKhann GM, van de Beek D. 3R: brain abscess. *N Engl J Med*. 2014. doi: 10.1056/NEJMra1301635.

72. Magill SS, Edwards JR, Fridkin SK. Emerging infections program: Healthcare-Associated Infections Antimicrobial Use Prevalence Survey Team. Survey of health care-associated infections. *N Engl J Med*. 2014;370:2542–2543.

73. Lepelletier D, Roquilly A, Demeure dit latte D, et al. Retrospective analysis of the risk factors and pathogens associated with early-onset ventilator-associated pneumonia in surgical-ICU head-trauma patients. *J Neurosurg Anesthesiol.* 2010;22:32–37.

74. Cinotti R, Dordonnat-Moynard A, Feuillet F, et al. Risk factors and pathogens involved in early ventilator-acquired pneumonia in patients with severe subarachnoid hemorrhage. *Eur J Clin Microbiol Infect Dis.* 2014;33:823–830.

75. American Thoracic Society (ATS) and Infectious Diseases Society of America (IDSA). Guidelines for the management of adults with hospital-acquired, ventilator-associated, and healthcare-associated pneumonia. *Am J Respir Crit Care.* 2005;171:388–416.

76. Kalil AC, Metersky ML, Klompas M, et al. Management of adults with hospital-acquired and ventilator-associated pneumonia: 2016 clinical practice guidelines by the Infectious Diseases Society of America and the American Thoracic Society. *Clin Infect Dis.* 2016;63:e61–e111.

77. Leroy O, Giradie P, Yazdanpanah Y et al. Hospital-acquired pneumonia: microbiological data and potential adequacy of antimicrobial regimens. *Eur Respir J.* 2012;20:432–439.

78. Leroy O, d'Escrivan T, Devos P, Dubreuil L, Kipnis E, Georges H. Hospital-acquired pneumonia in critically ill patients: factors associated with episodes due to imipenem-resistant organisms. *Infection.* 2005;33:129–135.

79. Fàbregas N, Ewig S, Torres A, et al. Clinical diagnosis of ventilator associated pneumonia revisited: comparative validation using immediate post-mortem lung biopsies. *Thorax.* 1999;54:867.

80. Torres A, Niederman MS, Chastre J, et al. International ERS/ESICM/ESCMID/ALAT guidelines for the management of hospital-acquired pneumonia and ventilator-associated pneumonia: guidelines for the management of hospital-acquired pneumonia (HAP)/ventilator-associated pneumonia (VAP) of the European Respiratory Society (ERS), European Society of Intensive Care Medicine (ESICM), European Society of Clinical Microbiology and Infectious Diseases (ESCMID) and Asociación Latinoamericana del Tórax (ALAT). *Eur Respir J.* 2017;50.

81. Luna CM, Alejandro V, Josue' M, et al. Blood cultures have limited value in predicting severity of Illness and as a diagnostic tool in ventilator-associated pneumonia. *Chest.* 1999;116:1075–1084.

82. McFarland LV. Epidemiology of infectious and iatrogenic nosocomial diarrhea in a cohort of general medicine patients. *Am J Infect Control.* 1995;23:295–305.

83. Larson HE, Borriello SP. Infectious diarrhea due to *Clostridium perfringens. J Infect Dis.* 1988;157:390–391.

84. Hongenauer C, Langner C, Beubler E, et al. Klebsiella oxytoca as a causative organism of antibiotic-associated hemorrhagic colitis. *N Engl J Med.* 2006;355:2418–2426.

85. McDonald LC, Gerding DN, Johnson S, et al. *Clostridium difficle. Clin Infect Dis.* 2018;66:e1–e48.

86. DeMaio J, Bartlett JG. Update on diagnosis of *Clostridium difficile*–associated diarrhea. *Curr Clin Top Infect Dis.* 1995;15:97–114.

87. McDonald LC, Gerding DN, Johnson S, et al. Clinical practice guidelines for clostridium difficile infection in adults and children: 2017 update by the Infectious Diseases Society of America (IDSA) and Society for Healthcare Epidemiology of America (SHEA). *Clin Infect Dis.* 2018;66:e1.

88. Hooton TM, Bradley SF, Cardenas DD, et al. Diagnosis, prevention, and treatment of catheter-associated urinary tract infections in adults: 2009 International Clinical Practice Guidelines from the Infectious Diseases Society of America. *Clin Infect Dis.* 2010;50:625.

89. Tambyah PA, Maki DG. Catheter-associated urinary tract infection is rarely symptomatic: a prospective study of 1,497 catheterized patients. *Arch Intern Med.* 2000;160:678–682.

90. Garibaldi RA, Burke JP, Britt MR, et al. Meatal colonization and catheter-associated bacteriuria. *N Engl J Med.* 1980;303:316.

91. Weld KJ, Dmochowski RR. Effect of bladder management on urological complications in spinal cord injured patients. *J Urol.* 2000;163:768.

92. Caplan ES, Hoyt NJ. Nosocomial sinusitis. *JAMA.* 1982;247:639–641.

93. Heffner JE. Nosocomial sinusitis. Den of multiresistant thieves? *Am J Respir Crit Care Med.* 1994;150:608.

94. Souweine B, Mom T, Traore O, et al. Ventilator-associated sinusitis: microbiological results of sinus aspirates in patients on antibiotics. *Anesthesiology.* 2000;93:1255–1260.

95. Baker CC, Petersen SR, Sheldon GF. Septic phlebitis: a neglected disease. *Am J Surg.* 1979;138:97–103.

96. Mertz D, Khanlari B, Viktorin N, et al. Less than 28 days of intravenous antibiotic treatment is sufficient for superficial thrombophlebitis in injection drug users. *Clin Infect Dis.* 2008;46:741–744.

97. Gillespie P, Siddiqui H, Clarke J. Cannula related suppurative thrombophlebitis in the burned patient. *Burns.* 2000;26:200–204.

98. Chatzinikolaou I, Hanna H, Hachem R, Alakech B, Tarrand J, Raad I. Differential quantitative blood cultures for the diagnosis of catheter-related bloodstream infections associated with short- and long-term catheters: a prospective study. *Diagn Microbiol Infect Dis.* 2004;50: 167–172.

99. Wang AJ, Wang TE, Lin CC, Lin SE, Shih SC. Clinical predictors of severe gallbladder complications in acute acalculous cholecystitis. *World J Gastroenterol.* 2003;9:2821–2823.

9 Diagnosis and Management of Sodium Disorders in the Neurosurgical Patient

Jesse Edwards, Sharad Sharma, and Rakesh Gulati

INTRODUCTION

Sodium disorders are common in neurosurgical patients and increase overall morbidity and mortality.[1] Hyponatremia develops in 2% of all hospitalized patients and in up to 50% of neurosurgical patients, including 30–50% of subarachnoid hemorrhages (SAH) and 10–20% of mass lesions and other intracranial hemorrhages (ICH).[1–3] Most commonly due to hypovolemia, cerebral salt wasting (CSW), the syndrome of inappropriate antidiuretic hormone secretion (SIADH), and adrenal insufficiency (AI), hyponatremia represents a complex phenomenon characterized by disruptions of physiologic water and sodium processing.[1–5] Regardless of the etiology or comorbidities, hyponatremia present at the time of admission or acquired during hospitalization is independently associated not only with increased risk of inpatient morbidity and mortality, but with higher rates of 1- and 5-year all-cause mortality.[2,5–7] According to Rahman et al.,[1] all-cause mortality among hospitalized patients is 25% when serum sodium is less than 120 mEq/L and sodium less than 130 mEq/L is associated with a "60-fold increase in fatality" when compared to eunatremic patients.[1] Hannon et al.[2] cite a similar mortality rate of 28% when sodium is less than 125 mEq/L, while Braun et al.[7] suggest that even mild hyponatremia in the outpatient setting is associated with increased rates of mortality.[2,7]

Hypernatremia is less common than its counterpoint, but equally important for neurosurgery hospitalists to understand and treat with proficiency. While only approximately 1% of all hospitalized patients are found to be hypernatremic, approximately 9% of neurosurgical patients develop hypernatremia in excess of 150 mEq/L.[8] Hypernatremia always represents hypertonicity due to a deficit of free water.[8–11] Neurosurgical patients are particularly susceptible to free water deficit due to unreplaced water losses in the setting of central (neurogenic) diabetes insipidus (DI), encephalopathy, and neurological deficits.[8–11] Even physiologic water losses (e.g., urine) can lead to hypernatremia in patients too frail or encephalopathic to compensate adequately for the ongoing deficit. Risk of morbidity and mortality is increased by hypernatremia, but this is often difficult to distinguish from the inherent morbidity and mortality of the causative pathology.[10,12,13] Nevertheless, hypernatremia itself is considered a poor prognostic indicator and often indicative of severe underlying disease.[8,12,13]

Although the harm associated with sodium abnormalities is evident, there are insufficient high-quality trials to guide management practices, and clinicians rely predominantly on retro-/prospective studies and expert consensus.[1,2] In this chapter we review the pathophysiology of sodium disorders, diagnostic features, and principles of treatment in the neurosurgical patient population. The discussion of hyponatremia will center on hypovolemia, CSW, SIADH, and AI as the most pertinent conditions for the neurosurgical hospitalist to understand. Next, hypernatremia caused by central DI and inadequate oral fluid intake will be discussed in detail, as these are especially common etiologies in the neurosurgical patient population.

HYPONATREMIA
Pathophysiology

While water freely crosses cell membranes and the blood-brain barrier through osmosis, sodium remains predominantly extracellular and its concentration is determined by water regulation and movement.[9,11,14] Thirst is the principal stimulant for water intake and antidiuretic hormone (ADH) the agent of water retention.[4,5,15] Normally, both are inhibited when serum sodium is less than 135 mEq/L, increasingly activated at higher concentrations, and maximally activated when sodium reaches 145 mEq/L.[11] Serum osmolality of greater than 280 mOsmol/kg stimulates hypothalamic osmoreceptors to increase thirst and ADH secretion, while carotid baroreceptors and the renin-aldosterone-angiotensin system (RAAS) work to increase water and sodium retention in response to decreased intravascular pressure.[4,5,15-20] Hyponatremia may develop when ADH production or activity is increased, pathologically un/responsive to osmotic fluctuations (e.g., ectopic production or reset osmostat), or when a primary sodium deficit exceeds free water excretion and net retention of water ensues.[3-5,21,22] While renal and extrarenal losses of sodium contribute significantly to the pathophysiology of hyponatremia, water regulation remains the primary determinant of serum sodium concentration.[2,3,5,15,18,19] Hypovolemic hyponatremia is caused by high-volume loss of water *and* sodium (e.g., vomiting, diarrhea, hemorrhage).[8,23] Decreased pressure-stimulation of carotid baroreceptors and increased activity of RAAS in response to hypovolemia stimulate ADH release and renal retention of sodium, but water retention predominates and sodium concentration falls.[8,18,19,23] The pathophysiology of CSW is a subject of debate, but it is believed to represent primary natriuresis stimulated by cerebral injury, followed by secondary release of ADH in response to mild hypovolemia, which only worsens hyponatremia by net retention of free water.[3,5,15] In contrast, SIADH is characterized by increased primary ADH secretion and water retention in a euvolemic state.[5,15] Finally, hyponatremia due to AI is thought to be associated with ADH overactivity, although variably characterized by features of increased natriuresis and hypovolemia, depending on the principal steroid deficiency (i.e., glucocorticoid vs. mineralocorticoid).[3,18,19,24]

Diagnosis

Hyponatremia is defined as serum sodium of less than 135 mEq/L.[1,11] Although even mild hyponatremia may be clinically significant by its association with increased morbidity and mortality, indications for further diagnostic evaluation are not clearly established. Generally, the risk of morbidity and symptomatology (directly proportional to the acuity and severity of hyponatremia) should inform the decision to investigate the causative disease process.[1,23] Early symptoms of hyponatremia may appear benign but signal clinically significant osmotic fluctuations and may include headache, nausea, malaise, altered cognition, lethargy, and restlessness.[9] Hyponatremia that is acute (<48 hours since onset) *or* severe is independently associated with increased risk of symptomatology, morbidity, and mortality.[1,2,8,9] Acute *and* severe hyponatremia rapidly widens the osmotic gradient and greatly increases risk of encephalopathy, cerebral edema, elevated intracranial pressure (ICP), seizure, and coma.[1,2,5,9,11,23] In contrast to acute disease, chronic hyponatremia (unknown duration or >48 hours since onset) may remain asymptomatic until very severe, especially when acquired over a prolonged period of time, and is less likely to cause acutely catastrophic morbidity.[2,9] In either scenario, patients almost always are asymptomatic while sodium is 125 mEq/L or higher, and seizure activity has been documented only when sodium is less than 121 mEq/L.[1,9,23] Fraser et al.[5] suggest that sodium of less than 130 mEq/L merits further testing, while Rahman et al.[1] assign a class II indication to evaluation of sodium at less than 131 mEq/L.[1,5] Since neurosurgical patients are uniquely susceptible to the adverse sequelae of osmotic fluid fluctuations, we concur with sodium of less than 131 mEq/L as an indication for further diagnostic testing.

Extracellular volume status is one of the most widely accepted paradigms for the subclassification of hyponatremia (Box 9.1).[3,7,18,19,25] Hypervolemic hyponatremia is characterized by a positive fluid balance and marked by symptoms of dyspnea, orthopnea, weight gain, and increasing abdominal girth in the setting of pulmonary and peripheral edema, anasarca, and ascites.[1,24–26] Hypervolemic hyponatremia may represent primary volume overload with high effective arterial blood volume (EABV) due to advanced renal failure or secondary volume overload with low EABV due to third-spacing of fluid in the setting of congestive heart failure (CHF), cirrhosis, and nephrotic syndrome.[3,5,18,19,23,25] Neurosurgical patients certainly may develop hypervolemic hyponatremia, but hypovolemia and euvolemia are the most frequently encountered conditions and will serve as a framework for the following discussion of hyponatremia due to hypovolemia, CSW, SIADH, and AI.

Hypovolemic hyponatremia develops because of baroreceptor-mediated secretion of ADH in response to intravascular volume depletion.[3,8,18,19,23] History alone predicts the diagnosis, as patients may present with vomiting, diarrhea, anorexia, hemorrhage, or recent diuretic therapy.[3,18,19,26] Physical examination reveals

Box 9.1 Etiologies of Hyponatremia in the Neurosurgical Patient

Hypovolemic

Renal

Cerebral salt wasting

Adrenal insufficiency (e.g., mineralocorticoid deficiency)

Osmotic diuresis (e.g., hyperglycemia, mannitol)

Thiazide diuretics

Extrarenal

Vomiting

Diarrhea

Hemorrhage

Decreased oral intake

Insensible losses

Euvolemic

Syndrome of inappropriate antidiuretic hormone secretion

Adrenal insufficiency (e.g., glucocorticoid deficiency)

Severe hypothyroidism

Inadequate dietary solute

Thiazide diuretics

Reset osmostat

Primary polydipsia

Hypervolemic

High Effective Arterial Blood Volume

Advanced renal failure

Low Effective Arterial Blood Volume

Congestive heart failure

Cirrhosis

---

tachycardia, orthostasis, hypotension, poor skin turgor, and dry oral mucous membranes.[2,3,5,26] Serum osmolality may be low or normal and associated with elevated creatinine, urea, hematocrit, protein, albumin, and urate.[1,3–5] Acidbase and potassium abnormalities may be caused directly by the primary disease process or represent significant intravascular volume depletion and inadequate tissue perfusion.[3–5] Urine findings reflect increased ADH and RAAS activity and include elevated osmolality (higher than serum osmolality and often >450 mOsm/kg), sodium of less than 25 mEq/L (<20 mEq/L nearly is diagnostic), and chloride of less than 20 mEq/L.[1,3-5] Fractional excretion of sodium (FENa) and urea (FEUrea) may be less than 1% or less than 35%, respectively.[3,7,27] Central venous pressure (CVP) typically is less than 6 cm H_2O, although invasive monitoring of CVP may be impractical and unnecessary for patients who do not require the intensive care unit.[1,5]

CSW manifests as mildly hypovolemic hyponatremia, and patients may present with commensurate physical examination findings, but the pathophysiology of CSW remains incompletely understood.[1,2] Up to 50% of patients with SAH develop transient hyponatremia, and it is believed that CSW accounts for the vast majority, although AI may coexist and confound the assessment.[1,2,8,28] Some experts, however, question whether SIADH or CSW is more common in patients with SAH. Hannon et al.[28] found hyponatremia in 49% of patients with mild to moderate SAH and suggest that 71.4% of those cases were primarily attributable to SIADH.[28] In contrast, Fraser et al.[5] and Rahman et al.[1] support CSW as the principal mechanism of hyponatremia in SAH and emphasize the importance of accurate volume assessment in the diagnostic distinction.[1,5] In fact, apart from esoteric biochemical pathophysiology, hypovolemia is the most consistent and significant clinical feature differentiating CSW from SIADH.[1,2,5,8,23] Given the risk of cerebral vasospasm and stroke associated with intravascular contraction in SAH, we support a diagnostic and therapeutic paradigm predicated on CSW as the most common etiology of hyponatremia in SAH and a substantial likelihood for coexistence in any patient who presents with SAH.[1-3,5]

CSW is thought to represent primary natriuresis provoked by cerebral injury (which can be related to traumatic brain injury [TBI] or intracranial aneurysm clipping in addition to SAH), resulting in reduction of total body sodium content and intravascular volume depletion.[3,5,8] Decreased EABV triggers baroreceptor-mediated secretion of ADH, but increased water retention fails to replete intravascular volume, does nothing to halt natriuresis, and ultimately worsens hyponatremia in the setting of ongoing sodium excretion.[2,3,5,8] Blood testing typically is characterized by low (sometimes normal) serum osmolality and may hint at intravascular contraction with elevated creatinine, urea, hematocrit, protein, albumin, and bicarbonate.[1-3,5,23] Urine osmolality is inappropriately elevated (100 mOsm/kg or higher) and often more concentrated than serum, consistent with ADH overactivity and net water retention in the context of pathologic natriuresis.[3,5,8] Despite hypovolemia—which normally stimulates RAAS and sodium retention—urine sodium levels are greater than 40 mEq/L (though >25 mEq/L may remain consistent with the diagnosis in some cases).[1,3,8]

Within the neurosurgical patient population, SIADH is the most common cause of euvolemic hyponatremia, which is characterized by normal vital signs and the absence of historical and clinical information that would otherwise suggest volume loss or overload.[1,2,5,9] Physical examination reveals moist oral mucous membranes, normal skin turgor, and absence of peripheral edema.[2,5,8] Serum analysis in euvolemic hyponatremia may be relatively normal aside from hypo-osmolality and disease-specific abnormalities, if applicable, such as low cortisol or elevated thyroid stimulating hormone (TSH).[1,2,4,24,29-31] Although most frequently associated with SIADH in the neurosurgical patient, clinically significant AI and hypothyroidism must be excluded when attributing euvolemic hyponatremia to SIADH.[24–26,29,30] SIADH is associated with numerous comorbidities, including neurological disease (e.g., intracranial masses, stroke, and ICH), TBI, malignancy, pulmonary disease (e.g., acute respiratory failure, pneumonia), surgery, pain, and nausea (Box 9.2).[1–3,9,11,26,32] Medications such as hydrochlorothiazide, carbamazepine, selective serotonin reuptake inhibitors (SSRI), opioid derivatives, nicotine, and antipsychotic agents can also cause euvolemic hyponatremia consistent with SIADH.[3,8,9,11,32,33]

SIADH may represent increased production of ADH, lower thresholds for ADH release, or impaired negative feedback inhibition of ADH secretion.[16,22] Regardless, inappropriate ADH secretion remains the consistent feature. Biochemically, SIADH is characterized by hypo-osmolar hyponatremia with serum osmolality nearly always less than 275 mOsm/kg, although less than 280 mOsm/kg also may be consistent with the diagnosis.[1–4,8] Urate often is low, but serum otherwise is notable for normal creatinine, urea, hematocrit, bicarbonate, protein, and potassium.[1,3–5,8] It is important to remember that cortisol and TSH may be equivocally or falsely abnormal in critically ill patients, though results should at least rule out clinically significant AI or hypothyroidism as an alternative or coexisting etiology.[2,8,34] Urine testing in SIADH reveals inappropriately elevated osmolality, defined as 100 mOsm/kg or higher (i.e., not maximally diluted in response to serum hypo-osmolality) and often more than 600 mOsm/kg.[1–4] While variability of laboratory findings is common, urine osmolality higher than hypo-osmolar serum convincingly verifies impaired

---

Box 9.2 Etiologies of Syndrome of Inappropriate Antidiuretic Hormone Secretion

Intracranial masses

Stroke

Traumatic brain injury

Intracranial/subarachnoid hemorrhage

Central nervous system infection

Pituitary surgery

Malignancy (e.g., small cell lung carcinoma)

Pulmonary disease (e.g., respiratory failure or pneumonia)

Reset osmostat

Postsurgical state

Pain

Nausea

Medications

    Opioid derivatives

    Nicotine

    Antipsychotic agents

    Carbamazepine

    Selective serotonin reuptake inhibitors

renal excretory mechanisms due to ADH overactivity.[3,4,8] Urine sodium typically is greater than 40 mEq/L, although this is a function of patients' oral intake of salt in the days prior to admission, and urine sodium of greater than 25 mEq/L may be consistent with SIADH in otherwise supportive clinical scenarios.[1-4] As an additional point of unique importance in the neurosurgical patient population, pituitary surgeries presenting postoperatively with hyponatremia suggestive of SIADH must be approached with caution. Hyponatremia affects 3–25% of patients following pituitary resection and may represent SIADH, CSW, acute AI, transient release of preformed ADH, and, in some cases, the second stage of a "triple-phase response" (discussed in greater detail under "Hypernatremia").[2,5,8,32]

AI is the final etiology of hyponatremia to be detailed and must always be included in the neurosurgical hospitalist's differential since it frequently develops as a coexisting disorder alongside numerous neurosurgical diseases. Hannon et al.[2] estimate that 15% of patients with TBI develop hyponatremia, and 87% of these cases are attributable to secondary AI due to transient adrenocorticotropic hormone (ACTH) deficiency arising because of acute pituitary dysfunction.[2] Similarly, hypothalamic-pituitary irritation from surgical manipulation may lead to acute nonprimary AI (typically transient), while adrenal suppression in the neurosurgical patient may arise due to prolonged or repeated exposure to exogenous steroids.[1,2] Finally, AI develops in 7.1–12% of all SAH and is suspected to be the primary etiology of hyponatremia in 8.2% of cases, although principal causality is difficult to establish because AI and CSW may coexist.[2,28]

Hyponatremia due to AI is euvolemic if glucocorticoid deficiency predominates.[2] However, mineralocorticoid-predominant deficiency impairs renal sodium retention and leads to hypovolemia, which may then be complicated by orthostasis or overt hypotension.[2,5,23] Disruption of physiologic water regulation and decreased renal sodium retention yields hypo-osmolar hyponatremia with urine osmolality typically greater than 200 mOsm/kg and urine sodium of greater than 40 mEq/L (as with SIADH, >25 mEq/L may be consistent with AI when accompanied by otherwise compelling biochemical and clinical data).[1,3] In theory, these findings may reflect oversecretion of ADH associated with glucocorticoid deficiency itself or triggered by mild volume contraction in the context of mineralocorticoid deficiency.[23,24] Additional serologic testing may be relatively normal, but hyperkalemia and hypoglycemia support the diagnosis of AI.[2,5,9,23] In light of the biochemical similarities between AI and SIADH, diagnostic findings consistent with SIADH should raise suspicion for AI, especially in patients at risk for pituitary injury.

The essential diagnostic criteria for AI is low serum cortisol.[2] Nonetheless, there is little consensus on a cortisol threshold for the definitive diagnosis of AI. Instead, physicians must rely heavily on their clinical suspicion for AI and take into consideration the patient's acute and chronic comorbidities, symptoms, medications, vital signs, and electrolyte abnormalities.[9] Given a constellation of findings that raise the pre-test probability of AI, low serum cortisol supports the diagnosis. Early morning cortisol levels of less than 10 μg/dL are supportive of the diagnosis when the clinical index of suspicion is high, while levels of less than 3 μg/dL are independently predictive of disease.[2,35,36] In clinical presentations with a very high likelihood of AI, early morning cortisol of less than 15 μg/dL may yet be compatible with the diagnosis, but cortisol 15 μg/dL or higher typically indicates normal function of the hypothalamic-pituitary-adrenal (HPA) axis.[2,37] While we do not recommend routine ACTH stimulation testing, it may be useful when AI is suspected but serum cortisol within an equivocal range. In this scenario, serum cortisol that increases by less than 9 μg/dL 3060 minutes after a single intravenous dose of ACTH 250 μg may support the diagnosis, although it does not specify the level of dysfunction along the HPA axis and a normal result does not rule out acute (<2 weeks duration) nonprimary disease.[2,37,38] For neurosurgical patients, the authors of this chapter adhere to a multifaceted diagnostic and therapeutic approach, including consideration of (1) historical, clinical, and biochemical features suggestive of AI; (2) likelihood of alternative etiologies; (3) severity of hyponatremia and associated symptoms; and (4) the relative risk of inappropriately withholding versus administering supplemental steroids. In most cases, serum cortisol of less than 10 μg/dL is an acceptable threshold for diagnosis in the appropriate clinical context. Diagnostic findings of hyponatremia in the neurosurgical patient are summarized in Table 9.1.

Management

Due to a shortage of high-quality trials to establish evidence-based guidelines, recommendations for the treatment of hyponatremia are largely derived from expert consensus.[1] Like the indications to pursue diagnostic testing, treatment modalities and suggested rates of sodium correction correspond to the risk of morbidity and mortality posed by the acuity and severity of disease. As previously noted, acute *or* severe hyponatremia is associated with increased risk for morbidity and mortality due to osmotic fluid shift and the combination of acute *and* severe hyponatremia magnifies this risk.[1,2,5,8,9,14,23,25] In cases of severe disease, clinicians must be prepared to intervene with prompt and precise corrective therapies in order to mitigate the risk of encephalopathy, seizure, cerebral edema, increased ICP, brainstem herniation, coma, and respiratory failure.[1,2,14,23] Unfortunately, the definition of severity itself lacks empiric standardization and interpractitioner variability may lead to inconsistent implementation of treatment methodologies. To a limited extent, the risk of symptomatology underlies the conception of disease severity, and, in that respect, it is important to recognize that nearly all patients remain asymptomatic while serum sodium is 125 mEq/L or greater.[9,23] Mild to moderate symptoms (e.g., headache, vomiting, confusion) manifest when sodium is less than 125 mEq/L and progress to more severe symptoms as sodium drops to less than 121 mEq/L (e.g., encephalopathy, seizure) and less than 115 mEq/L (e.g., cerebral edema, brainstem herniation, coma).[1,5,9,23]

Regardless of its etiology, the correction of acutely severe or symptomatic hyponatremia should target a total increase in serum sodium of 3–5 mEq/L over the first 2–4 hours of treatment.[1,2] In any scenario, clinicians should limit correction of hyponatremia to increasing sodium by 8 mEq/L over the first 24 hours and 18 mEq/L over the first 48 hours because raising sodium by more than 12 mEq/L in 24 hours and more than 18 mEq/L in 48 hours is associated with increased risk

Table 9.1 Hyponatremia: supportive diagnostics

Etiology	Serum Osmolality	Other	CVP	Urine Osmolality	Sodium
Hypovolemia	↓/↔	↑ creatinine, urea, hematocrit, protein, albumin, urate; severe anemia, hyperglycemia, acid-base disorder; ↑/↓ potassium	↓	↑ or > serum osm	<25 mEq/L[a]
CSW	↓/↔	↑ creatinine, urea, hematocrit, protein, albumin, bicarbonate	↓	↑	>40 mEq/L[b]
SIADH	↓[c]	↔ creatinine, urea, hematocrit, protein, acid-base, TSH, cortisol; ↓ urate	↔/↑	↑ or inappropriately concentrated[c]	>40 mEq/L[b]
Adrenal insufficiency	↓	↓ glucose, ↑ potassium, ↓ cortisol or ↓ response to ACTH[d]	↓/↔	↑ or inappropriately concentrated[e]	>40 mEq/L[b]

[a] Urine sodium <20 mEq/L nearly is diagnostic of hypovolemic hyponatremia; urine chloride <20 mEq/L is supportive.

[b] Urine sodium >25 mEq/L is supportive in otherwise compelling clinical scenarios.

[c] Serum osmolality typically is <275 mOsm/kg; urine osmolality always is ≥100 mOsm/kg, typically > serum osmolality, and often >600 mOsm/kg.

[d] Early morning cortisol <10 μg/dL or increase by <9 μg/dL after ACTH stimulation test.

[e] Urine osmolality almost always is >200 mOsm/kg and typically > serum osmolality.

From References 1-5, 8, and 9.

of morbidity.[1,2,7,9] Close monitoring of serum sodium is essential in all cases as "hypertonic stress" from rapid overcorrection of hyponatremia may induce osmotic water shift from the intra- to extracellular space, leading to osmotic demyelinating syndrome (ODS).[8,9,11] The risk of ODS is greatest when hyponatremia has been present for more than 48 hours, initial sodium was less than 110 mEq/L, or the concentration increased by more than 12 mEq/L within a 24-hour period.[1,2,9,23] High-risk patients with chronic or severe hyponatremia may benefit from even more conservative goals of correction, such as increasing by only 6 mEq/L in the first 24 hours.[2,9,11] In support of this approach, Adrogue et al.[9] and Sterns et al.[11] note that increasing the serum sodium concentration by as little as 5% significantly mitigates the risk of suffering acute sequelae, and an increase of 4–6 mEq/L can itself abort seizure activity and prevent brainstem herniation.[9,11] The following discussion will work through disease-specific principles of management for hyponatremia due to hypovolemia, CSW, SIADH, and AI.

Volume expansion and correction of causative pathologies (e.g., gastrointestinal distress, hemorrhage) are the principles of treatment for hypovolemic hyponatremia. Isotonic fluid such as 0.9% sodium chloride (NaCl) in water or lactated Ringer's solution (LR) is the mainstay of initial therapy.[8,9] Following partial resuscitation with isotonic fluid, increased EABV may reduce baroreceptor activity and decrease ADH secretion, resulting in rapid correction of hyponatremia due to relatively hypotonic diuresis.[8,9] For this reason, treatment of severe hypovolemic hyponatremia employs isotonic fluid until hemodynamics have stabilized and symptoms improved, at which point transition to 0.45% NaCl in water is recommended for slower correction of sodium and even 5% dextrose in water (D5W) when continued hydration is necessary, but further increasing the serum sodium concentration is undesirable.[8,9] It is important to remember, however, that D5W distributes physiologically and approximately 60% of the infusate will enter the intracellular compartment.[9] In neurosurgical patients at high risk for cerebral edema and catastrophic sequelae, clinicians often prefer to avoid large volumes of D5W and may opt for less hypotonic solutions, such as D5W-0.45% NaCl for continued hydration.

As previously discussed, CSW most commonly develops in patients with SAH.[1,2] Hyponatremia and intravascular contraction increase risk for cerebral vasospasm and infarction in cases of SAH.[1,2,5] Fraser et al.[5] note that patients with SAH suffer cerebral infarction at a rate of 21% when eunatremic and 61% when hyponatremic.[5] In order to minimize risk, treatment paradigms for CSW prioritize avoidance of hypovolemia, expansion of intravascular volume, and sodium load repletion.[1,2,5,8] As isotonic fluid alone may worsen hyponatremia due to increased ADH activity, clinicians must integrate volume and solute repletion in order to administer "hypertonic volume."[1,2,5,8,11] Isotonic fluid may be infused intermittently as low-volume boluses or at a slow continuous rate with simultaneous salt loading in the form of salt tablets or hypertonic fluid (such as 3% NaCl in water) depending on the acuity, severity, and symptomatology of disease.[5,8] Serum sodium should be monitored every 6 hours and treatment modified according to goal rates of correction.[5] In patients who appear euvolemic (especially when confirmed by CVP monitoring), clinicians may favor initial treatment with only salt tablets or sequential 100 mL boluses of

3% NaCl in water, reserving isotonic fluid for intermittent volume maintenance.[1,2,11] Given the propensity of CSW to cause intravascular contraction, its prevalence in SAH, and the increased risk of morbidity posed by worsened hypovolemia, fluid restriction is contraindicated in patients with CSW or SAH.[1,2,5]

Mineralocorticoid supplementation is recommended as a class I indication for treatment of hyponatremia in SAH and is particularly beneficial in patients at elevated risk for cerebral vasospasm.[1] Improved clinical outcomes with use of mineralocorticoids may reflect not only adaptive mechanisms of sodium and water retention in the setting of presumed CSW, but also, in some cases, concurrent treatment of undiagnosed coexisting AI.[1,2,28] While there are no universal guidelines establishing a dose and duration of mineralocorticoid therapy, multiple studies support their efficacy both independently and as an adjunct to volume and sodium repletion.[1,5] Fludrocortisone 0.1–0.4 mgday effectively promotes sodium retention and can be divided as 0.1 mg intravenouslythree times daily or 0.2 mg intravenouslytwice daily.[1,5,8] Some studies suggest improved sodium control and decreased risk of morbidity when fludrocortisone is initiated within 24–48 hours of hospitalization and continued for 7–12 days in all patients with SAH, even in the absence of hyponatremia.[1,5]

SIADH is treated by a combination of free water restriction and increased solute load.[5,9] Restricting fluid intake to 1,000 mL/day may itself result in net loss of free water and increased sodium concentration despite ADH overactivity.[1,5,8,25] In patients with more significant hyponatremia or inadequate response to fluid restriction, adding salt tablets raises the overall solute load, increases the volume of diuresis, and shifts the water-to-sodium retention ratio in favor of sodium.[1,5] Isotonic fluid should be strictly avoided, despite sodium equivalencies of 154 mEq/L in 0.9% NaCl in water and 130 mEq/L in LR, because the pathophysiology of SIADH results in net retention of free water and worsened hyponatremia in response to isotonic fluid.[5,9,39] Hypertonic fluid is recommended in cases of acute, moderate to severe, symptomatic, or persistent hyponatremia in which there is risk of suffering significant morbidity.[9,11,25] It can be administered as a 100 mL bolus of 3% NaCl in water, repeated twice at 10-minute intervals, or infused at 0.5–2 mL/kg/hr with close monitoring of sodium levels.[2,11] Last, patients at low risk for complications from volume contraction may benefit from furosemide, especially when used in combination with solute loading, as it stimulates hypotonic diuresis and thereby aids in correcting hypo-osmolar hyponatremia.[1,9] The class of medications known as vaptans (V_2-receptor antagonists) are more appropriately utilized in cases of persistent hyponatremia due to chronic disease processes as routine use in the context of acute neurological disease is limited by inadequate data and absence of guidelines.[1,2,5] Figure 9.1 depicts a treatment algorithm for CSW and SIADH, correlated to the severity and symptomatology of disease.

Treatment of AI as the etiology of hyponatremia is indicated for patients with clinical risk factors, consistent presentations, and early morning cortisol levels of less than 10 μg/dL.[2] The crux of treating hyponatremia of AI is timely recognition of disease and early initiation of appropriate mineralocorticoid replacement therapy, typically in the form of intravenous hydrocortisone administered two or three times daily.[1,2,9] Patients with acutely severe disease may also benefit from 3% NaCl in water

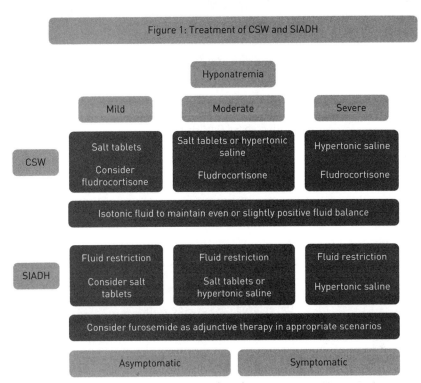

FIGURE 9.1 Treatment of cerebral salt wasting (CSW) and syndrome of inappropriate antidiuretic hormone (SIADH) secretion.

for rapid risk reduction, although intravenous hydrocortisone itself acts quickly to correct the disorder.[1,2] Consequently, AI first and foremost requires prompt treatment with steroid supplementation. When the pre-test probability of AI is high and accompanied by hypotension, hyperkalemia, and hypoglycemia, delay of treatment may be harmful and intravenous hydrocortisone should be administered empirically while serum cortisol results are in process.[2] In low-risk situations, however, treatment with hydrocortisone may be reserved for patients with serum cortisol of less than 10 μg/dL or an increase of less than 9 μg/dL following ACTH stimulation.[2] Depending on severity and symptomatology, hyponatremic patients in these scenarios may benefit from interim fluid restriction (when euvolemic), salt tablets, or hypertonic fluid while undergoing evaluation for AI.[1,2]

HYPERNATREMIA
Pathophysiology

Hypernatremia always implies a hypertonic state, and free water deficit is the fundamental principle of disease.[9–11] While the mechanisms of hypernatremia are less complex than those of hyponatremia, hypernatremia often is associated with severe comorbidities and underlying disease, summarized for reference in Box 9.3.[8] As discussed in relation to hyponatremia, hypothalamic osmoreceptors maintain serum sodium at 135–145 mEq/L and osmolality at approximately 280 mOsmol/

Box 9.3 Hypernatremia: Risk Factors in the Neurosurgical Population

Diabetes Insipidus

Central (i.e., neurogenic)

Nephrogenic

Decreased Oral Hydration

Encephalopathy

Elderly

Frailty

Limited mobility

Critically ill

Adipsia or hypodipsia

Dysphagia

Paresis/paralysis

Unreplaced Loss of Free Water

Vomiting

Diarrhea

Loop diuretics

Osmotic diuresis

Post-ATN diuresis

Insensible losses

Acute Salt Toxicity

Iatrogenic

Accidental/intentional oral ingestion

kg by regulating intake and retention of water through thirst and ADH, respectively.[4,5,8,10,32] This system normally remains compensated with great precision and even hypodipsia or inadequate access to water leads to hypernatremia only when maximum ADH activity is unable to offset the water deficit through renal retention of free water.[8,11,14,40,41] Conversely, even complete ADH deficiency (central DI) or resistance (nephrogenic DI) leads to hypernatremia only when thirst is impaired or water intake insufficient to counterbalance the ensuing hypotonic diuresis.[8,11,32]

Etiologies of free water deficit leading to hypernatremia include diarrhea, vomiting, loop diuretics, polyuria due to acute tubular necrosis (ATN) or osmotic diuresis, and inadequate ADH activity.[8,10,11] Neurosurgical patients may develop hypernatremia of any etiology, but are particularly at risk for unreplaced fluid losses in the setting of ADH deficiency, encephalopathy, and neurological deficits.[8,10] Central DI is characterized by ADH deficiency and may be due to traumatic insult or manipulation of the hypothalamic nuclei, hypothalamo-hypophyseal tract, or the posterior pituitary itself.[32] Injury to the hypothalamic-pituitary complex may arise as a consequence of TBI, ICH, brain tumors, ischemia, radiation, and aneurysms.[8,10,32] In each of these cases, central DI may be transient or permanent depending on the mechanism or location of injury and degree of hypothalamic neuronal degeneration.[32] Central DI caused by surgical manipulation of the hypothalamic-pituitary complex usually is transient and resolves upon recovery of pituitary function, typically within 10 days of onset.[32,42] Approximately 1–3% of pituitary surgeries experience a postoperative triple-phase response in which stunning of the pituitary leads to central DI within 24–48 hours, and this may last several days prior to spontaneous resolution at the outset of the second phase.[2,32] The second phase typically lasts a couple of days to 1 week and is marked by sudden release of preformed ADH from the posterior pituitary, rapidly correcting hypernatremia and potentially causing hyponatremia in a manner akin to SIADH.[2,32] Permanent DI may develop as the third and final phase, following depletion of ADH stores and inadequate recovery of productive or secretory capacity by the damaged hypothalamic-pituitary system.[2,32]

Encephalopathy and neurological deficits are common in the neurosurgical patient population and associated with hypernatremia when loss of free water is inadequately compensated by enteric intake (due to cognitive, volitional, or functional barriers).[8,10,11] In response to hyperosmolality, hypernatremia, and hypovolemia induced by inadequate hydration, ADH secretion is increased and acts to stimulate renal retention of free water.[8–11] Nevertheless, persistent and uncompensated free water loss exceeding the maximum retention capacity of ADH inevitably leads to hypernatremia.[10,11]

Diagnosis

Hypernatremia is defined as serum sodium of greater than 145 mEq/L.[8,10] Patients may or may not have obvious risk factors for free water deficit, and clinicians should work to identify the underlying etiology, such as those listed earlier. Calculating the total free water deficit is an important piece of the diagnostic evaluation, but represents only a cross-sectional assessment of the deficit and does not account for ongoing and fluctuating water loss.[10] Like hyponatremia, symptoms of hypernatremia primarily are neurologic (e.g., lethargy, impaired cognition, muscle weakness, ataxia, seizures, and coma) but may also include gastrointestinal and constitutional manifestations such as nausea, vomiting, restlessness, and malaise.[8,10,32] Patients with intact cognition may endorse thirst, provided that the underlying pathology does not include adipsia.[8,10,41] As hypernatremia is associated with dehydration and often hypovolemia, vital signs may include tachycardia and orthostasis, while physical examination may reveal dry oral mucus membranes and poor skin turgor.[4,8,10]

Central DI is associated with polyuria and polydipsia when thirst and access to water are preserved.[32] Confounding etiologies (e.g., hyperglycemia and diuretics) must be excluded, but it is important that neurosurgical hospitalists consider the possibility of central DI in any high-risk patient (e.g., recent pituitary surgery or TBI) presenting with polyuria and rising serum sodium. Serum osmolality is expected to be elevated in any case of hypernatremia—typically greater than 300 mOsm/kg—and distinction between central DI and alternative etiologies depends primarily on urine studies.[8] Central DI is characterized by urine osmolality that is inappropriately dilute in comparison to serum hyperosmolality.[4,8,32] Diagnostic guidelines include serum osmolality of greater than 300 mOsm/kg and urine osmolality of less than 300 mOsm/kg.[4,32] Urine specific gravity of less than 1.005 supports the diagnosis of central DI, and "high-volume" urine output is typical, although somewhat ill-defined.[8,32]

Patients with encephalopathy and neurological deficits develop hypernatremia when their cognition, volition, or functional capacity is prohibitive to adequate self-hydration, and insufficient water intake leads to free water deficit.[10] Serum osmolality is elevated and urine increasingly concentrated through the action of ADH, which appropriately manifests as urine osmolality that is higher than serum osmolality and often greater than 600 mOsm/kg when ADH activity is maximized.[4,10,43] Urine osmolality of 300–600 mOsm/kg does not exclude any diagnosis entirely, and urine osmolality should be monitored regularly during ongoing evaluation and treatment for changes that may clarify the diagnosis (e.g., decrease to <300 mOsm/kg suggesting underlying DI or increase to >600 mOsm/kg indicative of extrarenal water losses).[4]

Management

Like hyponatremia, treatment of hypernatremia is guided by the inherent risk for symptomatology and morbidity related to acuity and severity of disease.[11] Acute *and* severe disease (sodium >160 mEq/L) is understood to pose the greatest risk of harm, including ODS from relative "hypertonic stress" or ICH due to vascular injury.[7,10,11,44] Patients often remain asymptomatic or develop only mild symptomatology (e.g., nausea, restlessness, malaise) while serum sodium is 160 mEq/L or lower, but even mild hypernatremia merits corrective intervention, especially when there is high likelihood of ongoing free water deficit and progressive elevation of sodium concentration.[7,10] The core principles of treating hypernatremia include replacement of free water, identification of the cause, and correction of underlying pathology (e.g., resolution of gastrointestinal losses, osmotic diuresis, encephalopathy, or restoration of ADH activity).[8,10] Treatment paradigms for hypernatremia caution against excessively rapid correction of serum sodium, which may cause osmotic fluid shift and consequent cerebral edema, elevated ICP, seizures, or respiratory failure due to pulmonary edema.[8,10,11] Since neurosurgical patients are more susceptible than average to the detrimental sequelae of osmotic fluid shifts, clinicians may adopt a risk-averse strategy by targeting correction to serum sodium 145 mEq/L (rather than 140 mEq/L, for example, when calculating the rate and volume of hypotonic infusion necessary to lower sodium to the desired concentration) and directing management according to the acuity and etiology of disease.[10]

Hyperacute hypernatremia develops over the course of minutes to hours and should be treated urgently with free water supplementation or hemodialysis in cases of life-threatening sodium elevation.[11] Rapid correction of sodium concentration in this setting has not been associated with increased morbidity or mortality, and D5W may be infused intravenously without a 24-hour restriction, generally targeting a decrease of serum sodium by 1 mEq/L/hr[10,11] Less hypotonic fluids such as 0.2% or 0.45% NaCl in water may also be utilized, but a greater volume of fluid is required to lower the concentration of serum sodium.[10] Acute hypernatremia develops over 24–48 hours and similarly requires prompt correction through free water supplementation, whether via enteric or intravenous routes.[10,11] Although rapid correction also is not known to be harmful in this scenario, many experts recommend lowering serum sodium concentration by a maximum of 0.5 mEq/L/hr and 10 mEq/L/day[10,11] D5W, 0.2% NaCl, or 0.45% NaCl in water are acceptable intravenous treatment options, bearing in mind that high volume of infusate is a greater risk factor for cerebral edema and total body volume overload than fluid tonicity itself.[10] For this reason, 0.9% NaCl in water is not recommended apart from resuscitation of hemodynamic compromise—even when hypernatremia exceeds its intrinsic sodium concentration of 154 mEq/L—due to the massive volume of fluid required to achieve net water retention and sodium reduction, particularly in the context of ongoing free water loss.[10] When hypernatremia is chronic (i.e., unknown duration or >48 hours since onset), goals of decreasing serum sodium by 0.5 mEq/L/hr or less and 10 mEq/L/day or less are more relevant, and free water supplementation should be accompanied by frequent monitoring of serum sodium especially when intravenous infusions are utilized.[10,11] Reduction of serum sodium in excess of these limits is associated with a theoretical risk for cerebral edema, seizures, and coma.[10,11] Nonetheless, adverse consequences due to rapid correction of chronic hypernatremia have only been described in pediatric cases, and many adult patients suffer unnecessary morbidity due to undertreatment out of exaggerated concern for inadvertent overcorrection.[11,12]

Treatment modalities for hypernatremia due to central DI depend on the acuity and severity of disease, its distinctive pathophysiology, and the risk of water excretion fluctuations inherent to the postoperative triple-phase response observed in some cases of pituitary resections.[2,8,32] Increased enteric water intake is the preferred method of treatment for mild disease (orally or via nasogastric/gastric tubes), but hypotonic intravenous fluid may be necessary in cases of severe, persistent, or progressive disease refractory to enteric water supplementation.[8,32] Desmopressin is an ADH analog utilized to induce renal retention of free water in select cases of central DI.[32] It is available in numerous formulations, including oral tablets, intranasal spray, and intravenous or subcutaneous solutions.[32] When central DI responds inadequately to free water supplementation and its trajectory appears persistent or progressive, desmopressin may be administered while serum sodium is closely monitored.[32] Immediately following pituitary surgery, desmopressin should be used with caution because administration during the second stage (characterized by release of preformed ADH) of a triple-phase response may cause acutely severe hyponatremia and increase morbidity due to massive osmotic fluid shifts.[2,32] Oral desmopressin may be administered as 100–800 µg/day divided into two or three doses; intranasal spray as 10–40 µg/day divided into two doses; and intravenous or subcutaneous therapy as 2–4 µg/day in one or two doses.[32] In all scenarios, serum sodium, fluid intake, urine output, and body weight should be followed closely for appropriate titration of therapy.[32]

CONCLUSION

Neurosurgical patients are exceptionally susceptible to development of sodium abnormalities. Underlying neurological pathology predisposes to disordering of sodium and water regulation while simultaneously placing patients at greater risk for the morbidity and mortality associated with osmotic fluid shifts. Hyponatremia is common and most often attributable to hypovolemia, CSW, SIADH, and AI in the neurosurgical population. Diagnostic evaluation is recommended for serum sodium of less than 131 mEq/L and at minimum should include chem 7, serum osmolality, urine osmolality, and urine electrolytes.[1,2] Urate, hematocrit, and disease-specific assays such as cortisol and TSH should be tested as clinically indicated and for clarification of the diagnosis. Management decisions should be based on the acuity, severity, symptomatology, and pathophysiology of disease, accounting in each instance for comorbid conditions which may alter the patient's risk profile (e.g., SAH). Hypernatremia develops as a consequence of free water deficit.[10] Neurosurgical patients are at elevated risk for free water deficit due to central DI, encephalopathy, and neurological deficits.[32] Target rates of sodium correction in hypernatremia are less restrictive than those of hyponatremia, and clinicians must avoid undertreatment of disease.[12] Nevertheless, hypotonic intravenous fluid should be reserved for failure of enteric water supplementation and desmopressin administered only when absolutely indicated by the pathophysiology or severity of disease.[10,32] Sodium disorders are challenging to diagnose and treat but essential for the neurosurgical hospitalist to understand and manage with proficiency.

REFERENCES

1. Rahman M, Friedman WA. Hyponatremia in neurosurgical patients: clinical guidelines development. *Neurosurgery*. 2009;65(5):925–935; discussion 935–926.
2. Hannon MJ, Thompson CJ. Neurosurgical hyponatremia. *J Clin Med*. 2014;3(4):1084–1104.
3. Milionis HJ, Liamis GL, Elisaf MS. The hyponatremic patient: a systematic approach to laboratory diagnosis. *CMAJ*. 2002;166(8):1056–1062.
4. Rose BD, Post TW. *Clinical Physiology of Acid-Base and Electrolyte Disorders*. 5th ed. New York: McGraw-Hill, Medical Pub. Division; 2001.
5. Fraser JF, Stieg PE. Hyponatremia in the neurosurgical patient: epidemiology, pathophysiology, diagnosis, and management. *Neurosurgery*. 2006;59(2):222–229; discussion 222–229.
6. Waikar SS, Mount DB, Curhan GC. Mortality after hospitalization with mild, moderate, and severe hyponatremia. *Am J Med*. 2009;122(9):857–865.
7. Braun MM, Barstow CH, Pyzocha NJ. Diagnosis and management of sodium disorders: hyponatremia and hypernatremia. *Am Fam Physician*. 2015;91(5):299–307.
8. Tisdall M, Crocker M, Watkiss J, Smith M. Disturbances of sodium in critically ill adult neurologic patients: a clinical review. *J Neurosurg Anesthesiol*. 2006;18(1):57–63.

9. Adrogue HJ, Madias NE. Hyponatremia. *N Engl J Med.* 2000;342(21):1581–1589.

10. Adrogue HJ, Madias NE. Hypernatremia. *N Engl J Med.* 2000;342(20):1493–1499.

11. Sterns RH. Disorders of plasma sodium—causes, consequences, and correction. *N Engl J Med.* 2015;372(1):55–65.

12. Alshayeb HM, Showkat A, Babar F, Mangold T, Wall BM. Severe hypernatremia correction rate and mortality in hospitalized patients. *Am J Med Sci.* 2011;341(5): 356–360.

13. Vedantam A, Robertson CS, Gopinath SP. Morbidity and mortality associated with hypernatremia in patients with severe traumatic brain injury. *Neurosurg Focus.* 2017;43(5):E2.

14. Strange K. Regulation of solute and water balance and cell volume in the central nervous system. *J Am Soc Nephrol.* 1992;3(1):12–27.

15. Ellison DH, Berl T. Clinical practice. The syndrome of inappropriate antidiuresis. *N Engl J Med.* 2007;356(20):2064–2072.

16. Robertson GL, Aycinena P, Zerbe RL. Neurogenic disorders of osmoregulation. *Am J Med.* 1982;72(2):339–353.

17. Thompson CJ, Selby P, Baylis PH. Reproducibility of osmotic and nonosmotic tests of vasopressin secretion in men. *Am J Physiol.* 1991;260(3 Pt 2):R533–R539.

18. Anderson RJ, Chung HM, Kluge R, Schrier RW. Hyponatremia: a prospective analysis of its epidemiology and the pathogenetic role of vasopressin. *Ann Intern Med.* 1985;102(2):164–168.

19. Chung HM, Kluge R, Schrier RW, Anderson RJ. Clinical assessment of extracellular fluid volume in hyponatremia. *Am J Med.* 1987;83(5):905–908.

20. Verbalis JG, Goldsmith SR, Greenberg A, et al. Diagnosis, evaluation, and treatment of hyponatremia: expert panel recommendations. *Am J Med.* 2013;126(10 Suppl 1):S1–42.

21. Barlow ED, De Wardener HE. Compulsive water drinking. *Q J Med.* 1959;28(110): 235–258.

22. Fenske WK, Christ-Crain M, Horning A, et al. A copeptin-based classification of the osmoregulatory defects in the syndrome of inappropriate antidiuresis. *J Am Soc Nephrol.* 2014;25(10):2376–2383.

23. Cole CD, Gottfried ON, Liu JK, Couldwell WT. Hyponatremia in the neurosurgical patient: diagnosis and management. *Neurosurg Focus.* 2004;16(4):E9.

24. Schrier RW, Bichet DG. Osmotic and nonosmotic control of vasopressin release and the pathogenesis of impaired water excretion in adrenal, thyroid, and edematous disorders. *J Lab Clin Med.* 1981;98(1):1–15.

25. Yeates KE, Singer M, Morton AR. Salt and water: a simple approach to hyponatremia. *CMAJ.* 2004;170(3):365–369.

26. Schrier RW. Body water homeostasis: clinical disorders of urinary dilution and concentration. *J Am Soc Nephrol.* 2006;17(7):1820–1832.

27. Musch W, Thimpont J, Vandervelde D, Verhaeverbeke I, Berghmans T, Decaux G. Combined fractional excretion of sodium and urea better predicts response to saline in hyponatremia than do usual clinical and biochemical parameters. *Am J Med.* 1995;99(4):348–355.

28. Hannon MJ, Behan LA, O'Brien MM, et al. Hyponatremia following mild/moderate subarachnoid hemorrhage is due to SIAD and glucocorticoid deficiency and not cerebral salt wasting. *J Clin Endocrinol Metab.* 2014;99(1):291–298.

29. Derubertis FR, Jr., Michelis MF, Bloom ME, Mintz DH, Field JB, Davis BB. Impaired water excretion in myxedema. *Am J Med.* 1971;51(1):41–53.

30. Skowsky WR, Kikuchi TA. The role of vasopressin in the impaired water excretion of myxedema. *Am J Med.* 1978;64(4):613–621.

31. Allman RM, Walker JM, Hart MK, Laprade CA, Noel LB, Smith CR. Air-fluidized beds or conventional therapy for pressure sores. A randomized trial. *Ann Intern Med.* 1987;107(5):641–648.

32. Schreckinger M, Szerlip N, Mittal S. Diabetes insipidus following resection of pituitary tumors. *Clin Neurol Neurosurg.* 2013;115(2):121–126.

33. Van Amelsvoort T, Bakshi R, Devaux CB, Schwabe S. Hyponatremia associated with carbamazepine and oxcarbazepine therapy: a review. *Epilepsia.* 1994;35(1):181–188.

34. Hamrahian AH, Oseni TS, Arafah BM. Measurements of serum free cortisol in critically ill patients. *N Engl J Med.* 2004;350(16):1629–1638.

35. Jenkins D, Forsham PH, Laidlaw JC, Reddy WJ, Thorn GW. Use of ACTH in the diagnosis of adrenal cortical insufficiency. *Am J Med.* 1955;18(1):3–14.

36. Hagg E, Asplund K, Lithner F. Value of basal plasma cortisol assays in the assessment of pituitary-adrenal insufficiency. *Clin Endocrinol (Oxf).* 1987;26(2):221–226.

37. Marko NF, Gonugunta VA, Hamrahian AH, Usmani A, Mayberg MR, Weil RJ. Use of morning serum cortisol level after transsphenoidal resection of pituitary adenoma to predict the need for long-term glucocorticoid supplementation. *J Neurosurg.* 2009;111(3):540–544.

38. Cope CL. *Adrenal Steroids and Disease.* 2d ed. Philadelphia, PA: Lippincott; 1972.

39. Steele A, Gowrishankar M, Abrahamson S, Mazer CD, Feldman RD, Halperin ML. Postoperative hyponatremia despite near-isotonic saline infusion: a phenomenon of desalination. *Ann Intern Med.* 1997;126(1):20–25.

40. McIver B, Connacher A, Whittle I, Baylis P, Thompson C. Adipsic hypothalamic diabetes insipidus after clipping of anterior communicating artery aneurysm. *BMJ.* 1991;303(6815):1465–1467.

41. Mavrakis AN, Tritos NA. Diabetes insipidus with deficient thirst: report of a patient and review of the literature. *Am J Kidney Dis.* 2008;51(5):851–859.

42. Kristof RA, Rother M, Neuloh G, Klingmuller D. Incidence, clinical manifestations, and course of water and electrolyte metabolism disturbances following transsphenoidal pituitary adenoma surgery: a prospective observational study. *J Neurosurg.* 2009;111(3):555–562.

43. Latcha S, Lubetzky M, Weinstein AM. Severe hyperosmolarity and hypernatremia in an adipsic young woman. *Clin Nephrol.* 2011;76(5):407–411.

44. Chang L, Harrington DW, Milkotic A, Swerdloff RS, Wang C. Unusual occurrence of extrapontine myelinolysis associated with acute severe hypernatraemia caused by central diabetes insipidus. *Clin Endocrinol (Oxf).* 2005;63(2):233–235.

10 Blood Glucose Management in the Neurosurgical Patient

Kevin Furlong and Satya Villuri

INTRODUCTION

Hyperglycemia and diabetes are common in the neurosurgical population. Hyperglycemia in this setting has been associated with deleterious clinical sequelae that lead to increased postoperative complications, length of stay, mortality rates, and hospital costs.[1,2] The stress of neurological illness and surgery can activate a neuroendocrine response that antagonizes insulin activity.[3] This is mediated by an increase in hormones such as epinephrine and cortisol, as well as by an increase in proinflammatory cytokines.[4] This stress-induced hyperglycemia may cause deleterious effects. However, it is still debated whether hyperglycemia is a surrogate marker for worse outcomes or an underlying cause.[5]

While many studies have associated hyperglycemia with worse neurosurgical outcomes, there is a paucity of data showing that intensive glucose control provides benefit. In addition, the heterogeneity of pathology in the neurosurgical population calls for caution in generalizing study results from other surgical populations.

This chapter is meant to serve as a guide for glucose management in the neurosurgical population. It will provide practical tips for management with the intention of maximizing time in the appropriate glucose range while avoiding hypoglycemia.

We will first look at the available evidence in the various subpopulations of neurosurgery. We will then provide evidence-based goals where available. Finally, we will provide a practical approach for the management of hyperglycemia.

EVIDENCE AND RECOMMENDATIONS FOR BLOOD GLUCOSE GOALS IN THE NEUROSURGICAL PATIENT
Critical Care

Hyperglycemia is common in the critical care setting and has long been associated with adverse outcomes. There have been multiple trials comparing conventional glucose management (CGM) to intensive insulin therapy (IIT) in this setting. Differences in patient population, center experience, nutritional supplementation methods, severity of illness, and outcome measures make this a heterogeneous group of studies. Moreover, none of them focused specifically on the neurosurgical population.

Data from the original Van Den Berghe trial showed benefit to intensive glucose control in the surgical ICU patient who was receiving mechanical ventilation.[6] A total of 1,548 patients were enrolled and randomly assigned to either IIT with a goal blood glucose of 80–110 mg/dL or to CGM with a goal blood glucose level of 180–200 mg/dL. Only 4% of these patients were admitted to the ICU for neurologic disease, cerebral trauma, or brain surgery. IIT reduced mortality during intensive care from 8% to 4.6% (P <0.04). The benefit of IIT was attributable to its effect on mortality among patients who remained in the ICU for more than 5 days. ITT also reduced overall in-hospital mortality, bloodstream infections, acute renal failure requiring dialysis or hemofiltration, the medium number of red cell transfusions, and critical illness polyneuropathy. After this trial was published, many centers developed insulin protocols with more intensive glucose goals.

Subsequently, multicenter studies were performed in an attempt to investigate and verify these results. The Volume Substitution and Insulin Therapy in Severe Sepsis (VISEP) study and the Glucontrol study were multicenter prospective randomized trials that showed no significant difference in mortality in IIT versus CGM.[7,8] However, they did show increased episodes of severe hypoglycemia.

The NICE-SUGAR study was a large multicenter randomized control trial which enrolled 6,104 patients.[9] It compared an intensive glucose target of 80–108 mg/dL to a conventional target of 180 mg/dL or less. Mortality in the IIT group was 27.5% compared to 24.9% in the CGM group (p = 0.02). The incidence of severe hypoglycemia was 6.8% in the ITT group versus 0.5% in the CGM group (P <0.001). The bottom line is that the majority of these show no benefit to ITT and the possibility of increased harm.

The results of these subsequent trials have led to a more relaxed glucose goal in the critical care setting. Several major guidelines and consensus statements now recommend a glucose goal of 140–180 mg/dL in the ICU setting.[10] Given lack of data to the contrary, this range is appropriate in the neurosurgical ICU patient as well.

The data on IIT is scarce in the specific subsets of the neurosurgical population. The following sections provide a quick review of the latest literature.

Ischemic Stroke

Multiple studies have shown a correlation between increased blood glucose and increased infarct size, stroke severity, and poor outcome.[11,12] There have been several studies evaluating the effects of IIT in acute ischemic stroke patients with hyperglycemia. The THIS trial by Bruno et al. compared IIT with a goal blood glucose of less than 130 versus conventional therapy with a goal blood glucose of less than 200 mg/dL.[13] There was no difference at outcomes in 3 months; however, there was a 35% rate of hypoglycemia in the IIT group.

The Intensive versus Subcutaneous Insulin in Patients with Hyperacute Stroke (INSULINFARCT) trial, a prospective, randomized, unblinded trial including patients with hyperacute stroke, was designed to determine if IIT with continuous insulin infusion would improve glucose control and reduce subsequent infarct growth on MRI.[14] The authors found that patients in the IIT group had improved overall glucose control within the first 24 hours of stroke, but this was in fact associated with larger infarct growths.

The American Heart Association Stroke guidelines recommend that it is reasonable to obtain glucose levels between 140–180 mg/dL in acute ischemic stroke.[15]

Subarachnoid Hemorrhage

The data in this population have not shown universal benefit. A trial of 834 patients by Theile et al. showed no difference in mortality with IIT but a small increased risk of death with hypoglycemia in the IIT patients.[16] In another prospective observational follow-up study, 295 consecutive patients with intracranial hemorrhage (ICH) had extensive monitoring of blood glucose values and those with blood glucose values of greater than 150 mg/dL received a variable intravenous insulin dose to maintain blood glucose values between 60 and 150 mg/dL.[17] An 18 mg/dL increase in the blood glucose concentration at admission was associated with a 33% mortality increase. During the first 12 hours after ICH, the insulin treatment protocol reduced mortality, but this association was attenuated and no longer significant after that time period.

There are no specific guidelines on the appropriate glucose goal in this population.

Traumatic Brain Injury

There are several studies evaluating the use of IIT in the treatment of these patients. One study found no effect of IIT on sepsis rates, neurological outcome, or duration of ICU stay.[18] Another study showed IIT shortened ICU stays but had no effect on infection rates or mortality.[19] A further study found that IIT decreased infection rates, days spent in the ICU, and neurologic outcome at the 6-month follow-up.[20] Another small study by Wang et al. showed IIT decreased infection rate and reduced duration of ICU stay.[21] The mortality rates were similar between the two groups.

No formal guidelines exist for glucose management in the setting of acute brain trauma.

Spine Surgery

Diabetes has been shown to be an independent risk factor for postoperative infection in this population. Meng et al. showed an odds ratio (OR) of 2.04 in diabetic patients versus nondiabetic patients.[22] In another study, diabetics with an A1c of less than 7% had a 0% chance of infection, whereas patients with an A1c greater than 7% had a 35.5% infection rate.[23] Despite the association of hyperglycemia with increased infection, a recent systematic review reached the conclusion that there remains insufficient evidence that strict glucose control is advantageous over conventional management for the prevention of surgical site infection.[24]

Intracranial Tumors

In a retrospective study, McGirt et al. showed an association between persistent postoperative hyperglycemia and mortality in patients undergoing tumor resection.[25] However, there are no specific studies on perioperative glucose control and outcomes in this patient population.

Summary of Guidelines and Blood Glucose Goals

In conclusion, there are no specific data showing benefit in these specific neurosurgical populations. Therefore, it seems reasonable to follow one of the several established guidelines for the management of inpatient hyperglycemia and diabetes. They are meant to standardize processes of care based on the best available evidence.

In the noncritical care setting, most guidelines agree that a premeal blood glucose of less than 140 mg/dL and a random blood glucose of less than 180 mg/dL is recommended.[10] There is variability in recommendations in the critical care setting.[10] However, it seems reasonable to target a blood glucose between 140 and 180 mg/dL while avoiding hypoglycemia.[26]

Recent studies in surgical patients have reported that targeting perioperative blood glucose levels to less than 180 mg/dL is associated with lower rates of mortality and stroke compared with a target glucose of less than 200 mg/dL.[27,28] No significant additional benefit was shown with stricter glycemic control. These seem like reasonable goals for the neurosurgical population.

INSULIN

It is important for clinicians involved in the care of diabetic patients to understand the insulins available for the treatment of this disease. Table 10.1 shows the pharmacokinetics of subcutaneous insulin preparations.

An insulin regimen with basal, prandial, and correction components is the preferred treatment for noncritically ill hospitalized patients with good nutritional intake.[26] It is important to familiarize oneself with this insulin terminology.

Basal insulin is also known as *background insulin*. It is what is necessary to control glucose in the fasting state. It can be administered as an intermediate-acting insulin (NPH) twice daily or as a long-acting insulin once or twice daily.

The bolus or *prandial* component requires the administration of short- or rapid-acting insulin administered in coordination with meals or nutrient delivery.

Correction insulin refers to the administration of supplemental doses of short- or rapid-acting insulin together with the usual dose of bolus insulin for blood glucose above the target range. Correction-dose insulin should not be confused with *sliding scale insulin*, which usually refers to a set amount of insulin administered for hyperglycemia without regard to the timing of the food, the presence or absence of preexisting insulin administration, or even individualization of the patient's sensitivity to insulin.[29] Correction insulin is customized to match the insulin sensitivity for each patient.

Table 10.1 Pharmacokinetics of subcutaneous insulin preparations

Insulin	Onset	Peak (hours)	Duration (hours)
Rapid-Acting			
aspart with niacinamide	2–4 minutes	1–2	3–5
aspart	5–15 minutes	1–2	4–6
lispro	5–15 minutes	1–2	4–6
glulisine	5–15 minutes	1–2	4–6
Short-Acting			
regular insulin	30–60 minutes	2–3	6–10
Intermediate-acting			
NPH	2–4 hours	4–10	12–18
Long-acting			
Detemir	2 hours	variable	12–24
glargine	2 hours	none	20–24
degludec	2 hours	None	24+

PERIOPERATIVE MANAGEMENT OF THE NEUROSURGICAL PATIENT
Preoperative Evaluation

The preoperative evaluation of the diabetic patient can be complex given the co-morbid conditions that are often present in this patient population. Many of these patients have underlying cardiovascular disease and have a higher risk of silent ischemia.[30] They also have higher rates of comorbid conditions such as obesity, hypertension, chronic kidney disease, peripheral vascular disease, and neuropathy that can increase neurosurgical perioperative risk.

Patients with diabetes undergoing surgery should be evaluated for the type of diabetes they have, diabetic complications, antecedent pharmacological therapy, level of glucose control, hypoglycemic events, and the nature and extent of the surgical procedure.[29]

Admission and Perioperative Management

The American Diabetes Association recommends checking an A1c in any hospitalized patient with diabetes or hyperglycemia of greater than 140 mg/dL, if an A1c was not checked in the previous 3 months.[26] An A1c of 6.5% or higher suggests that the patient had diabetes before the hospital admission. It is also important that the initial inpatient orders clearly state if the patient has type 1 diabetes, type 2 diabetes, or no diabetes.[26,29] This distinction is important because type 1 diabetics can rapidly go into diabetic ketoacidosis if their insulin is withheld.

Hyperglycemia in hospitalized patients is defined as blood glucose levels of greater than 140 mg/dL.[26,29] The frequency of blood glucose monitoring depends on the patient's status. For patients who are eating, one should monitor blood glucose before meals.[26] For patients who are not eating, checking blood sugars every 4–6 hours is appropriate.[26]

Insulin therapy should be initiated for treatment of persistent hyperglycemia starting at a threshold of 180 mg/dL (10.0 mmol/L). Once insulin therapy is started, a target glucose range of 140–180 mg/dL is recommended for the majority of critically ill patients and noncritically ill patients, as reviewed earlier.

Critical Care

In the critical care setting, a continuous intravenous insulin infusion has been shown to be the best method for achieving glycemic targets. Intravenous insulin infusions should be administered based on validated protocols that allow for predefined adjustments in the infusion rate, accounting for glycemic fluctuations and insulin dose.[30,31] Several published insulin infusion protocols appear to be both safe and effective, with low rates of hypoglycemia, although most have been validated only in the ICU setting.[30,31]

When the patient is clinically stable, they can be converted over to a subcutaneous regimen. Converting over to subcutaneous insulin at 60–80% of the 24-hour insulin infusion dose has been shown to be effective.[31-33] The calculation should be made during a time period when the patient's glucose has been stable. It is also important to remember to give the subcutaneous insulin before stopping the insulin infusion to allow the subcutaneous insulin time to work. The amount of time overlap depends on the subcutaneous insulin preparation. Longer acting insulin needs a couple of hours to begin to work, whereas short- or rapid-acting insulin will only need about an hour. The preference is to convert over to a basal bolus regimen with a long-acting insulin and meal time insulin.[26] The majority of patients without a prior history of diabetes receiving an insulin infusion at a rate of 1 U/h or less at the time of transition may not require a scheduled subcutaneous insulin regimen.[34,35]

Differences in Diabetes Management Depending on Type of Diabetes Mellitus
Type 1 Diabetes Mellitus

Type 1 diabetics admitted to the hospital for a neurosurgical procedure should be continued on their outpatient regimen. It is important to remember that these patients require either a continuous insulin infusion or basal bolus insulin administration to prevent the development of diabetic ketoacidosis. This is imperative even when they are not eating. In a study of patients with type 1 diabetes, patients who received their full dose of long-acting insulin (glargine insulin) on a fasting day were compared with those obtained on a control day when the patients were eating their usual meals.[36] There were no significant differences in the mean blood glucose levels between the two days, suggesting it is safe to administer the full dose of basal insulin when the patient is NPO.

However, the Endocrine Society guidelines state that for type 1 diabetes who are well controlled, mild reductions of 10–20% in dosing of basal insulin are suggested to prevent hypoglycemia. For patients who are uncontrolled (blood glucose >200 mg/dL), full doses of basal insulin can be administered.[29] This is largely based on expert opinion and seems reasonable.

It is also important to recognize that there are slight pharmacokinetic differences in the long-acting and intermediate-acting (NPH) insulins. NPH insulin can peak and lead to hypoglycemia. Therefore, the patient on NPH insulin should have a 25–50% reduction of their NPH dose to prevent hypoglycemia.[29]

For short surgical procedures (<2 hours), patients can stay on their basal insulin. In addition, they require correctional dose insulin. For longer procedures, it is reasonable to use a continuous insulin infusion with frequent monitoring of blood sugars.

Patients on insulin pumps can remain on their pumps with self-management as long as they have the cognitive and physical skills needed to successfully self-administer insulin. For longer surgical procedures, it is appropriate that the patient be placed on a continuous insulin infusion.

Type 2 Diabetes Mellitus

Type 2 diabetics are a more heterogeneous and diverse population. Therefore there is a wide variation in the management of their disease. Some patients are only on diet modification, while others are on large doses of insulin.

For patients who are diet-controlled, it is reasonable to monitor their blood sugars before meals and start insulin therapy if they exceed the prespecified glucose targets outlined earlier. It is recommended that this be in the form of a long-acting basal insulin with rapid-acting meal time insulin.[26,29] For patients who are NPO or have poor oral intake, it is reasonable to use a long-acting basal insulin plus bolus correction insulin. If the patient is eating but the intake is poor or unpredictable, one can administer the rapid-acting insulin immediately after the meal.

A randomized controlled trial by Umpierrez et al. has shown that basal-bolus treatment improved glycemic control and reduced hospital complications compared with sliding scale insulin in general surgery patients with type 2 diabetes.[37] Therefore, most guidelines strongly recommend against the prolonged sole use of sliding scale insulin in the inpatient setting.[26,29]

Most guidelines argue against the use of oral diabetic medications in the inpatient setting. There are only a few small studies investigating their use. In addition, many of the agents have undesirable side effects that can be particularly deleterious in the inpatient setting. For example, metformin has been associated with lactic acidosis in the inpatient setting. It therefore must be discontinued in states associated with lactic acidosis, such as decompensated congestive heart failure, renal insufficiency, hypoperfusion, or chronic pulmonary disease.[38] It can also cause significant gastrointestinal side effects. Sulfonylureas have high potential to cause hypoglycemia, particularly the elderly, those with impaired hepatic or renal function, and in patients who have inconsistent oral intake.[39] There are also no data on the shorter acting insulin secretagogues repaglinide and nateglinide, however they certainly carry similar risks as sulfonylureas. SGLT-2 agents can cause diabetic ketoacidosis, urinary tract infections, and kidney injury. Thiazolidinediones can cause fluid retention and may precipitate heart failure. The onset of their glucose lowering action takes weeks and therefore limits their ability to lower glucose acutely.

DPP-IV inhibitors and GLP-1 analogues have been studied in the inpatient setting. For example, a small pilot study reported that a dipeptidyl peptidase 4 inhibitor alone or in combination with basal insulin was well tolerated and resulted in similar glucose control and frequency of hypoglycemia compared with a basal-bolus regimen.[40,41] However, proof of safety and efficacy in larger patient populations awaits the results of randomized controlled trials.

For type 2 diabetics admitted for surgery, it is recommended that they discontinue all their oral and non-insulin injectable agents before surgery with the initiation of insulin therapy in those who develop hyperglycemia as defined earlier.[29] For insulin-requiring type 2 diabetics, it is recommended that they reduce their basal insulin dose by approximately 50% when made NPO. This was shown to be safe in one nonrandomized study.[42] Postoperatively, they should remain on a basal bolus regimen until stable for discharge.

Medical Nutrition Therapy

Medical nutrition therapy (MNT) is an important component of inpatient glycemic management programs.[26,29] MNT is defined as a process of nutritional assessment and individualized meal planning in consultation with a nutrition professional.[29] The goals of inpatient MNT are to optimize glycemic control, to provide adequate calories to meet metabolic demands, and to create a discharge plan for follow-up care.[29] Consistent carbohydrate meal plans are preferred by many hospitals as they facilitate matching the prandial insulin dose to the amount of carbohydrate consumed.[43] Regarding enteral nutritional therapy, diabetes-specific formulas appear to be superior to standard formulas in controlling postprandial glucose, A1c, and the insulin response.[44]

Glucocorticoids

Glucocorticoids are commonly used in the neurosurgical patient, and they pose a significant challenge to the achievement of glucose goals. Hyperglycemia occurs in 20–50% of patients without a previous history of diabetes.[29,45] Glucocorticoids increase hepatic glucose production, stimulate the production of precursors for gluconeogenesis, and impair glucose uptake in the peripheral tissues.[46] They tend to induce mainly postprandial hyperglycemia, with peaks of glucose occurring in the afternoon and evening when given once daily.

Several approaches have been proposed for the treatment of glucocorticoid-induced hyperglycemia, but no published studies have investigated the efficacy of these approaches head to head.[26,29] It is important to consider which glucocorticoid

is being used, the dose, and the frequency of administration. For example, prednisone is short-acting and tends to peak in about 4–8 hours. If it is given daily, one can
use intermediate-acting NPH insulin in the morning to offset the hyperglycemic potential of this agent.[47] Longer acting glucocorticoids such as dexamethasone, or frequent administration of any glucocorticoid, often necessitate higher doses of longer
acting insulin.[48] Also, increasing doses of prandial and correctional insulin are often
necessary. The use of a continuous glucose infusion in patients on high glucocorticoid doses has been shown to result in rapid and sustained glycemic control.[49]

Whatever glucocorticoid is used, it is imperative to monitor glucose and adjust
the insulin dosages accordingly. This is particularly important during reductions or
discontinuation of glucocorticoid therapy which has been associated with increased
risk of developing hypoglycemia.[29]

Enteral/Parenteral Feedings

A significant percentage of critically ill patients require enteral tube (EN) feeding
or even parenteral feeding (PN). There are several retrospective and prospective
studies showing that the use of EN and PN is an independent risk factor for hyperglycemia independent of a prior history of diabetes.[50,51] In these cases, there is a paucity of data regarding the optimal method of glucose management. Diabetes-specific
formulations have been shown to lower blood glucose slightly, however, a majority
of patients will still need insulin therapy.

Insulin should be divided into basal, prandial, and correctional components.
It is very important that there is always a basal component for any type 1 diabetic to prevent diabetic ketoacidosis if EN is discontinued.[26,29] Several strategies
can be used. They should be tailored to the patient and the EN delivery method
(Table 10.2).

For patients on PN, regular insulin added to the PN solution has been shown
to be safe and effective (Table 10.2). In addition, subcutaneous correctional dose
insulin should be used.[26,29] The dose of insulin added to the PN solution can be
adjusted based on the correctional dose requirements. Endocrine Society guidelines
also state that the initial use of a separate insulin infusion can help estimate the total
daily dose of insulin that will be required.

Hypoglycemia

Hypoglycemia is associated with an increased risk of mortality in various hospitalized
patient populations.[52] It may be a marker of underlying disease rather than the cause
of increased mortality; however, it is prudent to avoid hypoglycemia in the management of hyperglycemia.[26,29]

The American Diabetes Association defines three levels of hypoglycemia. Level 1
is a glucose level of less than 70 mg/dL but greater than or equal to 54 mg/dL.
Level 2 is a glucose of less than 54 mg/dL, and level 3 is considered a severe event
characterized by altered mental and/or physical status requiring assistance.[26]

Table 10.2 Diabetes mellitus management in the neurosurgical patient receiving enteral tube feeding (TF) or parenteral nutrition

Type of nutrition	Basal insulin	Bolus insulin	Comments
Continuous TF	Continuous IV insulin infusion until patient reaches goal TF. This will be TDD* of insulin for that TF rate. Basal insulin will be 30–40% of the TDD in the form of glargine daily or NPH/detemir BID	Bolus: Regular insulin every 6 hours with regular insulin correction.	Patients with DM1 always require basal insulin. If TF is interrupted, DM1 patients will still require basal insulin. For DM2 patients, 5% or 10% dextrose should be given as infusion if TF interrupted, bolus insulin held, and basal insulin should be reduced. ADA recommends basal insulin plus rapid-acting correctional insulin every 4 hours for continuous TF.
Nocturnal TF	NPH and regular insulin given before TF	Can use correction dose rapid-acting insulin during TF.	Give an AM dose of NPH as well in insulin requiring DM2, DM1, and patients on glucocorticoids.
Bolus TF	Glargine daily or Detemir/NPH BID	Rapid-acting insulin with the TF bolus	
Parenteral	Add regular insulin to TPN bottle.	Rapid-acting correction dose insulin	

From Daniel R, Villuri S, Furlong K, et al. Management of hyperglycemia in the neurosurgery patient. *Hosp Pract.* 2017;45(4):150–157.

* TDD = total daily dose of insulin.

In one study, 84% of patient with an episode of hypoglycemia of less than 40 mg/dL had a prior episode of hypoglycemia of less than 70 mg/dL during the same admission.[54] In another study, 78% of patients with hypoglycemia were using basal insulin with the incidence of hypoglycemia peaking between midnight and 6 AM. Despite these episodes of hypoglycemia, 75% of patients did not have their dose of basal insulin adjusted.[55]

The key predictors of hypoglycemic events in hospitalized patients include older age, greater illness severity (presence of septic shock, mechanical ventilation, renal failure, malignancy, and malnutrition), diabetes, and the use of oral glucose-lowering medications and insulin.[56] There are preventable sources of iatrogenic hypoglycemia, such as improper prescribing of hypoglycemic medications, inappropriate management of the first episode of hypoglycemia, and nutrition–insulin mismatch.[26] Preventative therapies including proactive surveillance or glycemic outliers can reduce hypoglycemic episodes. Two such studies found that hypoglycemic events fell by 56% to 80%.[57,58]

Discharge Planning

The Agency for Healthcare Research and Quality and the American Diabetes Association recommend that discharge plans include the following[26,58]:

- The patient's medications must be cross-checked to ensure that no chronic medications were stopped and to ensure the safety of new prescriptions.
- Prescriptions for new or changed medication should be filled and reviewed with the patient and family at or before discharge.
- Information on medication changes, pending tests and studies, and follow-up needs must be accurately and promptly communicated to outpatient physicians.

The American Diabetes Association recommends that the following areas of knowledge be reviewed and addressed prior to hospital discharge[26]:

- Identification of the healthcare provider who will provide diabetes care after discharge.
- Level of understanding related to the diabetes diagnosis, self-monitoring of blood glucose, home blood glucose goals, and when to call the provider.
- Definition, recognition, treatment, and prevention of hyperglycemia and hypoglycemia.
- Information on making healthy food choices at home and referral to an outpatient registered dietitian nutritionist to guide individualization of meal plan, if needed.
- If relevant, when and how to take blood glucose-lowering medications, including insulin administration.
- Sick day management.
- Proper use and disposal of needles and syringes.

REFERENCES

1. Capes S, Hunt D, Malmberg K, et al. Stress hyperglycemia and prognosis of stroke in nondiabetic and diabetic patients: a systematic overview. *Stroke.* 2001;32(10):2426–2432.
2. Jeremitsky E, Omert L, Dunham C, et al. The impact of hyperglycemia on patients with severe brain injury. *J Trauma.* 2005;58(1):47–50.
3. McCowen K, Malhotra A, Bistrian B. Stress-induced hyperglycemia. *Crit Care Clin.* 2001;17(1):107–124.
4. Nylen E, Muller B. Endocrine changes in critical illness. *J Intensive Care Med.* 2004;19(2):67–82.
5. Atkins J, Smith D. A review of perioperative glucose control in the neurosurgical population. *J Diabetes Sci Technol.* 2009;3(6):1352–1364.
6. Van Den Berghe G, Wouters P, Weekers F, et al. Intensive insulin therapy in critically ill patients. *N Engl J Med.* 2001;345:1359–1367.
7. Brunkhorst F, Engel C, Bloos F, et al. Intensive insulin therapy and pentastarch resuscitation in severe sepsis. *N Engl J Med.* 2008;358(2): 125–139.
8. Preiser J, Devos P, Ruiz-Santana S, et al. A prospective randomised multi-centre controlled trial on tight glucose control by intensive insulin therapy in adult intensive care units: the Glucontrol study. *Intensive Care Med.* 2009;35(10): 1738–1748.
9. Finfer S, Chittock D, Su S, et al. Intensive versus conventional glucose control in critically ill patients. *N Engl J Med.* 2009;360(13):1283–1297.
10. Mathioudakis N, Golden S. A comparison of inpatient glucose management guidelines: Implications for patient safety and quality. *Curr Diab Rep.* 2015;15:13.
11. Pulsinelli W, Levy D, Sigsbee B, et al. Increased damage after ischemic stroke in patients with hyperglycemia with or without established diabetes mellitus. *Am J Med.* 1983;74(4):540–554.
12. Parsons M, Barber P, Desmond P, et al. Acute hyperglycemia adversely affects stroke outcome: a magnetic resonance imaging and spectroscopy study. *Ann Neurol.* 2002;52(1):20–28.
13. Bruno A, Kent T, Coull B, et al. Treatment of hyperglycemia in ischemic stroke (THIS): a randomized pilot trial. *Stroke.* 2008;39(2):384–389.
14. Rosso C, Corvol J, Pires C, et al. Intensive versus subcutaneous insulin in patients with hyperacute stroke: results from the randomized INSULINFARCT trial. *Stroke.* 2012;43(9):2343–2349.
15. Powers W, Rabinstein A, Ackerson T, et al. 2018 Guidelines for the early management of patients with acute ischemic stroke. *Stroke.* 2018;49. It is on page e79 accessed at https://www.ahajournals.org/doi/pdf/10.1161/STR.0000000000000158
16. Thiele R, Pouratian N, Zuo Z, et al. Strict glucose control does not affect mortality after aneurysmal subarachnoid hemorrhage. *Anesthesiology.* 2009;110(3):603–610.
17. Godoy D, Piñero G, Svampa S, et al. Hyperglycemia and short-term outcome in patients with spontaneous intracerebral hemorrhage. *Neurocrit Care.* 2008;9(2):217–229.
18. Coester A, Neumann C, Schmidt M. Intensive insulin therapy in severe traumatic brain injury: a randomized trial. *J Trauma.* 2010;68:904–911.
19. Bilotta F, Caramia R, Cernak I, et al. Intensive insulin therapy after severe traumatic brain injury: a randomized clinical trial. *Neurocrit Care.* 2008;9:159–166.
20. Yang M, Guo Q, Zhang X, et al. Intensive insulin therapy on infection rate, days in NICU, in-hospital mortality and neurological outcome in severe traumatic brain injury patients: a randomized controlled trial. *Int J Nurs Stud.* 2009;46:753–758.

21. Wang Y, Li J, Song Y, et al. Intensive insulin therapy for preventing postoperative infection in patients with traumatic brain injury. *Medicine*. 2017;96:13(e6458).

22. Meng F, Cao J, Meng X. Risk factors for surgical site infections following spinal surgery. *J Clin Neurosci*. 2015;22(12):1862–1866.

23. Hikata T, Iwanami A, Hosogane N, et al. High preoperative hemoglobin A1c is a risk factor for surgical site infection after posterior thoracic and lumbar spinal instrumentation surgery. *J Orthop Sci*. 2014;19(2):223–228.

24. Kao L, Meeks D, Moyer V, et al. Perioperative glycaemic control regimens for preventing surgical site infections in adults. *Cochrane Database Syst Rev*. 2009;(3):1–24.

25. McGirt M, Chaichana K, Gathinji M, et al. Persistent outpatient hyperglycemia is independently associated with decreased survival after primary resection of malignant brain astrocytomas. *Neurosurgery*. 2008;63(2):286–291.

26. American Diabetes Association.15. Diabetes care in the hospital: standards of medical care in diabetes–2019. *Diabetes Care*. 2019;42(Suppl. 1):S173–S181.

27. Sathya B, Davis R, Taveira T, et al. Intensity of perioperative glycemic control and postoperative outcomes in patients with diabetes: a meta-analysis. *Diabetes Res Clin Pract*. 2013;102:8–15.

28. Umpierrez G, Cardona S, Pasquel F, et al. Randomized controlled trial of intensive versus conservative glucose control in patients undergoing coronary artery bypass graft surgery: GLUCO-CABG trial. *Diabetes Care*. 2015;38:1665–1672.

29. Umpierrez G, Hellman R, Korytkowski M, et al. Management of hyperglycemia in hospitalized patients in non-critical care setting: an Endocrine Society clinical practice guideline. *J Clin Endocrinol Metab*. 2012;97:16–38.

30. Stamler J, Vaccaro O, Neaton J, Wentworth D. Diabetes, other risk factors, and 12-year cardiovascular mortality for men screened in the Multiple Risk Factor Intervention Trial. *Diabetes Care*. 1993;16(2):434.

31. Moghissi E, Korytkowski M, DiNardo M, et al.; American Association of Clinical Endocrinologists; American Diabetes Association. American Association of Clinical Endocrinologists and American Diabetes Association consensus statement on inpatient glycemic control. *Diabetes Care*. 2009;32:1119–1131.

32. Umpierrez G, Korytkowski M. Diabetic emergencies-ketoacidosis, hyperglycaemic hyperosmolar state and hypoglycaemia. *Nat Rev Endocrinol*. 2016;12:222–232.

33. Shomali M, Herr D, Hill P, et al. Conversion from intravenous insulin to subcutaneous insulin after cardiovascular surgery: transition to target study. *Diabetes Technol Ther*. 2011;13:121–126.

34. Maynard G, Lee J, Phillips G, et al. Improved inpatient use of basal insulin, reduced hypoglycemia, and improved glycemic control: effect of structured subcutaneous insulin orders and an insulin management algorithm. *J Hosp Med*. 2009;4:3–15.

35. Ramos P, Childers D, Maynard G, et al. Maintaining glycemic control when transitioning from infusion insulin: a protocol-driven, multidisciplinary approach. *J Hosp Med*. 2010;5:446–451.

36. Mucha G, Merkel S, Thomas W, Bantle J. Fasting and insulin glargine in individuals with type 1 diabetes. *Diabetes Care*. 2004;27:1209–1210.

37. Umpierrez G, Smiley D, Jacobs S, et al. Randomized study of basal-bolus insulin therapy in the inpatient management of patients with type 2 diabetes undergoing general surgery (RABBIT 2 surgery). *Diabetes Care*. 2011;34:256–261.

38. Calabrese A, Coley K, DaPos S, et al. Evaluation of prescribing practices: risk of lactic acidosis with metformin therapy. *Arch Intern Med*. 2002;162:434–437.

39. Bolen S, Feldman L, Vassy J, et al. Systematic review: comparative effectiveness and safety of oral medications for type 2 diabetes mellitus. *Ann Intern Med.* 2007;147:386–399.

40. Umpierrez G, Gianchandani R, Smiley D, et al. Safety and efficacy of sitagliptin therapy for the inpatient management of general medicine and surgery patients with type2 diabetes: a pilot, randomized, controlled study. *Diabetes Care.* 2013;36:3430–3435.

41. Pasquel F, Gianchandani R, Rubin D, et al. Efficacy of sitagliptin for the hospital management of general medicine and surgery patients with type 2 diabetes (Sita-Hospital): a multicentre, prospective, open-label, non-inferiority randomised trial. *Lancet Diabetes Endocrinol.* 2017;5:125–133.

42. DiNardo M, Donihi A, Forte P, et al. Standardized glycemic management improves perioperative glycemic outcomes in same day surgery patients with diabetes. *Endocr Pract.* 2011;17:404–411.

43. Curll M, Dinardo M, Noschese M, Korytkowski M. Menu selection, glycaemic control and satisfaction with standard and patient-controlled consistent carbohydrate meal plans in hospitalised patients with diabetes. *Qual Saf Health Care.* 2010;19:355–359.

44. Ojo O, Brooke J. Evaluation of the role of enteral nutrition in managing patients with diabetes: a systematic review. *Nutrients.* 2014;6:5142–5152.

45. Clore J, Thurby-Hay L. Glucocorticoid-induced hyperglycemia. *Endocr Pract.* 2009;15:469–474.

46. Schade D, Eaton R. The temporal relationship between endogenously secreted stress hormones and metabolic decompensation in diabetic man. *J Clin Endocrinol Metab.* 1980;50:131–136.

47. Kwon S, Hermayer K, Hermayer K. Glucocorticoid-induced hyperglycemia. *Am J Med Sci.* 2013;345:274–277.

48. Brady V, Thosani S, Zhou S, et al. Safe and effective dosing of basal bolus insulin in patients receiving high-dose steroids for hyper-cyclophosphamide, doxorubicin, vincristine, and dexamethasone chemotherapy. *Diabetes Technol Ther.* 2014;16:874–879.

49. Smiley D, Rhee M, Peng L, et al. 2010 Safety and efficacy of continuous insulin infusion in non- critical care settings. *J Hosp Med.* 2010;5:212–217.

50. Umpierrez G 2009 Basal versus sliding-scale regular insulin in hospitalized patients with hyperglycemia during enteral nutrition therapy. *Diabetes Care.* 2009;32:751–753.

51. Pancorbo-Hidalgo P, García-Fernandez F, Ramírez-Pe´rez C. Complications associated with enteral nutrition by nasogastric tube in an internal medicine unit. *J Clin Nurs.* 2001;10:482–490.

52. Daniel R, Villuri S, Furlong K, et al. Management of hyperglycemia in the neurosurgery patient. *Hosp Pract.* 2017;45(4):150–157.

53. Akirov A, Grossman A, Shochat T, Shimon I. Mortality among hospitalized patients with hypoglycemia: insulin related and noninsulin related. *J Clin Endocrinol Metab.* 2017;102:416–424.

54. Dendy JA, Chockalingam V, Tirumalasetty NN, et al. Identifying risk factors for severe hypoglycemia in hospitalized patients with diabetes. *Endocr Pract.* 2014;20:1051–1056.

55. Ulmer BJ, Kara A, Mariash CN. Temporal occurrences and recurrence patterns of hypoglycemia during hospitalization. *Endocr Pract.* 2015;21:501–507.

56. Krinsley JS, Grover A. Severe hypoglycemia in critically ill patients: risk factors and outcomes. *Crit Care Med.* 2007;35:2262–2267.

57. Maynard G, Kulasa K, Ramos P, et al. Impact of a hypoglycemia reduction bundle and a systems approach to inpatient glycemic management. *Endocr Pract.* 2015;21:355–367.

58. Milligan P, Bocox M, Pratt E, et al. Multifaceted approach to reducing occurrence of severe hypoglycemia in a large healthcare system. *Am J Health Syst Pharm.* 2015;72:1631–1641.

59. American Diabetes Association.15. Diabetes care in the hospital: standards of medical care in diabetes–2019. *Diabetes Care.* 2019;42(Suppl. 1):S173–S181.

11 Management of Pressure Injuries in Neurosurgical Patients

Rene Daniel and Babak Abai

INTRODUCTION

Pressure injury (PI) is a challenging problem for patients and physicians alike. It is a socioeconomic burden that plagues many patients with disabilities in the acute care setting and long-term care setting, as well as at home. Each year 2.5 million patients in US acute care facilities develop pressure injuries.[1,2] Since some will develop more than one PI, the incidence is likely higher. Per Joint Commission and other sources, PIs result in approximately 60,000 deaths per year.[2,3] There are about 17,000 lawsuits filed each year that cite hospital-acquired pressure injuries (HAPIs).[1,3] The economic cost of treatment of HAPIs is staggering and reaches $11 billion per year in the United States.[1,3] The cost ranges from $20,900 to $151,700[3] per patient, with average of $43,181. This adds significantly to the cost of hospital stay per Medicare.[1,3] In addition, there is an incalculable amount of human suffering involved as patients grapple with loss of integument, pain, infection, sepsis, and death. Given the human and economic costs, prevention is the number one approach to management of PI.

There are intrinsic and extrinsic risk factors to developing PI. The intrinsic factors include tissue hypoxemia, hypovolemia, older age, altered level of consciousness, and/or sensory impairment (due to stroke or spinal cord injury [SCI]) and others.[4] The extrinsic factors include immobility, hospital length of stay, and more.[4] The American College of Physicians (ACP) guideline on risk assessment and prevention of pressure ulcers also notes, among others, the risks of cognitive and physical impairment and comorbid conditions such as fecal or urinary incontinence and diabetes mellitus.[5]

Among SCI patients, a study by Margolis et al. found that between 30% and 50% of SCI patients develop PI during the first month post injury.[4,6] PIs are among the most common reasons for readmission among patients suffering from SCI.[7] A study by Han et al. that aimed to identify PI predictors among 34,287 admitted patients older than 65 years found that the level of consciousness was the most important variable and that drowsy patients were 3.77 times more likely to develop PIs than were alert patients.[8]

Patients with SCIs and brain injuries, both traumatic and nontraumatic, are the major focus of neurosurgeons and neurosurgery hospitalists. Sensory impairment and altered mental status are common conditions found among these patients. Brienza et al. demonstrated that SCI patients with a higher severity of injury are at increased risk of developing PI than are patients with a lower severity.[9] In addition, patients with a higher level of spinal cord lesion appear to be more at risk than patients with a lower level of lesion.[10,11]

Taken together, neurosurgery patients are at elevated risk for PI formation, and the presence of PI can lead to adverse outcome. A study published in 2015 demonstrated that the presence of preoperative PIs results in elevated risk of adverse effects following major surgery (e.g., septicemia, stroke, pneumonia, and urinary tract infection [UTI]).[12] Another retrospective study of stroke patients with preexisting PI showed increased poststroke mortality and increased risk for UTI, pneumonia, gastrointestinal bleeding, and epilepsy when compared to patients without PI.[13] Thus, PI presence and development among neurosurgery patients is a critical issue affecting the outcomes of neurosurgery patients.

In this chapter, we review prevention of and treatment approaches to PIs among patients admitted for neurosurgical procedure. The pathophysiology, staging, prevention, and management of PIs are addressed in general and also in regards to neurosurgical patients. In this way, we hope to provide a useful guide for neurosurgery hospitalists and other providers involved in the care of neurosurgery patients. Several guidelines for prevention and treatment of PIs have been developed. In this review, we focus on the National Pressure Ulcer Advisory Panel (NPUAP) guideline, the ACP guidelines for prevention and treatment of PIs, and an SCI guideline.[5,14–16] We point out similarities and differences among these guidelines, and we provide an update and recommendations as appropriate, based on the published studies.

DEFINITION OF PRESSURE INJURY

The NPUAP is responsible for the development of definitions and staging of pressure-related wounds in the United States. In 2016, NPUAP changed the terminology from the term "pressure ulcer" to "pressure injury."[15,17] PI is defined by NPUAP as "localized damage to the skin and/or underlying soft tissue usually over a bony prominence or related to a medical or other device. The injury can present as intact skin or an open ulcer and may be painful. The injury occurs as a result of intense and/or prolonged pressure or pressure in combination with shear." NPUAP made recent changes in staging terminology as well.

PATHOPHYSIOLOGY OF PRESSURE INJURY

Before we can discuss staging, prevention, and treatment, it is important to look at the pathophysiology of this type of skin and soft tissue damage. There are four components that lead to this type of injury: pressure, friction, shear, and moisture.

The external pressure on areas of bony prominence with small amounts of overlying tissue in an immobile patient causes ischemia to the tissues. The pressure can exceed capillary perfusion pressure, and it will stop the flow of blood, oxygen, and nutrients. The tissues are able to tolerate this for a short period of time, but sustained pressure between 30–240 minutes will lead to pressure injury.[18] A combination of soft tissue and skin ischemia as well as reperfusion injury leads to PI.

Friction occurs when the skin comes into rough contact with the bed sheets, gowns, or other clothing. The friction can help trigger PI by causing breaks in the epidermis. It can damage weakened skin and lead to further tissue injury.

Shear forces are created when two surfaces move in opposing directions. This usually occurs when the patient is placed on an incline or during moving the patient from bed to stretcher. As gravity pulls the patient's body down, the bed surface pulls the skin and soft tissue in the opposite direction. This added stress contributes to the formation of a PI.

Skin moisture is a less appreciated contributing factor. The skin can be compromised if it is wet. This is especially true if the fluid is urine or loose feces with incontinence. Perspiration can also have a similar but less caustic effect on the skin. These lead to skin maceration and can result in the initiation of ulceration.

STAGING OF PRESSURE INJURIES

Development of a PI is a progressive process, with the PI becoming deeper and more extensive if the cause is not addressed and the healing process and/or treatment does not commence. In order to determine PI severity, a staging classification was developed by NPUAP. NPUAP made recent changes in staging terminology: Arabic numbers replaced the Roman numbers which were used previously to describe states of pressure ulcers (now PI). NPUAP also removed the word "suspected" from the Suspected Deep Pressure Injury (see later discussion).[15,17]

Staging of PI is essential for both prevention and treatment. It is important to note that once PI is staged, its classification does not change. For example, Stage 3 PI will stay Stage 3 even if it starts improving and heals following initiation of treatment. The reason for this rule is the fact that different stages of PI heal in a different manner. For example, restoration of tissue layers occurs only in Stage 1 PIs, whereas Stage 3 PI heals by a process involving granulation and tissue remodeling.[14] Thus, relabeling of the stage of PI would lead to mischaracterization of the process and ultimately misunderstanding of the tissue composition at the base of the healed PI. This could eventually lead to improper evaluation of the site should PI or any other injury recur there.

Stages of Pressure Injury per NPUAP Staging System

Stage 1 PI is defined by NPUAP[15,17] as "non-blanchable erythema of intact skin." The full description is as follows: "Intact skin with a localized area of non-blanchable

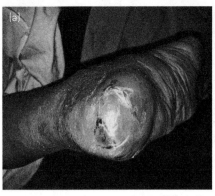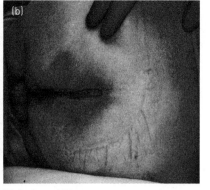

FIGURE 11.1 Stage 2 pressure injury (PI). A. Heel PI. B. Sacral PI.

erythema, which may appear differently in darkly pigmented skin. Presence of blanchable erythema or changes in sensation, temperature, or firmness may precede visual changes. Color changes do not include purple or maroon discoloration; these may indicate deep tissue pressure injury."

Stage 2 PI is defined as "partial-thickness loss of skin with exposed dermis (Figure 11.1). The wound bed is viable, pink or red, moist, and may also present as an intact or ruptured serum-filled blister. Adipose (fat) is not visible and deeper tissues are not visible. Granulation tissue, slough and eschar are not present. These injuries commonly result from adverse microclimate and shear in the skin over the pelvis and shear in the heel. This stage should not be used to describe moisture associated skin damage (MASD) including incontinence associated dermatitis (IAD), intertriginous dermatitis (ITD), medical adhesive related skin injury (MARSI), or traumatic wounds (skin tears, burns, abrasions)."

Stage 3 PI is defined as "full-thickness loss of skin, in which adipose (fat) is visible in the ulcer and granulation tissue and epibole (rolled wound edges) are often present (Figure 11.2). Slough and/or eschar may be visible. The depth of tissue damage varies by anatomical location; areas of significant adiposity can develop deep wounds. Undermining and tunneling may occur. Fascia, muscle, tendon, ligament, cartilage and/or bone are not exposed. If slough or eschar obscures the extent of tissue loss this is an Unstageable Pressure Injury."

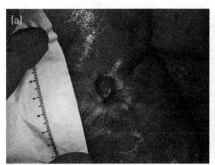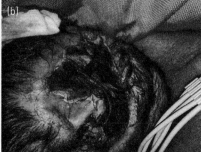

FIGURE 11.2 Stage 3 pressure injury (PI). A. Ischial PI. B. Scalp PI.

Stage 4 PI shows "Full-thickness skin and tissue loss with exposed or directly palpable fascia, muscle, tendon, ligament, cartilage or bone in the ulcer (Figure 11.3). Slough and/or eschar may be visible. Epibole (rolled edges), undermining and/or tunneling often occur. Depth varies by anatomical location. If slough or eschar obscures the extent of tissue loss this is an Unstageable Pressure Injury."

Unstageable PI is characterized as "full-thickness skin and tissue loss in which the extent of tissue damage within the ulcer cannot be confirmed because it is *obscured by slough or eschar* (Figure 11.3). If slough or eschar is removed, a Stage 3 or Stage 4 pressure injury will be revealed. Stable eschar (i.e., dry, adherent, intact without erythema or fluctuance) on the heel or ischemic limb should not be softened or removed."

Deep Tissue PI is defined as "intact or non-intact skin with localized area of persistent non-blanchable deep red, maroon, purple discoloration or epidermal separation revealing a dark wound bed or blood filled blister. Pain and temperature change often precede skin color changes. Discoloration may appear differently in darkly pigmented skin. This injury results from intense and/or prolonged pressure and shear forces at the bone-muscle interface. The wound may evolve rapidly to reveal the actual extent of tissue injury, or may resolve without tissue loss. If necrotic tissue, subcutaneous tissue, granulation tissue, fascia, muscle or other underlying structures are visible, this indicates a full thickness pressure injury (Unstageable, Stage 3 or Stage 4). Do not use DTPI to describe vascular, traumatic, neuropathic, or dermatologic conditions."

NPUAP guideline also notes *medical device–related PI*, which is due to a pressure exerted by a diagnostic or treatment device. It should be staged as above. Finally, *mucous membrane PI* is found on mucous membranes and is associated with the use of medical devices at its location. This PI cannot be staged due to its anatomy.

Staging is usually performed by the nursing staff, when patient is evaluated at admission, or in the emergency department. Nevertheless, the hospitalist must be

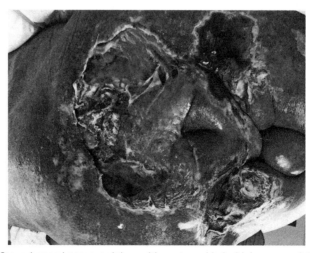

FIGURE 11.3 Stage 4 sacral pressure injury with unstageable ischial pressure injuries.

able to perform staging as well. This is particularly important if a doubt arises with respect to the staging. This latter occurrence is not uncommon, since later stage PIs may involve tunneling and other defects that may not be readily apparent to less experienced staff.

GENERAL RULES OF THE MANAGEMENT OF PRESSURE INJURIES
Risk Assessment

Management of PIs starts with identifying patients at high risk for PI development. NPUAP notes a role for comorbidities, perfusion, nutrition, and microclimate.[15] A number of additional risk factors were identified by multiple studies.[3,4,9–11] These are listed in the Table 11.1; they are, for the purpose of this chapter, divided between general and preoperative, intraoperative, and postoperative factors.[3] Neurosurgery patients are at a high risk for PI formation. This is due to the presence of general risk factors in these patients (immobility, altered consciousness) as well as to specific reasons, such as autonomous dysfunction and abnormalities of microcirculation in SCI patients.[4,14] In Table 11.1, we highlight those risk factors that are related to spinal cord and brain injured (altered cognition) patients.

Given the multiple risk factors, risk assessment tools have been developed to aid the clinical judgment of the PI-assessing healthcare provider. The general tools include the Braden scale, the Norton scale, and the Waterflow scale (see Table 11.2).[5] The widely used Braden scale measures mobility, activity, sensory perception, skin moisture, nutrition state, and friction/tear. The Braden scale ranges from 6 to 23 points, with a lower score indicating higher risk.[5]

In addition to general tools, a variety of scales were developed to evaluate PI risk in specific settings and patients. The Cubbin and Jackson scale is used to evaluate PI risk in intensive care patients.[5] The Braden scale does not fully measure PI risk for surgical patients since it does not assess certain perioperative risks.[3] Thus, the Munro scale and the Scott Triggers tool were developed to include the length of surgery and comorbidities.[3] These scales are also in wide use. Finally, for SCI patients, Salzberg et al. developed the Spinal Cord Injury Pressure Ulcer Scale (SCIPUS).[19] A further development of this scale is SCIPUS-A, which measures the risk of PI development in these patients in the acute hospital setting.[20] SCIPUS-A includes SCI-specific factors, such as the extent of paralysis.[19,20] The Cubbin and Jackson scale, the Munro scale, and the Scott Triggers are also described in Table 11.2.

The common issue linking the use of PI risk assessment tools is their validity. For the Braden scale, the ACP guideline on prevention of pressure ulcers notes a low level of evidence for sensitivity and specificity.[5] Similar findings were reported for other general scales.[5] Likewise, SCIPUS scales also seem to have only limited validity.[14] Nevertheless, the ACP guideline notes that risk assessment tools may be especially helpful if the PI-assessing provider has limited experience.[5]

Table 11.1 Risk factors for development of pressure injuries (PIs)

Preoperative	Intraoperative	Postoperative
Demographic	Manipulation (friction, shearing)	Vasopressors
Age[a]	Positioning and positioning devices	Immobility
		Mechanical Ventilation
Gender(male)[a]	Extended time in operating room	Sedatives
Ethnicity[a]	Anesthesia and sedation agents	Steroids
Marital status(single)[a]	Surgery-specific factors (type of surgery, multiple surgeries, instrumentation)	Length of stay >3 days
Education[a]		Extended stay in ICU
Environment/facility[a]		
	Other factors (hypotension, hypothermia, vasopressors)	
Physical		
SCI[a]		
Level of SCI[a]		
Severity of SCI[a]		
Previous PI		
Skin problems		
Hemodialysis		
Increased Creatinine		
Low Albumin		
Increased C-reactive protein		
Abnormal urea and electrolytes		
Anemia		
Lymphopenia		
Limited mobility[a]		
Decreased general ADLs		
Bladder, bowel and moisture control[a]		
Presence of urinary catheter		
Pain or pain detection impairment		
Diabetes mellitus		
Vascular disease		
Disorders of circulation		
Medications		
Smoking		
Edema		
Chronic wounds		
Malignant tumors		

Table 11.1 Continued

Preoperative	Intraoperative	Postoperative
Low BMI/weight		
Poor nutrition		
Infections		
American Society of Anesthesiologists		
Physical status Classification score of ≥3		
Psychosocial		
Psychological factors (depression/ anxiety,		
negative self-concept, anger, frustration)[a]		
Cognitive impairment[a,b]		
Social factors[a]		
Substance abuse[a]		
Adherence/compliance[a]		

ADL, activities of daily living; BMI, body mass index; SCI, spinal cord injury.

[a]Reported for SCI but likely not exclusive to SCI.

[b]Brain injury–related.

From References 3, 9, 10, 11, 14, and 15.

Table 11.2 PI risk assessment tools

Scale	Reference	Comment
General		
Braden	5	Widely used
Norton	5	
Waterflow	5	
Surgical		
Munro	3	
Scott Triggers	3	
Intensive Care		
Cubbin and Jackson	5	
Spinal Cord Injury		
SCIPUS	18	
SCIPUS-A	19	Acute setting

Prevention

Given the prevalence and incidence of PIs and the complex and often unsuccessful treatment after PIs develop, prevention is the number one approach to manage PIs in both outpatient and inpatient settings. Once risk assessment is done and patients at high risk are identified, several preventive methods are applied. There is a varying level of evidence for the efficacy of each method, as outlined in the following sections.

Pressure Redistribution

Because PIs are due to pressure on the body's surfaces, it is not surprising that pressure redistribution is a major tool of prevention. Two approaches are utilized.

Repositioning Currently, there is no consensus on how often repositioning should occur, although it does appear to depend on specific situations and patients.[5,14,17] The current practice is to turn a patient every 2 hours.[14] The common practice of raising the head of the bed to 30 degrees increases pressure on the sacral area, where most PIs occur.[14] The patient should not be dragged when repositioned, but always lifted, since dragging can increase shear, which may lead to PI.[14] The ACP guideline notes mixed results when repositioning intervals changed compared to usual care, so it does not make specific recommendations in regards to repositioning.[5] Thus, the evidence appears to be insufficient to recommend a change from the usual practice of turning every 2 hours. There are, however, specific concerns related to intraoperative positioning, which are discussed later.

Appropriate Support Surfaces Appropriate support surfaces include mattresses and various other surfaces. Given the supine position that most patients assume when in the hospital, bed mattresses are of major concern. Current evidence suggests that patients at risk of PI development benefit from the use of advanced static mattresses or advanced static overlays.[5] Alternating-air mattresses or overlays are also beneficial but do not appear to be better than advanced static mattresses or overlays, and they are more expensive.[5] Low air loss mattresses produced mixed results in several studies.[5] Therefore, advanced static mattresses or overlays are the preferred support surface for patients at risk of PI development.

Attention should be paid to heel supports, because heels are the second most common place for PI formation after the sacrum.[15] Ideally, heels should be free of the surface of the bed, for example by using foam-based supports under the calves.[15] Donut or ring-based surfaces are strongly discouraged because they increase pressure in certain small areas where they come in the contact with skin.[14,15,17]

For SCI patients, both the SCI guideline and NPUAP encourage the use of individualized seating pressure redistribution systems, although the ACP guideline notes mixed results with these support surfaces.[5,14,15,17]

Specific concerns about support surfaces during a surgical procedure are addressed later.

Inspection

Inspection of skin is crucial to detect early changes that may indicate the development of PI. This should be done twice daily, and more frequently in patients at a high risk of PI formation.[15] The areas of interest are places of bone protuberances, which include the ischium, sacrum, coccyx, greater trochanters, ankles, heels, knees, and occiput.[14] During examination, it is important to assess skin temperature, edema, and change in skin consistency.[15] Skin color is also important, but it may be difficult to assess in dark-skinned individuals,[14,15] so the first three parameters are preferred.

We noted earlier that most PIs occur at the sacrum and heels. However, in SCI patients, most PIs occur at the ischium (28%), followed by sacrum (21%), and trochanter (20%).[14] The areas of interest may thus slightly differ based on the nature of injury and the individual. If PI is detected, it is treated as outlined in the section "Treatment of Pressure Injuries" later in the chapter.

Nutritional Supplementation

Multiple studies demonstrated that malnutrition is associated with increased risk of PI formation.[14,15,21–27] However, there does not seem to be a benefit of adding nutritional supplementation to the standard hospital diet when nutrition is already adequate.[5] To assess nutritional status, several nutritional assessment tools exist. A generic nutrition screening tool, Malnutrition Universal Screening Tool (MUST), is used in acute care, long-term care, and community settings and has proved to be effective.[15] It has high sensitivity (87.3%) and a high negative predictive value (75%) for identifying nutritional risk.[15] However, PI-specific screening tools exist. The MNA tool is the only tool validated for PI patients. The Spinal Nutrition Screening Tool (SNST) was developed for SCI patients.[14] However, the SNST was found to be only marginally better compared to a generic screening tool.[14] In addition, we note that blood albumin levels are used in some risk assessment tools, but this does not correlate with healing in some studies.[14] To our knowledge, no comparison has yet evaluated the MNA, MUST, and SNST.

Thus, we conclude that whereas identification of malnutrition is important for PI prevention and the current tools are useful when assessing malnutrition, at present there is no clear advantage of using one tool over another. The assessment of nutritional status and ensuring adequate nutrition and fluid intake is effective in preventing PI formation and also helps with wound healing.

Dressings, Creams, Lotions, and Cleansers

Not surprisingly, all guidelines recommend keeping skin clean and dry,[15] but the ACP does not provide recommendation or evidence for one dressing over another.[5] Nevertheless, ACP notes that a fatty acid cream proved better than placebo and reduced risk for PIs in two studies.[5,28,29] Likewise, a skin cleanser reduced risk for PIs in patients with incontinence when compared to standard soap and water care.[5,30] Also, a pH-balanced cleanser was shown to be superior to standard hospital soap in some studies.[15] Finally, a continence management plan proved to be useful in some studies.[15] Thus, controlling skin cleanliness and moisture may have a role in prevention of PI development.

Exercise

The role of exercise is not addressed in ACP or NPUAP guidelines. However, it has been noted that participation in athletic activities is associated with less PI development in SCI patients. Thus, maintenance of joint range of motion, physical endurance, and mobility seems to be an appropriate goal for patients who are at risk of PI development.[14] If, through strengthening exercises, the patient can be conditioned to move and readjust body position naturally, he or she is less likely to develop a PI.

Education

At present, there is lack of studies that would indicate that educating patients and caregivers is important for prevention of PI formation. Yet the goal of appropriate education seems obvious.[14,15] Often patients are discharged from hospital with instructions and directions to prevent PI formation, yet they have little understanding of the underlying issues that lead to PI. Thus, readmission of patients due to new PIs is not uncommon.[7] We suggest that education with regards to PI risks and formation is crucial to maintain health status and prevent readmission.

Summary of the Principles of Prevention

Repositioning and appropriate support surfaces play a crucial role in PI prevention. Areas at risk of PI formation must be inspected frequently, and a prompt action should be taken when early signs of PI formation are detected. It is crucial to prevent or address malnutrition in patients at risk of PI formation. Cleansers and creams have a beneficial effect in prevention of PIs. Finally, it makes sense that exercise and appropriate education of patients and caregivers play important roles in preventing PIs, but more evidence is needed to better assess the role of these interventions in PI prevention.

TREATMENT OF PRESSURE INJURIES

The treatment methods of PIs can be roughly divided into medical and surgical methods. We first outline the medical methods, followed by a brief section on the surgical approach to PI treatment.

Removal of Intrinsic and Extrinsic Factors

PI occurs in response to the risk factors outlined earlier. The first step in treatment is addressing those factors that cause PI in the first place. These include both extrinsic factors (pressure, friction, tear) and intrinsic factors (e.g., nutrition, immobility, altered consciousness). Once a pressure ulcer has occurred, it is vital to eliminate the factors that led to its formation. The ACP guideline presents evidence for and against and a comparison of the various support surfaces that are commonly used to alleviate extrinsic factors.[16] However, ACP does not consider the presented evidence sufficient to provide recommendation for any specific support surface.[16] Nevertheless, air-fluidized beds were shown in some studies to reduce pressure ulcer size.[16,31–35] Other commonly used support surfaces include alternating-air beds and low air loss beds.[16]

Wound healing is a consumptive process that requires cellular building blocks that should come from good nutritional status and intake rather than internal catabolic processes. ACP, NPUAP, and SCI guidelines emphasize the importance of nutrition. Protein supplementation was reported to reduce PI size in multiple studies.[16] Positive nitrogen balance is considered crucial.[14,15] Nevertheless, there is not sufficient evidence to provide the optimal dose of proteins or amino acids (as per ACP guidelines). Several markers are used to evaluate nutritional status; these typically include albumin, prealbumin, and transferrin. Because of the long half-life of albumin (20 days), it remains a poor laboratory indicator in the acute setting, but it gives the clinician an indication of long-term nutritional status. Prealbumin and transferrin have a shorter half-life (3 days and 10 days, respectively) than albumin, and they can be used to monitor overall improvements in nutrition in the acute setting.[14] A full nutritional assessment including a diet-focused physical exam as well as a calorie count and consultation with a dietician is beneficial.

Local Wound Treatment

The first step in local wound treatment involves *cleansing the wound.* Normal saline (0.9% NaCl) is usually the agent of choice for this treatment step (as per SCI guidelines). In addition, many solutions with bactericidal properties are available. These are generally not recommended for cleansing of uninfected wound due to their potential cytotoxic effects that can hinder wound healing. However, these solutions are useful if the wound becomes infected (see later discussion).

Wound dressings are selected based on the overall healing objective, the most important being a reduction of wound size.[14,16] Other factors that are involved include, but are not limited to, the nature of the exudate, the presence or absence of infection and odor, and others.[15] ACP recommends two types of dressing: hydrocolloid and foam.[16] These dressings were shown to reduce wound size equally when compared to a plain gauze dressing.[16] Both have absorptive properties that can leach away wound exudate.[15,16] Most dressings should be changed daily, but in certain cases dressings may be changed three times per week.[14]

Adjunctive Therapies

In addition to wound cleansing and appropriate dressing, a number of adjunctive treatment modalities are available. These include electromagnetic therapy, electrical stimulation, light therapy, laser therapy, and negative pressure wound therapy

(NPWT). Based on available evidence, ACP recommends only electrical stimulation, which showed in some studies accelerated wound healing.[16] Interestingly, ACP does not recommend NPWT, which is widely used in treating wounds, including surgical wounds.[16] However, the NPUAP guideline states that NPWT can be useful when used in conjunction with wound debridement.[15] Finally, three recent clinical studies show improved wound healing when wounds are treated with platelet-derived growth factor (PDGF).[15] This evidence was also noted by ACP,[16] but the ACP guideline notes that hydrocolloid and foam dressings are also effective and less expensive than PDGF-soaked dressing.[16] Thus, ACP recommends the use of these dressings over PDGF.

Pain Management

PIs can be associated with severe pain. Changes in the pain level or quality can also indicate PI deterioration/infection or PI healing. Thus, pain assessment is an important part of PI evaluation. There is no specific pain scale when it comes to PIs. Nevertheless, in the neurosurgical populations, two factors need to be considered: first, many of these patients are cognitively impaired and thus may have difficulty in reporting pain. In certain cases, simple questions, such as "Does your pain keep you from sleeping?" can be employed.[15] Second some patients, particularly those with SCI, may have lost nociception in the affected area and have thus lost an important symptom by which to evaluate for PI.

If pain is present, it needs to be managed using both regular pain medications and other specialized approaches. These include less frequent dressing changes, repositioning, and limiting painful procedures, as well as nonmedical approaches such as distraction and conversation.[15]

Treatment of Infection and Osteomyelitis

Most chronic PIs contain bacterial microflora. The amount of bacteria in the wound is its *bioburden*. The presence of bacteria may not affect wound healing even if these bacteria live and proliferate in the wound (referred to as *colonization*). However, colonization may turn into infection, which is characterized by a lack of wound healing and damage to wound tissues.[14] The lack of wound healing may be the only symptom of wound infection.[14] Other signs of infection are malodor, friable granulation tissue, increased pain, heat and drainage, change in the quality of drainage, pocketing or bridging, expanding erythema, increase in wound size, and systemic symptoms such as enlarged lymph nodes, fever, malaise, delirium, and sepsis.[15] The presence of bacteria can be evaluated using a wound swab, but results are often polymicrobial and may reflect only colonization.[15] Treatment of the infected PIs can thus be challenging and is often considered only in cases of a heavy bioburden.[15] Treatment approaches are both local and systemic. At the local level, the PI must be cleansed. Here, antibacterial solutions are often used. One commonly used agent is Dakin solution (sodium hypochlorite). Sulfadiazine and medical-grade honey are also among the preferred agents.[15] However, evidence for each agent is limited, either due to the size of the trials or to its primary use for treatment of other types of wounds.[15]

PIs are a common source of bacteremia (second only to UTIs).[36] Systemic infection, such as bacteremia, cellulitis, or fasciitis or sepsis is an indication for the use of systemic antibiotic therapy according to appropriate guidelines for each type of infection. An infectious disease consult is warranted for more severe types of infection as well as for virulent causes of infection.

A question that often arises is whether to treat chronic osteomyelitis (OM), particularly in the patient with a stage IV sacral ulcer, with antibiotics. A systemic review of the literature by Wong et al. showed that it is crucial to identify sacral OM by bone biopsy before treatment is considered.[37] Even under these conditions, the available evidence supports systemic antibiotic therapy only if the wound can be surgically closed.[37] The length of therapy should be only 2 weeks if OM is limited to the superficial bony cortex, extending to 4–6 weeks if medullary bone is affected.[37] Interestingly, there is no evidence supporting intravenous over oral antibiotics in this case.[37] We note that more evidence is needed to address this issue for OM in other locations. Nevertheless, it seems that indications for use of antibiotics for treatment of PI-associated OM are limited, and an infectious diseases consult is warranted to advise on each individual case.

Debridement

Debridement is the removal of necrotic or devitalized tissue from the wound bed.[14,15] This is necessary to enable healing in underlying healthy tissues. The devitalized tissue also presents a focal point for bacterial growth and infection.[15] There are several methods of debridement.

- *Autolytic debridement* occurs through the action of the body's own autolytic enzymes and its own white blood cells. It typically occurs under an occlusive dressing.
- *Mechanical debridement* typically occurs in the setting of wet-to-dry dressing changes. It can be painful when the dressing is removed, and it may include removal of healthy tissue.[14,15] Once the base of the wound is clean, a wet-to-dry dressing change should be avoided to prevent removal of healing tissues.
- *Enzymatic debridement* utilizes commercially available enzymes that digest necrotic wound tissue. These include collagenase, which degrades collagen, and deoxyribonuclease, which digests DA papain and degrades fibrinous debris.[14,15]
- *Sharp surgical debridement* uses a scalpel, scissors, or a curette to excise necrotic tissues down to the level of healthy and viable tissue.[15] It usually requires anesthesia (see later discussion for more details on the surgical treatment of PIs).[15]
- *Sharp conservative debridement* involves only removal of the devitalized tissue using sharp instruments and does not involve pain or bleeding (unlike sharp surgical debridement).[15] Only devitalized tissue is removed.

- *Biological debridement* involves the use of maggots to eat away necrotic tissue. It is rarely used due to the undesirable factor of having living organisms inhabit a wound, but it is, however, very effective. These organisms are precise in their debridement and ingest only devitalized tissue.[14] Use of maggots is restricted and not recommended when there are exposed vessels, acute infection, circulatory impairment, and other factors.[15]

Assessment of Healing and Reassessment

An important aspect of PI treatment is assessment, which should be done daily in an acute care facility. A formal reevaluation should occurs after 2–4 weeks of treatment, when PI is expected to improve.[14,15] It is important to use consistent methods of evaluation. These include wound size, the presence of healing (i.e., granulation tissue), stage (although this does not change if the original stage was assessed to be "better" than the current stage), presence of infection, and other factors.[15] Assessment/reassessment should be performed at least weekly.[17] Photographs of PIs should be used to assess treatment effectiveness.[15] In the era of electronic medical records, it is essential to record the progress or lack thereof of wound healing with a photographic record. If a PI deteriorates, the treatment approach should be changed immediately.[17]

Surgical Treatment of Pressure Injuries

One important part of PI management is making the decision to refer to or consult with a surgery team. In general, there are several indications for this referral:

1. If there is a presence of a systemic infection (sepsis, advancing cellulitis)
2. If there is extensive necrotic tissue and/or tunneling that cannot be addressed with conservative debridement methods
3. If there is stage III PI that does not improve using conservative treatment methods
4. If the wound is stage IV; all stage IV wounds by definition have exposure and infection of the underlying bony structures.

An important aspect is the presence of OM, which needs to be addressed if the surgery is to be successful. The surgery itself usually involves debridement and creation of a flap.[15] Following surgery, the flap and the surgery site need to be closely monitored for any signs of flap failure.

In certain ischial and sacral wounds, and in patients who have recurrent loose stools and incontinence, other auxiliary procedures may be performed, such as a diverting colostomy to keep stool from contaminating the wound and causing recurring infections

Summary of Pressure Injury Treatment

Nutrition and removal of those factors that caused a PI are the first steps in PI management. Local wound care is focused on maintaining a healing microenvironment. Infection is managed both at the local and systemic levels, depending on the extent and symptoms. Removal of necrotic tissue is crucial since it prevents healing. Finally, surgical approaches that involve extensive debridement and wound closure may be necessary for stage II to stage IV PIs.

PERIOPERATIVE CONCERNS REGARDING PRESSURE INJURIES IN NEUROSURGICAL PATIENTS
Preoperative Concerns and Managing Patients Undergoing Neurosurgical Procedures

The presence or absence of PIs is not included in the two major indexes that are used to evaluate the cardiovascular risk of patients undergoing a procedure (i.e., the Revised Cardiac Risk Index [RCRI] and the Gupta Cardiac Index; see Chapter 2). Nevertheless, a retrospective study of 334 patients who underwent spinal cord surgery in southwest China showed that preoperative stage III and stage IV PIs were associated with increased risk of UTIs, surgical site infections, pneumonia, and other postoperative infections, and with readmission for infections within 30 days.[38] A retrospective study of 3,002 Taiwanese patients who had a preexisting PI and a first-ever stroke showed that the presence of a PI is associated with a higher risk for UTIs, pneumonia, gastrointestinal bleeding, epilepsy, and poststroke mortality compared to controls.[13]

Thus, the presence of PI likely constitutes an additional risk factor that should be taken into consideration when an elective neurosurgical procedure is planned. It is not, however, an absolute contraindication to surgery.

Another significant concern is perioperative factors that increase the risk for postoperative PIs. Two scales that are used perioperatively are the Scott Triggers and the Munro Pressure Ulcer Risk Assessment Scale for Perioperative Patients. The Scott Triggers evaluates several factors and includes the ASA score as used in the Gupta Cardiac Index and the estimated surgery time (Table 11.2). Two "yes" answers indicate a high-risk patient.[3] The Munro Scale is a complex tool that also takes into consideration intraoperative factors as they occur (e.g., hypotension, positioning) and post-anesthesia care unit events (e.g., bleeding).[39] Taken together, these scales can help in risk-stratification and can direct intraoperative and postoperative management if the patient is determined to be at high risk of PI development. Finally, the SCIPUS-A scale, noted earlier, measures the risk of PI development in SCI patients in the acute setting and thus can be used at this point and throughout hospitalization. Neurosurgery patients must be evaluated for the risk of PI development in the preoperative phase.

Intraoperative Concerns and Management

During a procedure in an operating room, patients remain in an immobile position for an extended period. Not surprisingly, this puts surgery patients at an increased risk of PIs. The intraoperative incidence of PIs is high, although studies indicate a wide range, from 4% to 66%.[15,40] A general approach that is used to reduce the risk of PI includes, first, minimizing the length of surgery. Second, risk factors such as hypotension and/or hypothermia should be avoided, if possible. Third, proper support surfaces should be used to minimize pressure on PI-prone areas. Fourth, the patient must be properly positioned. Finally, the position and the areas at PI risk in the given position need to be properly documented.[15]

The ACP guideline does not provide recommendations with respect to the intraoperative support surfaces. Nevertheless, a review by Reddy et al. noted that dynamic support surfaces appear to decrease the risk of PIs.[3] Consistently, NPUAP recommends use of alternating pressure or high specification reactive support surfaces.[15] These support surfaces should be used particularly for high-risk patients who have been identified preoperatively.[3]

In addition, patients should not be subjected to sliding or pulling when moved to and from the operating table and during the procedure.[3,14]

An important factor that influences PI formation is positioning of patients during surgery. Various positions include supine, prone (which is often employed in spinal procedures), and lateral decubitus. Different body areas are at risk of PI depending on the used surgical position.[41] A recent study shows that the body areas most at risk for intraoperative PI development are the coccygeal/sacral area, the buttocks, genitalia, and heels (Figure 11.4).[41] These results correlate with the supine position, which was used in 85.1% of the cases in this study.[41] In contrast, in the "park bench position," which is used to access the cerebellopontine angle, PIs were observed to develop at the lateral thorax, greater trochanter, iliac, lateral knee, and lateral malleolus areas.[42] Consequently, specialized support surfaces are often used to unload pressure in the areas at risk. A hospitalist in conjunction with the nursing team should be aware of intraoperative PI risk that is associated with various operating table positions and postoperatively monitor closely those areas at risk. PIs are then treated according to the principles outlined earlier in this chapter.

At present, there is no specific guideline that would suggest that preexisting PIs should be managed differently intraoperatively than preoperatively. Thus, PIs in the OR should be dressed and managed as in the preoperative period.

Postoperative Pressure Injury Management

Prevention of PI formation is an indicator of the quality of postoperative care. PI develops over a period of time and thus may not be detected immediately after a procedure even if intraoperative factors played a role in its etiology. Thus, PI which appears within 72 hours after surgery can be considered to occur either during the intraoperative period or in the period immediately preceding or succeeding the operation.[3] Finding such a PI should be communicated to the relevant teams, and

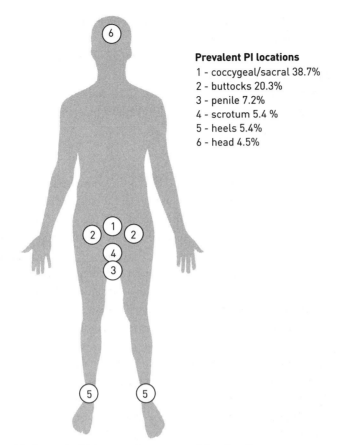

Prevalent PI locations
1 - coccygeal/sacral 38.7%
2 - buttocks 20.3%
3 - penile 7.2%
4 - scrotum 5.4 %
5 - heels 5.4%
6 - head 4.5%

FIGURE 11.4 Most prevalent intraoperative pressure injury locations.
From Yoshimura et al.[40]

causes should be determined.[3] Treatment of existing PIs then proceeds according to the established guidelines.

An important factor in wound healing is the use of corticosteroids. It has been shown that less than 40 mg/d of prednisone for more than 3 days does not adversely affect fibroplasia and collagen remodeling.[14,43,44] However, many neurosurgery patients are taking dexamethasone at doses which exceed the equivalent 40 mg/d of prednisone. Corticosteroids may affect healing of neurosurgery patient, and, if possible, the dose should be tapered off. Other immunosuppressants, such as methotrexate, do not appear to inhibit wound healing.[14,43,44]

For SCI patients, as in the earlier phase of care, the SCIPUS-A scale may help to evaluate the risk of PI. SCIPUS-A includes seven factors: extent of paralysis, moisture, serum creatinine, incontinence, albumin, mobility, pulmonary disease, and the level of activity.[20] Similar, NPUAP notes the immobility risk factor and also includes decreased sensation and altered pathophysiology.[15]

A completely separate topic is support surfaces for wheelchair-bound SCI patients.[14,15] As expected, the bony prominences of wheelchair-bound patients are at risk of PI formation. Ischial ulcers are the most common PIs found in these patients, followed by trochanteric and sacral ulcers.[14] Thus, frequent repositioning is encouraged. Wheelchair-support surfaces should be individualized according to the posture and needs of each patient.[14]

Finally, SCI patients often use various support braces. This is an often-neglected source of PIs. For example, application of a C-collar creates a significant risk of PI formation, particularly in the occipital region.[45] Care should be taken to apply and possibly custom-create braces that uniformly distribute pressure on the body.

CONCLUSION

In this chapter we present current approaches to the prevention and treatment of PIs. We also point out concerns which are unique to surgery and neurosurgery patients. Taken together, current guidelines focus on PI prevention, which includes multiple steps. The emphasis is on pressure redistribution using appropriate support surfaces and repositioning, close monitoring, prevention of malnutrition, and education. The treatment of PIs involves both medical and surgical approaches.

Currently, many if not most prevention and treatment methods are based on limited evidence and sometimes on expert opinion. There is a need for evidence-based research, including randomized double-blinded clinical trials.

From the standpoint of the neurosurgery hospitalist, preexisting PI is known to increase the postoperative risk of infections and/or mortality in spinal injury and stroke patients.[12,13,38] Likewise, the presence of preexisting PI-related osteomyelitis increases the risk of postoperative complications. The presence or absence of PI should play an important role in preoperative risk stratification. However, in contrast to cardiovascular surgery patients, at present we do not have a nomogram that would allow the clinician to weigh the significance of PI and/or osteomyelitis when evaluating preoperative risk for neurosurgery patients. We hope that future studies will allow the development of such a nomogram/algorithm.

Unlike medical patients, surgery patients are exposed to the risk of PI formation during the operating room procedure. Neurosurgery procedures use a number of unique positions that create risk for PI formation in uncommon places. These include, for example, the chin in the prone position and others as already mentioned. It is important that neurosurgery hospitalist in conjunction with the whole treatment team monitor these sites and be aware of the risk of PI development.

Finally, SCI patients are at high risk of PI during the postoperative period. This is secondary to immobility, which can be lengthy. Some of these patients will require braces; some become wheelchair-bound. These patients will require close monitoring and tailored approaches to PI prevention. More evidence is needed to establish the best methods to prevent and treat PI in these patients.

In summary, PI prevention and treatment is crucial to the well-being of neurosurgery patients. We would welcome more studies and trials to refine the current methods and approaches to prevention and treatment of these patients. Based on the current evidence, we propose an algorithm for prevention and treatment of PIs in neurosurgery patients (Figure 11.5).

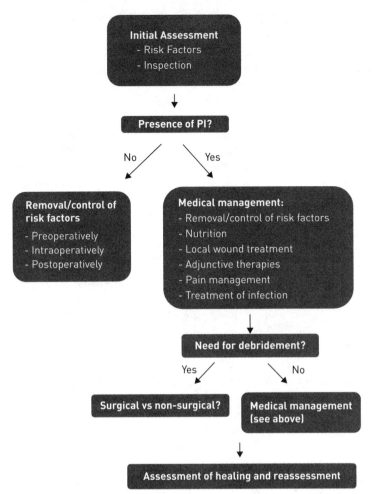

FIGURE 11.5 Algorithm for prevention of treatment of pressure injuries in neurosurgery patients.

REFERENCES

1. Agency for Healthcare Research and Quality, Rockville, MD. Preventing Pressure Ulcers in Hospitals. Agency for Healthcare Research and Quality, Rockville, MD. Content last reviewed October 2014. http://www.ahrq.gov/professionals/systems/hospital/pressureulcertoolkit/index.html.

2. King, M. Identifying Root Causes and Solutions for Hospital Acquired Pressure Injuries. Nov 19, 2018. https://www.jointcommission.org/high_reliability_healthcare/identifying_root_causes_and_solutions_for_hospital_acquired_pressure_injuries/.

3. Spruce L. Back to basics: preventing perioperative pressure injuries. *AORN J.* 2017;105(1):92–99.

4. Edsberg LE, Langemo D, Baharestani MM, Posthauer ME, Goldberg M. Unavoidable pressure injury: state of the science and consensus outcomes. *J Wound Ostomy Continence Nurs.* 2014;41(4):313–334.

5. Qaseem A, Mir TP, Starkey M, Denberg TD; Clinical Guidelines Committee of the American College of Physicians. Risk assessment and prevention of pressure ulcers: a

clinical practice guideline from the American College of Physicians. *Ann Intern Med.* 2015;162(5):359–369.

6. Margolis DJ, Knauss J, Bilker W, Baumgarten M. Medical conditions as risk factors for pressure ulcers in an outpatient setting. *Age Ageing.* 2003;32(3):259–264.

7. Cardenas DD, Hoffman JM, Kirshblum S, McKinley W. Etiology and incidence of rehospitalization after traumatic spinal cord injury: a multicenter analysis. *Arch Phys Med Rehabil.* 2004;85(11):1757–1763.

8. Han SH, Kim YS, Hwang J, Lee J, Song MR. Predictors of hospital-acquired pressure ulcers among older adult inpatients. *J Clin Nurs.* 2018;27(19-20):3780–3786.

9. Brienza D, Krishnan S, Karg P, Sowa G, Allegretti AL. Predictors of pressure ulcer incidence following traumatic spinal cord injury: a secondary analysis of a prospective longitudinal study. *Spinal Cord.* 2018;56(1):28–34.

10. Fuhrer MJ, Garber SL, Rintala DH, Clearman R, Hart KA. Pressure ulcers in community-resident persons with spinal cord injury: prevalence and risk factors. *Arch Phys Med Rehabil.* 1993;74(11):1172–1177.

11. Kruger EA, Pires M, Ngann Y, Sterling M, Rubayi S. Comprehensive management of pressure ulcers in spinal cord injury: current concepts and future trends. *J Spinal Cord Med.* 2013;36(6):572–585.

12. Chou CL, Lee WR, Yeh CC, Shih CC, Chen TL, Liao CC. Adverse outcomes after major surgery in patients with pressure ulcer: a nationwide population-based retrospective cohort study. *PLoS One.* 2015;10(5):e0127731.

13. Lee SY, Chou CL, Hsu SP, et al. Outcomes after stroke in patients with previous pressure ulcer: a nationwide matched retrospective cohort study. *J Stroke Cerebrovasc Dis.* 2016;25(1):220–227.

14. Consortium for Spinal Cord Medicine. Pressure Ulcer Prevention and Treatment Following Spinal Cord Injury: A Clinical Practice Guideline for Health-Care Professionals. Second Edition. 2014. http://www.pva.org/media/pdf/CPG_Pressure%20Ulcer.pdf.

15. National Pressure Ulcer Advisory Panel, European Pressure Ulcer Advisory Panel and Pan Pacific Pressure Injury Alliance. Prevention and Treatment of Pressure Ulcers: Clinical Practice Guideline. Emily Haesler (Ed.). Cambridge Media: Osborne Park, Western Australia; 2014.

16. Qaseem A, Humphrey LL, Forciea MA, Starkey M, Denberg TD; Clinical Guidelines Committee of the American College of Physicians. Treatment of pressure ulcers: a clinical practice guideline from the American College of Physicians. *Ann Intern Med.* 2015;162(5):370–379.

17. National Pressure Ulcer Advisory Panel (NPUAP). National Pressure Ulcer Advisory Panel (NPUAP) announces a change in terminology from pressure ulcer to pressure injury and updates the stages of pressure injury. April 13, 2016. https://www.npuap.org/national-pressure-ulcer-advisory-panel-npuap-announces-a-change-in-terminology-from-pressure-ulcer-to-pressure-injury-and-updates-the-stages-of-pressure-injury/.

18. Harris AG, Leiderer R, Peer F, Messmer K. Skeletal muscle microvascular and tissue injury after varying durations of ischemia. *Am J Physiol.* 1996;271(6 Pt 2):H2388–H2398.

19. Salzberg CA, Byrne DW, Cayten CG, van Niewerburgh P, Murphy JG, Viehbeck M. A new pressure ulcer risk assessment scale for individuals with spinal cord injury. *Am J Phys Med Rehabil.* 1996;75(2):96–104.

20. Spinal Cord Research Evidence Professional. Spinal Cord Injury Pressure Ulcer Scale – Acute (SCIPUS-A). Mar 2, 2017. https://scireproject.com/outcome-measures/outcome-measure-tool/spinal-cord-injury-pressure-ulcer-scale-acute-scipus-a/

21. Iizaka S, Okuwa M, Sugama J, Sanada H. The impact of malnutrition and nutrition-related factors on the development and severity of pressure ulcers in older patients receiving home care. *Clin Nutr.* 2010;29(1):47–53.

22. Yamamoto T, Fujioka M, Kitamura R, et al. Evaluation of nutrition in the healing of pressure ulcers: are the EPUAP nutritional guidelines sufficient to heal wounds? *Wounds.* 2009;21(6):153–157.

23. Guenter P, Malyszek R, Bliss DZ, et al. Survey of nutritional status in newly hospitalized patients with stage III or stage IV pressure ulcers. *Adv Skin Wound Care.* 2000;13(4 Pt 1):164–168.

24. Banks M, Bauer J, Graves N, Ash S. Malnutrition and pressure ulcer risk in adults in Australian health care facilities. *Nutrition.* 2010;26(9):896–901.

25. Wojcik A, Atkins M, Mager DR. Dietary intake in clients with chronic wounds. *Can J Diet Pract Res.* 2011;72(2):77–82.

26. Thomas DR, Verdery RB, Gardner L, Kant A, Lindsay J. A prospective study of outcome from protein-energy malnutrition in nursing home residents. *JPEN J Parenter Enteral Nutr.* 1991;15(4):400–404.

27. Verbrugghe M, Beeckman D, Van Hecke A, et al. Malnutrition and associated factors in nursing home residents: a cross-sectional, multi-centre study. *Clin Nutr.* 2013;32(3):438–443.

28. Torra i Bou JE, Segovia Gomez T, Verdu Soriano J, Nolasco Bonmati A, Rueda Lopez J, Arboix i Perejamo M. The effectiveness of a hyperoxygenated fatty acid compound in preventing pressure ulcers. *J Wound Care.* 2005;14(3):117–121.

29. Declair V. The usefulness of topical application of essential fatty acids (EFA) to prevent pressure ulcers. *Ostomy Wound Manage.* 1997;43(5):48–52, 54.

30. Cooper P, Gray D. Comparison of two skin care regimes for incontinence. *Br J Nurs.* 2001;10(6 Suppl):S6, S8, S10 passim.

31. Allman RM, Walker JM, Hart MK, Laprade CA, Noel LB, Smith CR. Air-fluidized beds or conventional therapy for pressure sores. A randomized trial. *Ann Intern Med.* 1987;107(5):641–648.

32. Jackson BS, Chagares R, Nee N, Freeman K. The effects of a therapeutic bed on pressure ulcers: an experimental study. *J Enterostomal Ther.* 1988;15(6):220–226.

33. Munro BH, Brown L, Heitman BB. Pressure ulcers: one bed or another? *Geriatr Nurs.* 1989;10(4):190–192.

34. Ochs RF, Horn SD, van Rijswijk L, Pietsch C, Smout RJ. Comparison of air-fluidized therapy with other support surfaces used to treat pressure ulcers in nursing home residents. *Ostomy Wound Manage.* 2005;51(2):38–68.

35. Strauss MJ, Gong J, Gary BD, Kalsbeek WD, Spear S. The cost of home air-fluidized therapy for pressure sores. A randomized controlled trial. *J Fam Pract.* 1991;33(1):52–59.

36. Muder RR, Brennen C, Wagener MM, Goetz AM. Bacteremia in a long-term-care facility: a five-year prospective study of 163 consecutive episodes. *Clin Infect Dis.* 1992;14(3):647–654.

37. Wong D, Holtom P, Spellberg B. Osteomyelitis complicating sacral pressure ulcers: whether or not to treat with antibiotic therapy. *Clin Infect Dis.* 2018.

38. Yang LL, Peng WX, Wang CQ, Li Q. Elevated risk of infections after spinal cord surgery in relation to preoperative pressure ulcers: a follow-up study. *Sci Rep.* 2018;8(1):14027.

39. Munro CA. The development of a pressure ulcer risk-assessment scale for perioperative patients. *AORN J.* 2010;92(3):272–287.

40. Yoshimura M, Iizaka S, Kohno M, et al. Risk factors associated with intraoperatively acquired pressure ulcers in the park-bench position: a retrospective study. *Int Wound J.* 2016;13(6):1206–1213.

41. Lumbley JL, Ali SA, Tchokouani LS. Retrospective review of predisposing factors for intraoperative pressure ulcer development. *J Clin Anesth.* 2014;26(5):368–374.

42. Furuno Y, Sasajima H, Goto Y, et al. Strategies to prevent positioning-related complications associated with the lateral suboccipital approach. *J Neurol Surg B Skull Base.* 2014;75(1):35–40.

43. Karukonda SR, Flynn TC, Boh EE, McBurney EI, Russo GG, Millikan LE. The effects of drugs on wound healing: part 1. *Int J Dermatol.* 2000;39(4):250–257.

44. Karukonda SR, Flynn TC, Boh EE, McBurney EI, Russo GG, Millikan LE. The effects of drugs on wound healing—part II. Specific classes of drugs and their effect on healing wounds. *Int J Dermatol.* 2000;39(5):321–333.

45. Jacobson TM, Tescher AN, Miers AG, Downer L. Improving practice: efforts to reduce occipital pressure ulcers. *J Nurs Care Qual.* 2008;23(3):283–288.

12 Perioperative Optimization of Pain Control in Patients Undergoing Spinal Surgery Using Multimodal Analgesia

Newton Mei and Ashwini D. Sharan

GENERAL PRINCIPLES

Adequate control of postoperative pain is a shared goal among providers and their patients. Patients with controlled postoperative pain are shown to have better surgical outcomes, decreased hospital stay, increased satisfaction, and improved functional status.[1-7] Conversely, uncontrolled postoperative pain has been linked to higher readmission rates, increased usage of healthcare resources, and development of hospital complications including venous thromboembolism, pneumonia, and development of chronic pain conditions.[3,4,8-10] Therefore, it is important for healthcare providers caring for surgical patients to be well versed in addressing and treating pain in the perioperative setting.

In the past, opioids were the choice agent to treat acute postoperative pain.[11] In the United States, oxycodone and methadone sales in 2002 were almost four times as much as the sales in 1997.[12,13] However, increasing literature is showing that opioids are not the all-encompassing panacea hoped for. Patients still report uncontrolled pain despite being placed on opioids. This is likely because a patient's individual experience of pain is often affected by a complex mix of nociceptive and neuropathic pain, which may further be aggravated by a patient's psychosocial factors.[14]

Furthermore, with the rampant prescription of opioids for pain control in the recent past, an opioid epidemic is currently afflicting the United States. In 2015, more than 90 million people in the US were estimated to be using opioids, and more than 10 million of these individuals reported misuse.[15] The rate of opioid-related deaths was also estimated at 1 death every 35 minutes in the United States.[16] Moreover, opioids have a myriad of adverse side effects including nausea, vomiting, sedation, pruritus, constipation, ileus, urinary retention, respiratory depression, and delayed wound healing.[8,17–20] Chronic opioid use also leads to addiction, tolerance, dependence, hypothalamic-pituitary-adrenal (HPA) axis suppression leading to sexual dysfunction, and increased risk of bone fractures.[9,18,21] Studies show that even short-term use of opioids prior to a surgery can decrease the effectiveness of opioids used postoperatively.[22,23] Chapman et al. reported that patients on chronic opioids experienced hyperalgesia and reported higher levels of acute pain. The time required to achieve adequate pain control in patients on chronic opioids was also longer.[24] Therefore, the opioid epidemic has propelled providers and researchers to identify and use nonopioid agents for pain control.

Increasing research is recommending multimodal analgesia (MMA) to treat perioperative pain given its effectiveness in providing patients with pain relief and its opioid-sparing ability. MMA utilizes a combination of different pharmacologic agents and nonpharmacologic modalities to optimize pain control in the patient while minimizing side effects.[8,25] Theoretically, different classes of pain medications effect pain relief using different pathways in the body, and, in combination, these different classes could have a synergistic or additive effect, allowing for lower doses of each agent and thus decreasing the risk of overall side effects.[13,26] The strategy of MMA has been shown to provide significant pain relief in patients undergoing various surgeries. However, the medications used and their effectiveness varied with the type of surgery, highlighting that MMA should be tailored to the particular surgery.[14,22] To develop the appropriate MMA, the provider should incorporate medications that demonstrate significant effectiveness as shown by the latest evidence for the particular surgery type. The provider should then further customize the MMA to best suit each patient, using a patient-centered approach that takes into account the patient's allergies, age, and possible interactions with the patient's other medications and medical comorbidities to minimize complications and adverse effects. Thus, as Schwenk suggests, an MMA regimen should be more of a checklist rather than a recipe.[14] The use of MMA is on the rise, and increasing research is promoting its use in the perioperative setting for many surgeries including spine surgery.

PAIN AND SPINE SURGERY

Spinal pathology and spinal surgery produce a complex array of neuropathic and nociceptive pain, making postoperative pain management particularly challenging for healthcare providers caring for this patient population.[22] Providers caring for spine patients in the perioperative setting should become familiar with (1) the difference between neuropathic and nociceptive pain, (2) the different tissues that make up the spine and how their pain manifests in patients after injury or surgical manipulation of those tissues, and (3) the medications that can best treat neuropathic and nociceptive pain.

Neuropathic pain results from injury to the nerve itself resulting in abnormal signaling in the somatosensory pathway.[27,28] Therefore, neuropathic pain often presents as an altered sensation. Patients may describe their pain as a burning, pins and needles, numbness, icy or cold sensation, electric, or shooting type of pain that often runs along the distribution of the affected nerve. The pain may also be associated with weakness and motor deficits of the surrounding innervated muscles.[29] Neuropathic pain may persist even after the insult is removed as evidenced in phantom limb syndrome and persistence of paresthesias postoperatively despite successful spinal decompression.[30–32]

In contrast, *nociceptive pain* usually results from acute injury to other tissues and organs. Structures that make up the spine, such as vertebral discs, muscle, and bone, are highly vascularized and innervated with nociceptive fibers or pain neurons.[22] These nociceptive neurons warn the body of any acute insult to the tissue they are innervating. The injury can be mechanical, such as trauma or surgical manipulation, ischemic from insufficient oxygen supply to the tissue or organ, or chemical from medications or toxins. Nociceptive pain signaling often is through inflammatory biomolecules such as bradykinin, prostaglandins, cytokines, and hydrogen ions.[22] The clinical presentation of nociceptive pain is generally more localized around the injured tissue, and the associated inflammation may be described by patients as a sharp or throbbing pain with associated warmth or heat in the affected region. Nociceptive pain from muscle injury is generally described as a tearing or cramping quality in a broad area around the affected muscle with possible associated spasms.[33] Bone pain affecting the facet joint or vertebral body and vertebral disc pain are generally more focal and can be localized with palpation over that area. The pain can be described as a sharp or dull ache.[34]

However, both prolonged neuropathic or nociceptive pain can lead to peripheral and central sensitizations leading to increased pain sensitivity in patients. This neurochemical phenomenon is known as *hyperalgesia*. Altered pain pathways can also lead to *allodynia* in which previously nonpainful stimuli now trigger a pain response. Therefore, it is important for providers to adequately treat the acute pain and prevent this downstream negative effect resulting from persistent uncontrolled pain.[22] In particular, spine patients are more susceptible to central sensitization as a study showed increased expression of cyclooxygenase (COX2) mRNA in the spinal cord.[35] Fortunately, the body of literature in pain management after spine surgery has been growing rapidly. The following paragraphs will review medication classes that recent evidence has shown to be effective in perioperative pain management in patients receiving spine surgery.

GABAPENTINOIDS

Gabapentinoids are increasingly being used in MMA regimens across all surgeries and have shown effectiveness in perioperative pain control in patients receiving spine surgery. Gabapentinoids such as gabapentin and pregabalin are well-known neuromodulatory agents that bind to the alpha-2-delta-1 (α2-δ1) subunit of N-type voltage-gated calcium channels in the presynaptic neurons and function to inhibit the release of excitatory neurotransmitters.[8,36] They were originally prescribed to treat seizures, but, over time, their use has expanded to treat multiple neuropathic conditions such as diabetic neuropathy and postherpetic neuralgia.[27,37,38] They have also been incorporated in the treatment of postoperative pain. A significant decrease in postoperative pain and morphine consumption in patients who underwent lower extremity orthopedic surgery was noted.[39]

Recent spine literature demonstrates the effectiveness of gabapentinoids in improving pain control in spine patients. An earlier meta-analysis by Yu et al. in 2013 reviewed 7 studies and concluded that patients who received gabapentin and pregabalin had decreased opioid use and significant pain reduction when compared to placebo.[40] Han et al. showed that gabapentin preoperatively reduced cumulative morphine consumption and reduction of visual analog scale (VAS) scores in all time points.[41] A meta-analysis performed by Liu et al. in 2017 evaluating 16 randomized control trials further validated these results and concluded that patients who received gabapentinoids versus placebo prior to lumbar spine surgery had significantly decreased VAS at 6, 12, 24, and 48 hours after surgery. Pregabalin was also shown to significantly decrease morphine consumption at 24 and 48 hours postoperatively. Patients who received gabapentinoids were also interestingly noted to have decreased nausea, vomiting, and pruritus.[42] Khurana et al. also demonstrated improved VAS modified Prolo score and Oswestry Disability Index score at 3 months suggesting long-term improvements in functionality in patients who received gabapentin when compared to placebo.[43] Other studies noted other benefits of using gabapentinoids in the perioperative setting. Patients who received pregabalin demonstrated reduced anxiety, better sleep, decreased myalgias and fasciculations associated with succinylcholine, and increased pain relief from spinal anesthesia and nerve blocks.[44–47]

However, the multiple studies evaluating gabapentinoids had heterogeneous doses for gabapentin and pregabalin and different administration schedules, some only preoperatively while others continued gabapentinoids postoperatively for 2–7 days; thus it was difficult to achieve a unified conclusion on the optimal dosing and administration timing relative to surgery. Gabapentinoids' analgesic effect, however, appears to be dose dependent. A single dose of 150 mg of pregabalin given preoperatively was more effective at reducing pain when compared to the 75 mg dose.[48,49] After lumbar fusion, Kim et al. also showed that patients who received 150 mg of pregabalin but not those who received 75 mg of pregabalin had a significant decrease in patient-controlled analgesia (PCA) use when compared to placebo at 24 and 48 hours after surgery. However at 300 mg of pregabalin, there was a statistically significant increase in dizziness and blurry vision.[50] Khan et al. showed a dose-dependent effect with gabapentin. The time for first demand analgesia was longer in patients who received higher doses of gabapentin 900–1,200 mg compared to those who received 600 mg.[51]

Regarding administration schedules for gabapentinoids, Puvanesarajah et al. suggest a single preoperative dose with continued postoperative administration.[22] Pitchon agrees and reports that continuation of gabapentin and pregabalin are likely more effective than a single preoperative dose.[27]

In comparing pregabalin versus gabapentin, pregabalin appears to be more effective.[42,52] Pregabalin compared to gabapentin has increased bioavailability and is faster to achieve therapeutic levels, but there is also increased sedation noted.[53,54] In a study by Khetarpal, patients who underwent lower extremity orthopedic surgery either received 300 mg pregabalin, 1,200 mg gabapentin, or placebo. Patients who received pregabalin had longer periods of being pain-free compared to those who received gabapentin.[55] More studies, however, are needed to compare the two in terms of analgesic efficacy in spine patients. It is also important to note that pregabalin is associated with a higher cost. A 300 mg capsule of gabapentin costs less than 15 cents while a 75 mg capsule of pregabalin costs more than 7 dollars.[27] Pregabalin is not generic, and certain insurance companies may not cover its cost. Furthermore, given the higher risk of sedation associated with pregabalin, some patients, such as those with obstructive sleep apnea or elderly patients who receive pregabalin concomitantly with other sedating medications including opioids, are found to have a greater risk for respiratory depression.[56]

Therefore, based on the literature, gabapentinoids are effective in improving pain in patients having spine surgery and should be incorporated in MMA for spine patients barring contraindications such as an allergy. Common side effects of gabapentin and pregabalin include sedation, dizziness, and peripheral edema.[13] The analgesic property of gabapentinoids increases in a dose-dependent manner, and doses should be titrated up gradually to optimize pain control while monitoring for adverse effects. Special attention should be placed on patients who have underlying kidney disease as gabapentinoids are cleared by kidneys. Patients who are elderly or those with sleep apnea are at a higher risk for oversedation when placed on gabapentinoids.[56] Choosing between gabapentin and pregabalin should be an informed decision made between the clinician and his or her patient. Prescribers should take into account their patient's insurance as pregabalin is more expensive. Some patients may also have a better response with one drug or the other.

NONSTEROIDAL ANTI-INFLAMMATORY DRUGS

Nonsteroidal anti-inflammatory drugs (NSAIDs) block COX-1 and -2 isoenzymes and inhibit prostaglandin synthesis.[36] NSAIDs are commonly prescribed in the outpatient setting for pain control given their anti-inflammatory properties. However, providers are more hesitant to use NSAIDs in patients undergoing spinal surgery and in particular spinal fusion given the concern for increased perioperative bleeding and past studies showing increased risk for nonunion, failure of fusion, and pseudoarthrosis.[36] A study by Glassman et al. showed increased nonunion rates in patients who had lumbar spine fusion and received intramuscular ketorolac.[57]

However, recent studies have challenged these concerns. A meta-analysis of 27 studies showed that ketorolac use did not increase perioperative bleeding.[58] A different meta-analysis also found no association between nonunion and NSAID exposure.[59] Sivaganesan et al. performed a systematic review of five retrospective studies to evaluate the effect of NSAIDs on spinal fusion and noted NSAIDs to have dose-dependent and duration-dependent effects on fusion rates. The study showed that *high* doses of ketorolac at 120 mg/d did increase the risk of spinal nonunion, but short-term (<14 days) use at normal doses of ketorolac, diclofenac, celecoxib, or rofecoxib did not exhibit increased rates of nonunion.[60]

Furthermore, the use of selective COX-2 inhibitors such as celecoxib may be able to provide improved analgesia without affecting fusion rates. Long et al. showed that rabbits who received celecoxib had reduced nonunion rates compared to those that received indomethacin.[61] Selective COX-2 inhibitors use will also minimize the side effects related to COX-1 blockade by preserving platelet function and gastrointestinal mucosa.[8] Celecoxib remains the only COX-2 inhibitor on the US market. All others were removed because of cardiovascular complications. In addition to cardiovascular complications such as myocardial infarction, all NSAIDs increase the risk of kidney injury, GI ulceration, and bleeding.[8,14,54] These side effects are also thought to be dose- and time-dependent, so short term use up to 2–5 days post discharge was recommended.[54]

However, after accounting for all possible risks and side effects which can be controlled with dosing and duration of treatment, the analgesic benefit of NSAIDs is significant. Jirarattanphochai et al. showed that 40 mg intravenous parecoxib given 30 minutes before lumbar discectomy followed by additional doses every 12 hours for 48 hours postoperatively resulted in improved pain control and increased patient satisfaction.[62] Furthermore, a meta-analysis of 17 studies of patients who received NSAIDs showed improved pain scores and decreased opioid use in patients who underwent lumbar spine surgery.[63] Moonla et al. performed a prospective randomized double-blind controlled trial and compared parecoxib versus placebo. Patients in the parecoxib arm received 40 mg intravenously or intramuscularly followed by 20 or 40 mg every 6 to 12 hours for a maximum of 80 mg/d. A significant improvement in VAS scores was noted in the parecoxib group when compared to control. There was also a significant decrease in morphine consumption over 24 hours in the parecoxib group when compared to control.[20] Furthermore, it is interesting to note that in Japan few patients are prescribed narcotic pain medications after spine surgery and instead receive oral or suppository NSAIDs.[64]

Therefore, in conclusion, NSAIDs should be incorporated in the MMA regimen for patients receiving spine surgery after taking into account a patient's medical comorbidities and allergies. Studies have shown no increase in NSAID-associated perioperative bleeding, and the concern for fusion failure can be mitigated with regular dosing and short-term use of NSAIDs. Celecoxib, a selective COX-2 inhibitor, has an even better side-effect profile given its reduced effect on platelet function and GI prostaglandin production. Timing of NSAID administration is unclear. Moonla et al. noted no significant differences between patients who were initiated on parecoxib prior to surgery versus those who stared parecoxib after surgery.[20] The initial dose of celecoxib can be started at 200 mg twice a day and can be titrated up to optimize pain control.

ACETAMINOPHEN

Acetaminophen provides effective analgesia in the perioperative period and is particularly favorable because of its limited side effects. Acetaminophen's mechanism of action has been thought to be related to activating serotonergic pathways in the central nervous system and inhibiting prostaglandin production.[27,36] Intravenous acetaminophen has been extensively studied for perioperative pain control in hip and knee surgery; however, limited studies were done regarding spine surgery. In a randomized, controlled study of patients who had total hip and total knee replacements, patients who received intravenous acetaminophen reported improved pain control and decreased opioid use compared to placebo.[27,65,66] Similar results were noted in the Khalili study, which showed that preemptive intravenous acetaminophen had decreased overall opioid demand and extended time to rescue in lower extremity surgery.[67] Cakan et al. demonstrated improved pain scores and greater patient satisfaction in patients who received intravenous acetaminophen but no difference in narcotic use when compared to the placebo group.[68] Yang et al. performed a meta-analysis that concluded that intravenous acetaminophen in total joint procedures decreased pain and opioid consumption in postoperative days 1–3.[69]

Extrapolating to spine surgery, acetaminophen is expected to provide similar analgesic effects. A study by Hansen et al. showed that patients who received intravenous acetaminophen had shorter lengths of stay, less resource use, and improved clinical status at time of discharge.[70] Morwald et al. also found that intravenous acetaminophen did not decrease opioid prescription among hospitalized spine patients.[71] More research is necessary to further validate its use in spine surgery.

Despite studies showing benefit of intravenous acetaminophen, its use in clinical practice is limited by its cost. A 1 g oral acetaminophen costs around 3 cents whereas its intravenous counterpart costs approximately 40 dollars.[72] A systematic review also noted no difference in analgesic efficacy between oral and intravenous formulations.[27,73] The maximum dose of acetaminophen is 4 g in 24 hours. However, US Food and Drug Administration (FDA) guidelines recommend up to 3 g in 24 hours. Acetaminophen is metabolized in the liver, so in patients who have cirrhosis, severe liver disease, or heavy alcohol use disorder, a reduced dose is recommended. For a more conservative approach, a cap of 2 g over 24 hours is suggested.[74]

More studies evaluating acetaminophen and its efficacy in patients undergoing spine surgery are needed. However, with the substantial literature supporting its benefit in lower extremity orthopedic surgery and its relatively low risk of side effects, it is suggested to incorporate acetaminophen in MMA for spine surgery patients at the appropriate doses based on underlying medical comorbidities. New studies are suggesting no significant differences in efficacy between intravenous and oral formulations, and, given the higher cost of the intravenous formulation, it is suggested to use an oral formulation if possible.

KETAMINE

Ketamine is an N-methyl-D-aspartic acid (NMDA) receptor antagonist and blocks the formation of pro-inflammatory cytokines such as tumor necrosis factor-alpha (TNF-α) and interleukin-6 (IL-6).[75] At higher doses, ketamine may be used as an anesthetic, however, at subanesthetic doses, it has been shown to provide significant analgesia and reduce peripheral and central sensitization of pain.[8,25,76] Ketamine may also modulate opioid receptors and have opioid sparing effects in addition to its analgesic properties, making it a useful option to treat patients who have underlying opiate or opioid dependency.[25,77] This medication is often under the jurisdiction of anesthesiologists and pain specialists. Therefore, it is prudent to screen patients for opioid dependence and consult the specialist early on to incorporate ketamine in a patient's MMA. Side effects of ketamine include sedation, hallucination and nightmares, dizziness, blurry vision, nausea, and vomiting.[25,27,54,77]

Ketamine is an effective analgesic and opioid-sparing agent for patients undergoing spine surgery. In patients who underwent spinal fusion, chronic pain and opioid-dependent patients who received ketamine had decreased pain and postoperative opioid use when compared to placebo. At 6 months, patients in the ketamine group continued to report decreased pain.[76,78] In a different trial, opioid-dependent patients undergoing lumbar spine surgery had reduced postoperative opioid demand after receiving ketamine intraoperatively. Loftus showed that patients in the ketamine group had decreased morphine use and decreased pain intensity both immediately and 6 weeks after surgery when compared to placebo. There was no difference in nausea, vomiting, or hallucinations.[79] Lumbar spine fusion patients who received intraoperative ketamine reported less pain at rest and with physical therapy on postoperative day 1.[80]

Therefore ketamine is recommended to be incorporated in the MMA regimen for patients on chronic opioids or who have a history of opiate use, such as intravenous heroin. Ketamine may be given intraoperatively as a bolus with infusion and continued postoperatively. Its management is often initiated and managed by a trained specialist in anesthesiology, pain medicine, or palliative care. Intranasal ketamine is another recently available option. More research is needed to determine the appropriate use of this formulation.

DEXAMETHASONE

Dexamethasone is a glucocorticoid that reduces inflammation and may provide analgesia after surgery.[81] In a systematic review, 0.1 mg/d of dexamethasone was able to decrease postoperative pain across different types of surgery.[82] In a different study, dexamethasone use reduced pain and narcotic use in 24 hours after lumbar surgery.[83] No significant differences in wound healing and wound infection were noted.[25,82,83] In lumbar discectomy, patients who received 16 mg dexamethasone prior to surgery had significantly decreased pain with mobilization in the first 24 hours compared to placebo. However no significance was noted with pain at rest or pain after 48 hours.[25] With all glucocorticoids, providers should watch for side effects such as hyperglycemia, GI bleeding, and myocardial infarction.[25]

More research needs to be done with dexamethasone to determine its utility in MMA for spine patients.

NEURAXIAL AND LOCAL ANALGESIA

Since the neuraxial and local analgesia modality is done primarily by anesthesiologists in the intraoperative setting, this chapter will provide a general overview and will defer further discussion to the anesthesiology literature. Neuraxial pain relief involves epidural or intrathecal infusion of opioids such as morphine or fentanyl. Two randomized controlled trials using intrathecal opioids have resulted in decreased postoperative VAS and opioid use in patients who had lumbar spine surgery.[84,85] Epidural injections of steroids were also shown to improve pain after lumbar discectomy.[36]

Local anesthesia is usually injected into the surgical site. Local lidocaine and bupivacaine inhibit voltage-gated sodium channels and decreases neurotransmission of sensory nerves. Patients who received bupivacaine infusions had significant postoperative analgesia and decreased opioid consumption postoperatively.[36] Intravenous lidocaine infusions were noted to decrease pain and opioid consumption, reduce length of stay, and allow earlier return of bowel function.[86]

The optimal doses and timing of neuraxial analgesia and local anesthesia have yet to be elucidated, and the decision for their use rests on the comfort level of the anesthesiologist. However nonanesthesiologist providers should be aware of these options and discuss them with the anesthesiologist on the case. The safer transdermal lidocaine patch is also an alternative to consider. Although there is lack of evidence supporting its effectiveness, its low risk profile makes it an attractive adjunct.

OPIOIDS

With the ongoing opioid epidemic, providers are increasingly wary of using opioids for pain relief; however, the significant analgesic effect of opioids is undeniable, and judicious use of opioids in the acute postoperative setting is appropriate and useful. A variety of prescription opioids are available with different formulations and duration of action. Providers who prescribe opioids are expected to undergo training for appropriate prescription and use of opioids. Therefore, further discussion regarding mechanism of action, opioid equianalgesic conversion, morphine equivalents, and indications for long-acting versus short-acting opioids will be deferred to the extensive existing body of literature. Instead, this section will focus on how to incorporate opioids in MMA regimens for spine patients for short-term use to adequately treat acute postoperative pain.

Patients who have underlying opioid dependence and those who are unable to take oral pain medications in the immediate postoperative setting may benefit from PCA, which allows for a patient-controlled bolus dose of an intravenous opioid for pain relief with an optional continuous basal dose if necessary. PCA is recommended to be continued for 12–24 hours postoperatively or until the patient is able to take oral doses. Then, based on opioid requirements as collected on the PCA, the equianalgesic dose for an oral formulation can be calculated. Of note, any comorbid medical condition that would limit the patient from being able to activate the PCA pump would bar its use. Therefore, patients who have organic brain pathology, those who are overly sedated, and those with limited hand dexterity would require an alternative form of analgesia.[22]

Regarding oral opioids, the literature suggests choosing tramadol or oxycodone. Tramadol is a weak mu receptor opioid agonist and also inhibits serotonin and norepinephrine reuptake. Tramadol has a lower risk of addiction, constipation, cardiovascular side effects, and depression.[13,87] Side effects of tramadol include lowering the seizure threshold and serotonin syndrome.[13,87] Oxycodone is a semisynthetic opioid and is a weak mu opioid agonist but a strong kappa opioid receptor.[11,88,89] Oral bioavailability of oxycodone is superior to that of morphine, 60% compared to 30% or less.[11,90,91] Oxycodone is also noted to be better at crossing the blood–brain barrier which is particularly beneficial in patients undergoing spine surgery.[11,92] It is estimated to have a rapid onset of analgesic in less than 30 minutes.[11,93] Side effects of nausea, hallucinations, and pruritus were also noted be less when compared to morphine.[11,94] Blumenthal et al. evaluated patients undergoing lumbar discectomy and noted that patients who received oxycodone extended release had improved pain control, decreased morphine use, improved satisfaction with pain control, and faster return of GI function.[95]

Therefore, opioids should still be incorporated in managing moderate to severe pain in the acute postoperative setting. In patients with expected high opioid requirements or inability to take oral doses, the recommendation is to use PCA and subsequently convert to oral opioids based on calculated requirements. For oral opioids, tramadol and oxycodone are recommended with their better side-effect profile compared to morphine and oxycodone's improved pharmacodynamics. Active titration off or down to baseline doses should discussed and agreed among patients and their providers. If opioids are required at time of discharge, a prescription with the shortest duration possible, preferably 7 days or less, is recommended because the risk of opioid dependence increases with the length of initial prescription after surgery.[14]

OTHER MEDICATIONS TO LOOK FOR IN THE FUTURE

As the literature regarding pain medications for spine surgery continues to grow, other agents may be added to the MMA regimen. Medications to look out for include methadone, magnesium, amantadine, and muscle relaxants. Future studies may further reveal the appropriate timing, dosing, and formulation of these agents and allow for the continued fine tuning of the optimal MMA regimen for spinal surgery.

GUIDELINES FOR DEVELOPING AN MMA REGIMEN FOR SPINE SURGERY PATIENTS
Preoperative Management

Patients undergoing spine surgery should have a full pain assessment as part of their initial admission history and physical. The pain assessment should delineate onset, precipitating factors, palliating or exacerbating factors, quality, radiation, severity, and timing. An easy acronym by which to remember these elements is OPQRST. There is also a validated form, the McGill Pain Questionnaire, that may be given to the patient to fill out.[8,96] The patient's baseline pain score should be assessed using a validated tool such as the VAS or Numeric Rating Scale (NRS).[8,97] The VAS and

NRS rate pain on a scale from 1 to 10, and the same scale should be used to assess pain severity postoperatively and with the introduction of each additional pain medication or up-titration of a medication. A baseline functional assessment such as Roland Morris Low Back Pain and Disability and the Brief Pain Inventory should be incorporated to assess the patient's ability to ambulate and work, their mood, sleep quality, and their enjoyment of life.[98–100] These tools provide an objective measure that allows the provider and patient to identify any progress in pain and functionality after surgery and the introduction of a pain regimen. It will also allow for adjustment of pain medications to optimize analgesia.[8]

Since a large of number of patients with spinal pathology have chronic back pain and may be opioid dependent, it is important to assess for opioid use in all patients.[8] Early identification of patients with opioid dependence will alert providers to consult pain specialists for possible use of ketamine and PCA.

All of the patient's medical comorbidities should be taken into consideration, and special attention should be paid to comorbid cardiovascular, renal, or liver diseases as these conditions may preclude the usage of certain analgesics discussed in this chapter. Special attention should also be given to elderly patients, patients who are chronic benzodiazepine users, patients who have alcohol use disorder, and patients who have obstructive sleep apnea as they are at higher risk for oversedation and its complications. The patient's list of allergies and the associated reactions should be up to date.

Puvanesarajah et al. recommend continuing home pain medications, especially opioids, in the preoperative setting. Patients who are gabapentinoid-naïve should receive either 600–1,200 mg of gabapentin or 150 mg pregabalin.[22] If the patient is on a gabapentinoid, that home medication may be continued with dose titration up as needed. Acetaminophen, given its benign profile, may be given 1 g preoperatively but consider dose adjustment or holding if the patient has a history of cirrhosis, severe liver disease, or significant alcohol use disorder.[27,74] NSAIDs such as celecoxib may also be given preoperatively as the literature does not note any associated increased bleeding. The initial dose of celecoxib is 400 mg total preoperatively. NSAIDs should be avoided in stroke, severe heart disease, acute or chronic kidney disease, patients who had recent bleeding, and in patients with dysfunctional platelets or thrombocytopenia, etc.[14]

Intraoperative Management

The anesthesiologist in charge of the case should consider neuraxial analgesia, local anesthesia in the incision site, and ketamine bolus followed by a ketamine infusion, especially in opioid tolerant patients.

Postoperative Pain Management

Depending on the duration of surgery, how extensive it was, the patient's prior opioid use history, and expected severity of pain, providers can consider placing patients on a PCA for 12–24 hours. Patients with opioid tolerance should also be started on intravenous ketamine. Acetaminophen, celecoxib, and gabapentinoids should be continued postoperatively. Titration is based on patient's symptoms, teasing out the more predominant complaint. If there is primarily a neuropathic component, consider increasing gabapentinoids. If there is more of a nociceptive component, consider increasing acetaminophen or celecoxib, or adding adjuncts such as lidocaine patches. Muscle relaxants should be considered for signs or symptoms consistent with muscle spasms. Slow and gradual up-titration of pain medications will minimize the risk of side effects. All patients should work with physical and occupational therapy and be encouraged for early mobilization. Opioid-tolerant patients should be converted to oral opioids based on their PCA requirements. Opioid naïve-patients should be started on the lowest dose of oral opioid and titrated up. Short-acting opioids should be given on an as-needed schedule and uptitrated. Tramadol and oxycodone are suggested, but the choice of opioid can be determined based on the patient's current medications, possible interactions, and patient-reported prior history of effectiveness with a particular agent. The provider and patient should have a unified goal to titrate opioids off or down as soon as possible, preferably by the time of discharge or within 7 days post discharge. The risk for long-term opioid use after surgery increases with the length of the initial prescription.[14] NSAIDs should not be continued for greater than 14 days, particularly in patients who underwent spinal fusion. For patients with opioid use disorder, initiation of methadone or Suboxone may be beneficial, with a patient's commitment and agreement.[10] Consults for social work, addiction specialists, and/or psychiatry will facilitate this process.

Taken together, our proposed algorithm for pain management in neurosurgical patients is outlined in Figure 12.1.

CONCLUSION

The rate of spinal surgery continues to grow each year across the United States and worldwide. Therefore, it is vital for healthcare providers to be well-versed in managing perioperative pain in patients undergoing spinal surgery. Uncontrolled pain carries with it a myriad of negative effects for both the patient and the healthcare system. The patient with uncontrolled pain is afflicted with increased hospital complications, development of heightened pain sensitivity, and decreased functional status. The healthcare system is negatively impacted by increased hospital readmissions and increased utilization of healthcare resources.[3,4,8–10]

MMA has been shown to be effective in controlling perioperative pain across multiple surgeries including spine surgery. The appropriate MMA should be surgery specific, using medications and modalities that have demonstrated evidence-based effectiveness in providing analgesia for that particular surgical patient population. It also needs to be patient specific, customized to take into account of the patient's age, allergies, and comorbidities. Current spine literature suggests significant analgesic effectiveness in the use of gabapentinoids such as gabapentin and pregabalin, NSAIDs, ketamine, neuraxial analgesia, and local anesthesia. More research needs to be done to further validate the efficacy of dexamethasone and acetaminophen. As the body of evidence continues to grow, more medications or modalities will likely

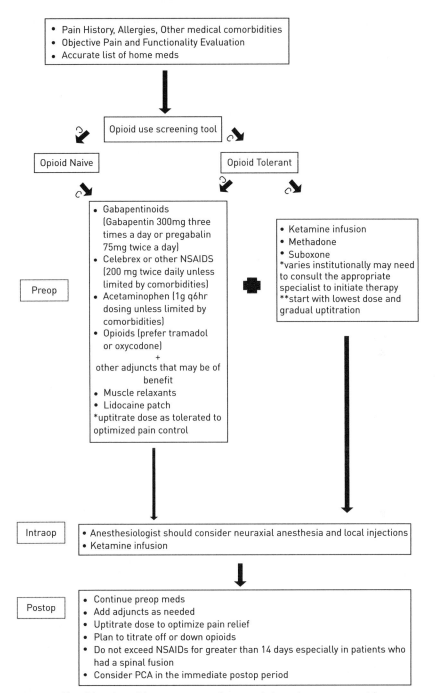

FIGURE 12.1 Algorithm describing our proposed approach for pain management in neurosurgical spine patients.

be added to the MMA checklist. For the time being, it is recommended that patients be started preoperatively on home doses of opioids or low doses of opioids on an as-needed basis, gabapentinoids, celecoxib, and acetaminophen. Despite acetaminophen not exhibiting strong evidence of efficacy in spine surgery, it is a common agent in most MMA regimens and has a limited side-effect profile, with its benefits likely outweighing its risks. Intraoperatively, the patient's anesthesiologist should consider intravenous ketamine, neuraxial analgesia, and/or local anesthesia. Postoperatively, patients should be evaluated for PCA and continuation of intravenous ketamine. Gabapentinoids, celecoxib, and acetaminophen should be continued postoperatively, and their respective doses titrated up slowly, with a follow-up pain and functionality assessment with each pain medication adjustment. Agents that have no strong literature support, such as muscle relaxants or lidocaine patches, may serve as adjuncts. Patients who are opioid-tolerant should be converted to an oral opioid regimen based on their PCA requirements. Patients who are opioid-naïve should start with a low dose of oral opioids on an as-needed basis and be uptitrated to optimize pain control. Tramadol and oxycodone are recommended given their reduced side-effect profile compared to other opioids. Opioids should be titrated down and off actively with a goal of no opioids prior to discharge or within 7 days from discharge. The side effects of NSAIDs, including fusion failure, are time dependent and therefore NSAIDs should be used in a short-term basis of less than 14 days.

FUTURE DIRECTIONS

Research in pain management for spinal surgery patients is still in its infancy. More research is needed to identify new medications or modalities that are effective in treating perioperative spinal surgery pain, to delineate the optimal dose and administration timing of these medications, and to evaluate the effectiveness and possible synergism/additive effect of different MMA backbone regimens. Furthermore, the spine literature generally focuses on lumbar surgery, so it would be interesting to evaluate if there are any differences in the pain management of cervical or thoracic spine patients.

REFERENCES

1. Carli F, Kehlet H, Baldini G, et al. Evidence basis for regional anesthesia in multidisciplinary fast-track surgical care pathways. *Reg Anesth Pain Med.* 2011;36(1):63–72. doi: 10.1097/AAP.0b013e31820307f7.

2. Abou-Setta AM, Beaupre LA, Rashiq S, et al. Comparative effectiveness of pain management interventions for hip fracture: a systematic review. *Ann Intern Med.* 2011;155(4):234–245. doi: 10.7326/0003-4819-155-4-201108160-00346.

3. Borghi B, D'Addabbo M, White PF, et al. The use of prolonged peripheral neural blockade after lower extremity amputation: the effect on symptoms associated with phantom limb syndrome. *Anesth Analg.* 2010;111(5):1308–1315. doi: 10.1213/ANE.0b013e3181f4e848.

4. Boezaart AP, Davis G, Le-Wendling L. Recovery after orthopedic surgery: techniques to increase duration of pain control. *Curr Opin Anaesthesiol.* 2012;25(6):665–672. doi: 10.1097/ACO.0b013e328359ab5a.

5. Lenart MJ, Wong K, Gupta RK, et al. The impact of peripheral nerve techniques on hospital stay following major orthopedic surgery. *Pain Med.* 2012;13(6):828–834. doi: 10.1111/j.1526-4637.2012.01363.x.

6. Pugely AJ, Martin CT, Gao Y, Mendoza-Lattes S. Causes and risk factors for 30-day unplanned readmissions after lumbar spine surgery. *Spine (Phila Pa 1976)*. 2014;39(9):761–768. doi: 10.1097/BRS.0000000000000270.

7. Lemos P, Pinto A, Morais G, et al. Patient satisfaction following day surgery. *J Clin Anesth*. 2009;21(3):200–205. doi: 10.1016/j.jclinane.2008.08.016.

8. Devin CJ, McGirt MJ. Best evidence in multimodal pain management in spine surgery and means of assessing postoperative pain and functional outcomes. *J Clin Neurosci*. 2015;22(6):930–938. doi: 10.1016/j.jocn.2015.01.003.

9. Dunn LK, Durieux ME, Nemergut EC. Non-opioid analgesics: novel approaches to perioperative analgesia for major spine surgery. *Best Pract Res Clin Anaesthesiol*. 2016;30(1):79–89. doi: 10.1016/j.bpa.2015.11.002.

10. Gottschalk A, Durieux ME, Nemergut EC. Intraoperative methadone improves postoperative pain control in patients undergoing complex spine surgery. *Anesth Analg*. 2011;112(1):218–223. doi: 10.1213/ANE.0b013e3181d8a095.

11. Cheung CW, Ching Wong SS, Qiu Q, Wang X. Oral oxycodone for acute postoperative pain: a review of clinical trials. *Pain Physician*. 2017;20(2S):SE33–SE52.

12. Okie S. A flood of opioids, a rising tide of deaths. *N Engl J Med*. 2010;363(21):1981–1985. doi: 10.1056/NEJMp1011512.

13. Wick EC, Grant MC, Wu CL. Postoperative multimodal analgesia pain management with nonopioid analgesics and techniques: a review. *JAMA Surg*. 2017;152(7):691–697. doi: 10.1001/jamasurg.2017.0898.

14. Schwenk ES, Mariano ER. Designing the ideal perioperative pain management plan starts with multimodal analgesia. *Korean J Anesthesiol*. 2018;71(5):345–352. doi: 10.4097/kja.d.18.00217.

15. Compton PA, Wu SM, Schieffer B, Pham Q, Naliboff BD. Introduction of a self-report version of the prescription drug use questionnaire and relationship to medication agreement noncompliance. *J Pain Symptom Manage*. 2008;36(4):383–395. doi: 10.1016/j.jpainsymman.2007.11.006.

16. Manchikanti L, Helm S, 2nd, Fellows B, et al. Opioid epidemic in the United States. *Pain Physician*. 2012;15(3 Suppl):ES9–E38.

17. Buvanendran A, Thillainathan V. Preoperative and postoperative anesthetic and analgesic techniques for minimally invasive surgery of the spine. *Spine (Phila Pa 1976)*. 2010;35(26 Suppl):S274–S280. doi: 10.1097/BRS.0b013e31820240f8.

18. Garimella V, Cellini C. Postoperative pain control. *Clin Colon Rectal Surg*. 2013;26(3):191–196. doi: 10.1055/s-0033-1351138.

19. Inturrisi CE. Clinical pharmacology of opioids for pain. *Clin J Pain*. 2002;18(4 Suppl):S3–S13.

20. Moonla R, Threetipayarak A, Panpaisarn C, et al. Comparison of preoperative and postoperative parecoxib administration for pain control following major spine surgery. *Asian Spine J*. 2018;12(5):893–901. doi: 10.31616/asj.2018.12.5.893.

21. Chou R, Turner JA, Devine EB, et al. The effectiveness and risks of long-term opioid therapy for chronic pain: a systematic review for a national institutes of health pathways to prevention workshop. *Ann Intern Med*. 2015;162(4):276–286. doi: 10.7326/M14-2559.

22. Puvanesarajah V, Liauw JA, Lo SF, Lina IA, Witham TF, Gottschalk A. Analgesic therapy for major spine surgery. *Neurosurg Rev*. 2015;38(3):407–418; discussion 419. doi: 10.1007/s10143-015-0605-7.

23. Guignard B, Bossard AE, Coste C, et al. Acute opioid tolerance: intraoperative remifentanil increases postoperative pain and morphine requirement. *Anesthesiology*. 2000;93(2):409–417.

24. Chapman CR, Davis J, Donaldson GW, Naylor J, Winchester D. Postoperative pain trajectories in chronic pain patients undergoing surgery: the effects of chronic opioid pharmacotherapy on acute pain. *J Pain*. 2011;12(12):1240–1246. doi: 10.1016/j.jpain.2011.07.005.

25. Nielsen RV. Adjuvant analgesics for spine surgery. *Dan Med J*. 2018;65(3):B5468. doi: B5468 [pii].

26. De Jong R, Shysh AJ. Development of a multimodal analgesia protocol for perioperative acute pain management for lower limb amputation. *Pain Res Manag*. 2018;2018:5237040. doi: 10.1155/2018/5237040.

27. Pitchon DN, Dayan AC, Schwenk ES, Baratta JL, Viscusi ER. Updates on multimodal analgesia for orthopedic surgery. *Anesthesiol Clin*. 2018;36(3):361–373. doi: S1932-2275(18)30051-X [pii].

28. Song KS, Cho JH, Hong JY, et al. Neuropathic pain related with spinal disorders: a systematic review. *Asian Spine J*. 2017;11(4):661–674. doi: 10.4184/asj.2017.11.4.661.

29. Kehlet H, Jensen TS, Woolf CJ. Persistent postsurgical pain: risk factors and prevention. *Lancet*. 2006;367(9522):1618–1625. doi: S0140-6736(06)68700-X [pii].

30. Hall N, Eldabe S. Phantom limb pain: a review of pharmacological management. *Br J Pain*. 2018;12(4):202–207. doi: 10.1177/2049463717747307.

31. Cohen SP, Mao J. Neuropathic pain: mechanisms and their clinical implications. *BMJ*. 2014;348:f7656. doi: 10.1136/bmj.f7656.

32. Daniell JR, Osti OL. Failed back surgery syndrome: a review article. *Asian Spine J*. 2018;12(2):372–379. doi: 10.4184/asj.2018.12.2.372.

33. Mense S. Muscle pain: mechanisms and clinical significance. *Dtsch Arztebl Int*. 2008;105(12):214–219. doi: 10.3238/artzebl.2008.0214.

34. Yang KH, King AI. Mechanism of facet load transmission as a hypothesis for low-back pain. *Spine (Phila Pa 1976)*. 1984;9(6):557–565.

35. Samad TA, Moore KA, Sapirstein A, et al. Interleukin-1beta-mediated induction of cox-2 in the CNS contributes to inflammatory pain hypersensitivity. *Nature*. 2001;410(6827):471–475. doi: 10.1038/35068566.

36. Kurd MF, Kreitz T, Schroeder G, Vaccaro AR. The role of multimodal analgesia in spine surgery. *J Am Acad Orthop Surg*. 2017;25(4):260–268. doi: 10.5435/JAAOS-D-16-00049.

37. Rullan M, Bulilete O, Leiva A, et al. Efficacy of gabapentin for prevention of postherpetic neuralgia: study protocol for a randomized controlled clinical trial. *Trials*. 2017;18(1):24–016–1729-y. doi: 10.1186/s13063-016-1729-y.

38. Snyder MJ, Gibbs LM, Lindsay TJ. Treating painful diabetic peripheral neuropathy: an update. *Am Fam Physician*. 2016;94(3):227–234. doi: d12555 [pii].

39. Montazeri K, Kashefi P, Honarmand A. Pre-emptive gabapentin significantly reduces postoperative pain and morphine demand following lower extremity orthopaedic surgery. *Singapore Med J*. 2007;48(8):748–751.

40. Yu L, Ran B, Li M, Shi Z. Gabapentin and pregabalin in the management of postoperative pain after lumbar spinal surgery: a systematic review and meta-analysis. *Spine (Phila Pa 1976)*. 2013;38(22):1947–1952. doi: 10.1097/BRS.0b013e3182a69b90.

41. Han C, Kuang MJ, Ma JX, Ma XL. The efficacy of preoperative gabapentin in spinal surgery: a meta-analysis of randomized controlled trials. *Pain Physician*. 2017;20(7):649–661.

42. Liu B, Liu R, Wang L. A meta-analysis of the preoperative use of gabapentinoids for the treatment of acute postoperative pain following spinal surgery. *Medicine (Baltimore)*. 2017;96(37):e8031. doi: 10.1097/MD.0000000000008031.

43. Khurana G, Jindal P, Sharma JP, Bansal KK. Postoperative pain and long-term functional outcome after administration of gabapentin and pregabalin in patients undergoing spinal surgery. *Spine (Phila Pa 1976)*. 2014;39(6):E363–E368. doi: 10.1097/BRS.0000000000000185.

44. Shimony N, Amit U, Minz B, et al. Perioperative pregabalin for reducing pain, analgesic consumption, and anxiety and enhancing sleep quality in elective neurosurgical patients: a prospective, randomized, double-blind, and controlled clinical study. *J Neurosurg*. 2016;125(6):1513–1522. doi: 10.3171/2015.10.JNS151516.

45. Srivastava VK, Agrawal S, Nimbhorkar VK, Mishra A, Sharma S, Panda PK. Prophylactic use of pregabalin for prevention of succinylcholine-induced fasciculation and myalgia: a randomized, double-blinded, placebo-controlled study. *Braz J Anesthesiol*. 2016;66(2):165–170. doi: 10.1016/j.bjane.2014.08.004.

46. Park M, Jeon Y. Preoperative pregabalin prolongs duration of spinal anesthesia and reduces early postoperative pain: a double-blind, randomized clinical CONSORT study. *Medicine (Baltimore)*. 2016;95(36):e4828. doi: 10.1097/MD.0000000000004828.

47. Cegin MB, Soyoral L, Yuzkat N, Baydi V, Goktas U. Pregabalin administered as an anxiolytic agent in ultrasound-guided infraclavicular block: a controlled, double-blind, dose-ranging trial. *Eur Rev Med Pharmacol Sci*. 2016;20(3):568–574. doi: 10297 [pii].

48. Hetta DF, Mohamed MA, Mohammad MF. Analgesic efficacy of pregabalin in acute postmastectomy pain: placebo controlled dose ranging study. *J Clin Anesth*. 2016;34:303–309. doi: 10.1016/j.jclinane.2016.05.007.

49. Fujita N, Tobe M, Tsukamoto N, Saito S, Obata H. A randomized placebo-controlled study of preoperative pregabalin for postoperative analgesia in patients with spinal surgery. *J Clin Anesth*. 2016;31:149–153. doi: 10.1016/j.jclinane.2016.01.010.

50. Kim JC, Choi YS, Kim KN, Shim JK, Lee JY, Kwak YL. Effective dose of perioperative oral pregabalin as an adjunct to multimodal analgesic regimen in lumbar spinal fusion surgery. *Spine (Phila Pa 1976)*. 2011;36(6):428–433. doi: 10.1097/BRS.0b013e3181d26708.

51. Khan ZH, Rahimi M, Makarem J, Khan RH. Optimal dose of pre-incision/post-incision gabapentin for pain relief following lumbar laminectomy: a randomized study. *Acta Anaesthesiol Scand*. 2011;55(3):306–312. doi: 10.1111/j.1399-6576.2010.02377.x.

52. Bruhn J, Scheffer GJ, van Geffen GJ. Clinical application of perioperative multimodal analgesia. *Curr Opin Support Palliat Care*. 2017;11(2):106–111. doi: 10.1097/SPC.0000000000000267.

53. White PF, Tufanogullari B, Taylor J, Klein K. The effect of pregabalin on preoperative anxiety and sedation levels: a dose-ranging study. *Anesth Analg*. 2009;108(4):1140–1145. doi: 10.1213/ane.0b013e31818d40ce.

54. Cao X, Elvir-Lazo OL, White PF, Yumul R, Tang J. An update on pain management for elderly patients undergoing ambulatory surgery. *Curr Opin Anaesthesiol*. 2016;29(6):674–682. doi: 10.1097/ACO.0000000000000396.

55. Khetarpal R, Kataria AP, Bajaj S, Kaur H, Singh S. Gabapentin vs pregabalin as a premedication in lower limb orthopaedics surgery under combined spinal epidural technique. *Anesth Essays Res*. 2016;10(2):262–267. doi: 10.4103/0259-1162.172339.

56. Toth C. Pregabalin: Latest safety evidence and clinical implications for the management of neuropathic pain. *Ther Adv Drug Saf*. 2014;5(1):38–56. doi: 10.1177/2042098613505614.

57. Glassman SD, Rose SM, Dimar JR, Puno RM, Campbell MJ, Johnson JR. The effect of postoperative nonsteroidal anti-inflammatory drug administration on spinal fusion. *Spine (Phila Pa 1976)*. 1998;23(7):834–838.

58. Gobble RM, Hoang HL, Kachniarz B, Orgill DP. Ketorolac does not increase perioperative bleeding: a meta-analysis of randomized controlled trials. *Plast Reconstr Surg.* 2014;133(3):741–755. doi: 10.1097/01.prs.0000438459.60474.b5.

59. Dodwell ER, Latorre JG, Parisini E, et al. NSAID exposure and risk of nonunion: a meta-analysis of case-control and cohort studies. *Calcif Tissue Int.* 2010;87(3):193–202. doi: 10.1007/s00223-010-9379-7.

60. Sivaganesan A, Chotai S, White-Dzuro G, McGirt MJ, Devin CJ. The effect of NSAIDs on spinal fusion: a cross-disciplinary review of biochemical, animal, and human studies. *Eur Spine J.* 2017;26(11):2719–2728. doi: 10.1007/s00586-017-5021-y.

61. Long J, Lewis S, Kuklo T, Zhu Y, Riew KD. The effect of cyclooxygenase-2 inhibitors on spinal fusion. *J Bone Joint Surg Am.* 2002;84-A(10):1763–1768.

62. Jirarattanaphochai K, Thienthong S, Sriraj W, et al. Effect of parecoxib on postoperative pain after lumbar spine surgery: a bicenter, randomized, double-blinded, placebo-controlled trial. *Spine (Phila Pa 1976).* 2008;33(2):132–139. doi: 10.1097/BRS.0b013e3181604529.

63. Jirarattanaphochai K, Jung S. Nonsteroidal antiinflammatory drugs for postoperative pain management after lumbar spine surgery: a meta-analysis of randomized controlled trials. *J Neurosurg Spine.* 2008;9(1):22–31. doi: 10.3171/SPI/2008/9/7/022.

64. Yoshihara H. Pain medication use after spine surgery: is it assessed in the literature? A systematic review, january 2000-december 2009. *BMC Res Notes.* 2015;8:323–015–1287–5. doi: 10.1186/s13104-015-1287-5.

65. Sinatra RS, Jahr JS, Reynolds L, et al. Intravenous acetaminophen for pain after major orthopedic surgery: an expanded analysis. *Pain Pract.* 2012;12(5):357–365. doi: 10.1111/j.1533-2500.2011.00514.x.

66. Sinatra RS, Torres J, Bustos AM. Pain management after major orthopaedic surgery: current strategies and new concepts. *J Am Acad Orthop Surg.* 2002;10(2):117–129.

67. Khalili G, Janghorbani M, Saryazdi H, Emaminejad A. Effect of preemptive and preventive acetaminophen on postoperative pain score: a randomized, double-blind trial of patients undergoing lower extremity surgery. *J Clin Anesth.* 2013;25(3):188–192. doi: 10.1016/j.jclinane.2012.09.004.

68. Cakan T, Inan N, Culhaoglu S, Bakkal K, Basar H. Intravenous paracetamol improves the quality of postoperative analgesia but does not decrease narcotic requirements. *J Neurosurg Anesthesiol.* 2008;20(3):169–173. doi: 10.1097/ANA.0b013e3181705cfb.

69. Yang L, Du S, Sun Y. Intravenous acetaminophen as an adjunct to multimodal analgesia after total knee and hip arthroplasty: a systematic review and meta-analysis. *Int J Surg.* 2017;47:135–146. doi: S1743-9191(17)31259-1 [pii].

70. Hansen RN, Pham AT, Boing EA, Lovelace B, Wan GJ, Miller TE. Comparative analysis of length of stay, hospitalization costs, opioid use, and discharge status among spine surgery patients with postoperative pain management including intravenous versus oral acetaminophen. *Curr Med Res Opin.* 2017;33(5):943–948. doi: 10.1080/03007995.2017.1297702.

71. Morwald EE, Poeran J, Zubizarreta N, Cozowicz C, Mazumdar M, Memtsoudis SG. Intravenous acetaminophen does not reduce inpatient opioid prescription or opioid-related adverse events among patients undergoing spine surgery. *Anesth Analg.* 2018;127(5):1221–1228. doi: 10.1213/ANE.0000000000003344.

72. Gallipani A, Mathis AS, Lee Ghin H, Fahim G. Adverse effect profile comparison of pain regimens with and without intravenous acetaminophen in total hip and knee arthroplasty patients. *SAGE Open Med.* 2017;5:2050312117699146. doi: 10.1177/2050312117699146.

73. Jibril F, Sharaby S, Mohamed A, Wilby KJ. Intravenous versus oral acetaminophen for pain: systematic review of current evidence to support clinical decision-making. *Can J Hosp Pharm.* 2015;68(3):238–247.

74. Chandok N, Watt KD. Pain management in the cirrhotic patient: the clinical challenge. *Mayo Clin Proc.* 2010;85(5):451–458. doi: 10.4065/mcp.2009.0534.

75. Kaye AD, Cornett EM, Helander E, et al. An update on nonopioids: intravenous or oral analgesics for perioperative pain management. *Anesthesiol Clin.* 2017;35(2):e55–e71. doi: S1932-2275(17)30011-3 [pii].

76. Nielsen RV, Fomsgaard JS, Siegel H, et al. Intraoperative ketamine reduces immediate postoperative opioid consumption after spinal fusion surgery in chronic pain patients with opioid dependency: a randomized, blinded trial. *Pain.* 2017;158(3):463–470. doi: 10.1097/j.pain.0000000000000782.

77. Bell RF, Dahl JB, Moore RA, Kalso E. Perioperative ketamine for acute postoperative pain. *Cochrane Database Syst Rev.* 2006;(1):CD004603. doi(1):CD004603. doi: 10.1002/14651858.CD004603.pub2.

78. Mitra S, Carlyle D, Kodumudi G, Kodumudi V, Vadivelu N. New advances in acute postoperative pain management. *Curr Pain Headache Rep.* 2018;22(5):35–018–0690–8. doi: 10.1007/s11916-018-0690-8.

79. Loftus RW, Yeager MP, Clark JA, et al. Intraoperative ketamine reduces perioperative opiate consumption in opiate-dependent patients with chronic back pain undergoing back surgery. *Anesthesiology.* 2010;113(3):639–646. doi: 10.1097/ALN.0b013e3181e90914.

80. Urban MK, Ya Deau JT, Wukovits B, Lipnitsky JY. Ketamine as an adjunct to postoperative pain management in opioid tolerant patients after spinal fusions: a prospective randomized trial. *HSS J.* 2008;4(1):62–65. doi: 10.1007/s11420-007-9069-9.

81. Rhen T, Cidlowski JA. Antiinflammatory action of glucocorticoids: new mechanisms for old drugs. *N Engl J Med.* 2005;353(16):1711–1723. doi: 353/16/1711 [pii].

82. De Oliveira GS, Jr, Almeida MD, Benzon HT, McCarthy RJ. Perioperative single dose systemic dexamethasone for postoperative pain: a meta-analysis of randomized controlled trials. *Anesthesiology.* 2011;115(3):575–588. doi: 10.1097/ALN.0b013e31822a24c2.

83. Waldron NH, Jones CA, Gan TJ, Allen TK, Habib AS. Impact of perioperative dexamethasone on postoperative analgesia and side-effects: systematic review and meta-analysis. *Br J Anaesth.* 2013;110(2):191–200. doi: 10.1093/bja/aes431.

84. Ziegeler S, Fritsch E, Bauer C, et al. Therapeutic effect of intrathecal morphine after posterior lumbar interbody fusion surgery: a prospective, double-blind, randomized study. *Spine (Phila Pa 1976).* 2008;33(22):2379–2386. doi: 10.1097/BRS.0b013e3181844ef2.

85. Chan JH, Heilpern GN, Packham I, Trehan RK, Marsh GD, Knibb AA. A prospective randomized double-blind trial of the use of intrathecal fentanyl in patients undergoing lumbar spinal surgery. *Spine (Phila Pa 1976).* 2006;31(22):2529–2533. doi: 10.1097/01.brs.0000241135.79983.52.

86. Sun Y, Li T, Wang N, Yun Y, Gan TJ. Perioperative systemic lidocaine for postoperative analgesia and recovery after abdominal surgery: a meta-analysis of randomized controlled trials. *Dis Colon Rectum.* 2012;55(11):1183–1194. doi: 10.1097/DCR.0b013e318259bcd8.

87. Beakley BD, Kaye AM, Kaye AD. Tramadol, pharmacology, side effects, and serotonin syndrome: a review. *Pain Physician.* 2015;18(4):395–400.

88. Ross FB, Smith MT. The intrinsic antinociceptive effects of oxycodone appear to be kappa-opioid receptor mediated. *Pain.* 1997;73(2):151–157. doi: S0304-3959(97)00093-6 [pii].

89. Nielsen CK, Ross FB, Lotfipour S, Saini KS, Edwards SR, Smith MT. Oxycodone and morphine have distinctly different pharmacological profiles: radioligand binding and behavioural studies in two rat models of neuropathic pain. *Pain.* 2007;132(3):289–300. doi: S0304-3959(07)00135-2 [pii].

90. Poyhia R, Seppala T, Olkkola KT, Kalso E. The pharmacokinetics and metabolism of oxycodone after intramuscular and oral administration to healthy subjects. *Br J Clin Pharmacol.* 1992;33(6):617–621.

91. Thirlwell MP, Sloan PA, Maroun JA, et al. Pharmacokinetics and clinical efficacy of oral morphine solution and controlled-release morphine tablets in cancer patients. *Cancer.* 1989;63(11 Suppl):2275–2283.

92. Bostrom E, Hammarlund-Udenaes M, Simonsson US. Blood-brain barrier transport helps to explain discrepancies in in vivo potency between oxycodone and morphine. *Anesthesiology.* 2008;108(3):495–505. doi: 10.1097/ALN.0b013e318164cf9e.

93. Gammaitoni AR, Galer BS, Bulloch S, et al. Randomized, double-blind, placebo-controlled comparison of the analgesic efficacy of oxycodone 10 mg/acetaminophen 325 mg versus controlled-release oxycodone 20 mg in postsurgical pain. *J Clin Pharmacol.* 2003;43(3):296–304.

94. Ordonez Gallego A, Gonzalez Baron M, Espinosa Arranz E. Oxycodone: a pharmacological and clinical review. *Clin Transl Oncol.* 2007;9(5):298–307. doi: 946 [pii].

95. Blumenthal S, Min K, Marquardt M, Borgeat A. Postoperative intravenous morphine consumption, pain scores, and side effects with perioperative oral controlled-release oxycodone after lumbar discectomy. *Anesth Analg.* 2007;105(1):233–237. doi: 105/1/233 [pii].

96. Melzack R. The McGill pain questionnaire: major properties and scoring methods. *Pain.* 1975;1(3):277–299. doi: 0304-3959(75)90044-5 [pii].

97. Gallagher EJ, Liebman M, Bijur PE. Prospective validation of clinically important changes in pain severity measured on a visual analog scale. *Ann Emerg Med.* 2001;38(6):633–638. doi: S0196-0644(01)04166-X [pii].

98. Roland M, Morris R. A study of the natural history of back pain. Part I: development of a reliable and sensitive measure of disability in low-back pain. *Spine (Phila Pa 1976).* 1983;8(2):141–144.

99. Cleeland CS, Ryan KM. Pain assessment: global use of the brief pain inventory. *Ann Acad Med Singapore.* 1994;23(2):129–138.

100. Keller S, Bann CM, Dodd SL, Schein J, Mendoza TR, Cleeland CS. Validity of the brief pain inventory for use in documenting the outcomes of patients with noncancer pain. *Clin J Pain.* 2004;20(5):309–318. doi: 00002508-200409000-00005 [pii].

13 Rehabilitation Medicine in the Neurosurgical Patient

Catriona M. Harrop, Kristin Gustafson, Swathi Maddula, James Bresnehan, and Philip Koehler

THE PATIENT WITH BRAIN INJURY
Introduction

The Demographics and Clinical Assessment Working Group of the International and Interagency Initiative Toward Common Data Elements for Research on Traumatic Brain Injury and Psychological Health position statement defines traumatic brain injury (TBI): "TBI is defined as an alteration in brain function, or other evidence of brain pathology, caused by an external force."[1]

Alteration in brain function is defined as one of the following signs:

- Any period or loss of or a decreased level of consciousness
- Any loss of memory for events immediately before (retrograde amnesia) or after the injury (posttraumatic amnesia)
- Neurologic deficits (weakness, loss of balance, change in vision, dyspraxia, paresis/plegia, sensory loss, aphasia, etc.)
- Any alteration in mental state at the time of injury (confusion, disorientation, slowed thinking, etc.)

Evidence of brain pathology may include:

- Visual
- Neuroradiologic
- Laboratory confirmation

An external force may include any of the following events:

- The head being struck by an object
- The head striking an object

233

- The brain undergoing an acceleration/deceleration movement without direct external trauma to the head
- A foreign body penetrating the brain
- Forces generated from events such as a blast or explosion
- Or other force yet to be defined.

Patients with TBI represent a significant percentage of the neurosurgical population; therefore their medical management is important. We will examine the clinical consequences of TBI in relation to their impact on rehabilitation by organ system.

Neurologic System Disorders

Because TBI represents an injury to the neurologic system, we review here the most common clinical issue aside from cognitive dysfunction.

Sleep–Wake Disorders

Sleep disturbance is common after TBI,[2] most often represented by excessive daytime sleepiness,[3] and can persist for years post injury. A study by Kempf et al. demonstrated that 67% of patients studied had sleep–wake disturbances (SWD) that persisted up to 3 years after TBI. The most common SWD were excessive daytime sleepiness, fatigue, posttraumatic hypersomnia, and insomnia.[3] Animal models underscore the potential significance of sleep disturbance in the recovery of the brain-injured patient. One study found that 3 days of sleep deprivation and sleep disruption worsened injury patterns and impaired recovery after simulated stroke in rat models.[4–6] Another study compared sleep-deprived animals to non–sleep deprived and found that the sleep-deprived animals did significantly worse on behavioral tasks. And at autopsy, the sleep-deprived animals were found to have lower evidence of brain repair such as axonal sprouting and vasogenesis compared to the control group.[4,6]

Human studies also show a causal relationship between non–brain injured patient's sleep disruption and negative health effects. There is sufficient evidence in patients with obstructive sleep apnea (OSA) to show that there are higher rates of hypertension, myocardial infarction, stroke, and insulin resistance.[7–9] It is reasonable to infer that there is an association between the brain-injured patient's sleep disruption and negative health consequences. In the brain-injured population, patients have been studied during inpatient rehabilitation after TBI, and there is a negative association with total sleep time and neurobehavioral impairment.[2] Therefore early recognition and management of SWD is important to overall patient outcomes.

Identifying Sleep–Wake Disorders

The first step in treating the TBI patient is to identify a SWD and treat any of its potential reversible causes. Identification of a SWD can be challenging as the gold standard for diagnosis is polysomnography, which can be difficult to attain in rehabilitation settings. A through history and physical can identify bowel and/ or bladder disorders such as incontinence or urgency that prevent a patient from sleeping through the night. Additional screening tools such as the STOP-BANG questionnaire can identify patients with underlying OSA.[10] Sources of pain should be identified and controlled, as well as any psychiatric disorders such as anxiety or depression, which can interfere with the sleep–wake cycle.

Environmental Regulation

Environmental factors play extensive roles in the maintenance of sleep–wake cycles. After the identification of treatable causes of SWD, the patient's environment needs to be modified to ensure successful sleep–wake regulation. Shades should be up and lights on during the day, and the disruptions at night with vital signs, blood draws, etc. need to be kept to a minimum. For patients with TBI who have transitioned to home, educate the patient and caregivers about proper sleep hygiene. Caffeinated drinks should be limited to the early part of the day, and the use of electronics at bedtime should be avoided.[7]

Adjunctive Treatment

There are adjunctive therapies that have been found to help with the regulation of SWD which could be helpful in the patient with SWD and TBI. Cognitive behavioral therapy (CBT) is now considered first-line treatment for chronic insomnia,[11] yet there are only a handful of studies that have investigated CBT in TBI patients. One small study by Ouellet and Morin showed a benefit for CBT and insomnia in 8 out of 11 participants with TBI.[12] Acupuncture has been theorized to improve sleep in patients with TBI and insomnia, and there is a study showing that the patient's perception of sleep quality was improved after acupuncture despite sleep times being unchanged.[13]

Blue light therapy is another area of emerging research for treatment of SWD in patients with TBI. Blue light, also known as shortwave length light (430–475 nm), triggers photosensitive retinal ganglion cells which transmit to the hypothalamic nuclei, which in turn regulates the secretion of melatonin.[14] The hypothesis is that exposure to blue light in the morning leads to suppression of melatonin production and stabilization of circadian rhythms.[15] Blue light lamps and kits are sold commercially, are relatively affordable, and may provide a low-risk option for improving sleep quality.

Pharmacologic Therapy

Depending on the type of SWD, there are pharmacologic agents that can help ameliorate the symptoms of SWD in the brain-injured patient. For those with hypersomnolence as a symptom, stimulant agents such as methylphenidate, amantadine, and modafinil have been used.[7] Because these agents are stimulants, caution must be used in patients with hypertension and arrhythmias. For the patient in whom insomnia is the major symptom, agents such as benzodiazepines and nonbenzodiazepine receptor agonists have been used. These agents run the risk of cognitive dysfunction and dependence, so caution must be exercised when using them.

Musculoskeletal System Disorders

Musculoskeletal complications are common sequelae of TBI. In a retrospective study performed by Brown et al.[16] it was found that 79% of individuals in the study complained of musculoskeletal symptoms within 30 days of injury. Spasticity is a common complication after TBI, and it can present in a focal or generalized pattern. It can be a response to damage of the pyramidal system in the brain or spinal cord.[17] Long-term effects of spasticity can be debilitating, leading to great pain and disability, as well as making overall recovery cumbersome for a patient who has suffered TBI.[18]

In a study performed by Perez et al.,[17] goals of therapy were defined as improvement in functionality, quality of life and comfort, and body aesthetics; ability to provide care and perform activities of daily living; and prevention and treatment of musculoskeletal complications.

Gordon et al.[16] performed a review of several studies that explored the various treatment modalities that should be considered in the post-TBI patient suffering from spasticity. It was noted that oral muscle relaxants such as tizanidine and baclofen were effective in treating lower limb spasticity; however, tizanidine was also effective for upper limb spasticity. Caution should be exercised when administering either medication as they are both associated with sedative effects.

Additional proposed pharmacologic agents include antiepileptics such as pregabalin and gabapentin, immunomodulators, cannabinoid receptor agonists, and cannabis.[17] Injection therapies include intrathecal baclofen, which exhibits overall less systemic side effects although frequent dose adjustments must be made. Botulinum type A injection has been considered the optimal treatment for spasticity because it is focal, and phenol injection is another option.[16,17]

Adjuvant therapy with specialized stretches and ambulation have been shown to improve strength and balance.[16,17] Alternative modalities have been identified in the form of orthopedic management with selective surgical procedures, splinting, ultrasound thermotherapy, and neuromuscular electrical stimulation.

Cardiovascular System Disorders

The cardiovascular effects of TBI can be viewed in terms of the chronicity of the injury. In the acute phase, the catecholamine surge that accompanies a TBI can cause tachycardia, hypertension, arrhythmia, and myocardial ischemia. The chronic cardiovascular consequences are the most relevant to the rehabilitation setting and are discussed here.

Hypotension

Hypotension is the most common cardiovascular complication of TBI; it occurs after the initial catecholamine surge[19] and can be an issue in the rehabilitation setting. It is considered a symptom of overall autonomic instability that can accompany TBI. Treatment includes compression stockings, abdominal binders, and medications to elevate blood pressure. These medications include fludrocortisone and midodrine. Fludrocortisone acts by enhancing sodium retention by the renal tubules, thereby increasing blood volume. Midodrine is an alpha-1 receptor agonist which acts on the alpha receptors in the vasculature to increase tone, thereby increasing blood pressure.

Paroxysmal Sympathetic Hyperactivity

There are many clinical consequences of TBI, but few are as dramatic as paroxysmal sympathetic hyperactivity (PSH) or "sympathetic storming." The syndrome was first described in 1929 by Wilder Penfield who described it as "diencephalic autonomic seizures."[20] This state is characterized by episodic symptoms of sympathetic hyperactivity such as tachycardia, hypertension, hyperthermia, diaphoresis, and motor posturing.

There have been many different names for this condition, as well as differing diagnostic criteria; therefore, in 2014, Baguley et al. simplified nomenclature and unified classification with a consensus paper.[21] The authors established an 11-point scale known as the Paroxysmal Sympathetic Hyperactivity-Assessment Measure (PSH-AM; see Table 13.1). The higher the score, the greater the probability that the patient has PSH.

Clinical Outcomes Some studies demonstrate that patients with TBI and PSH do worse clinically than patients without PSH. Another study by Baguley et al. in 1999 reported that patients with PSH had worse clinical outcomes and longer hospital stays than their matched controls.[22] In a review of PSH published in *Lancet* in 2018, the authors agreed that "the overall clinical impression is that PSH is an independent risk factor for poorer Neurologic outcomes in patient who have had brain injury."[23] Therefore the identification and treatment of patients with PSH in the rehabilitation setting is vitally important.

Pharmacologic Therapy Meyfroidt et al.[23] described three goals in the treatment of PSH in their review. The first is to avoid triggers that provoke the episodes, the second is to mitigate sympathetic response, and the third is to limit the effects of PSH on other organ systems through supportive therapy. Table. 132 shows the different classes of pharmacologic agents that are used to mitigate sympathetic response in PSH. In clinical practice it is observed that most patients need multiple therapies with overlapping therapeutic targets to control their symptoms.[23] Currently there is no one drug or protocol that is considered a standard of care in treatment of PSH.[24]

Table 13.1 Paroxysmal sympathetic hyperactivity-assessment measure (PSH-AM)

Clinical Feature Scale (CFS)

	0	1	2	3	Score
Heart rate	<100	100–119	120–139	≥140	
Respiratory rate	<18	18–23	24–29	≥30	
Systolic blood pressure	<140	140–159	160–179	≥180	
Temperature	<37	37–37.9	38–38.9	≥39.0	
Sweating	Nil	Mild	Moderate	Severe	
Posturing during episodes	Nil	Mild	Moderate	Severe	
			CFS subtotal		
Severity of clinical features			Nil	0	
			Mild	1–6	
			Moderate	7–12	
			Severe	≥13	

Diagnosis Likelihood Tool (DLT)

Clinical features occur simultaneously

Episodes are paroxysmal in nature

Sympathetic overreactivity to normally nonpainful stimuli

Features persist ≥3 consecutive days

Features persist ≥2 weeks post brain injury

Features persist despite treatment of alternative differential diagnoses

Medication, administered to decrease sympathetic features

≥2 episodes daily

Absence of parasympathetic features during episodes

Absence of other presumed cause of features

Antecedent acquired brain injury

(Score 1 point for each feature percent)   DLT subtotal

Combined total (CFS + DLT)

PSH diagnostic likelihood	Unlikely		<8
	Possible		8–16
	Possible		>17

Table 13.2 Classes of drugs used for treatment and prevention of paroxysmal sympathetic hyperactivity (PSH)

	Prevention or treatment: dose and route	Site of action	Clinical features targeted	Evidence of efficacy	Cautionary notes
Opioids					
Morphine ‡ 40	Prevention: intravenous infusion, titrate to effect Treatment: 1–10 mg intravenous bolus	Opioid receptors in brain and spinal cord (and possibly in peripheral tissue)	Most features, particularly hypertension, allodynia, and tachycardia	Consistent	Respiratory depression, tolerance, and need for dose escalation
Fentanyl 41	Prevention: patch 12–100 μg/h	Opioid receptors in brain and spinal cord (and possibly in peripheral tissue)	Most features, particularly hypertension, allodynia, and tachycardia	Consistent	Respiratory depression, tolerance, and need for dose escalation
Intravenous anaesthetics					
Propofol	Prevention: intravenous infusion; maximum <4 mg/kg/h Treatment: 10–20 mg intravenous bolus	GABA A receptors in brain	Most features	Consistent	Only if mechanically ventilated, and in acute phase
β-adrenergic blockers					
Propranolol 42–44	Prevention: 20–60 mg q4–6h, orally (rectal administration also described)	Nonselective β adrenoceptors (central, cardiac, and peripheral)	Tachycardia, hypertension, and diaphoresis; might help with dystonia	Consistent	Bradycardia, hypotension, bradyarrhythmia, sleep disturbances, and masked hypoglycemia, especially with oral antidiabetics

(continued)

Table 13.2 Continued

	Prevention or treatment: dose and route	Site of action	Clinical features targeted	Evidence of efficacy	Cautionary notes
Labetalol 45	Prevention: 100–200 mg q12h, orally	β and α adrenoceptors	Tachycardia, hypertension, and diaphoresis; might help with dystonia	Limited	Bradycardia, hypotension, bradyarrhythmia, sleep disturbances, and masked hypoglycemia, especially with oral antidiabetics
Metoprolol	Prevention: 25 mg q8h, orally	Cardioselective β adrenoceptors	Limited or no impact on any features	Ineffective	Bradycardia, hypotension, bradyarrhythmia, sleep disturbances, and masked hypoglycemia, especially with oral antidiabetics
α2 agonists					
Clonidine 46	Prevention: 100 µg q8–12h, orally; titrate to a maximum of 1,200 µg/d Prevention: intravenous infusion; titrate to effect	α2 adrenoceptors in brain and spinal cord	Hypertension and tachycardia	Intermediate	Hypotension, bradycardia, and sedation; intravenous infusions are not a long-term solution
Dexmedetomidine 47,48	Prevention: intravenous infusion; titrate to effect Prevention and treatment: 0.2–0.7 µg/kg/h	α2 adrenoceptors in brain and spinal cord	Hypertension and tachycardia	Intermediate	Hypotension, bradycardia, and sedation; intravenous infusions are not a long-term solution

Neuromodulators

Drug	Dosing	Mechanism	Clinical target	Duration	Adverse effects
Bromocriptine 34,46	Prevention: 1.25 mg q12h, orally; titrate to a maximum of 40 mg/d	Dopamine D 2 receptors	Temperature and sweating	Intermediate	Confusion, agitation, dyskinesia, nausea, and hypotension
Gabapentin 49	Prevention: 100 mg every q8h, orally; titrate to a maximum of 4,800 mg/d	$\alpha2\delta$ presynaptic voltage-gated Ca 2+ channels in brain and spinal cord	Spasticity and allodynic responses	Consistent	Well tolerated
Baclofen 50–52	Prevention: 5 mg q8h, orally; titrate to a maximum of 80 mg/d Prevention: intrathecal (specialist use only)	GABA B receptors	Spasticity and dystonia	Orally: limited; intrathecal: consistent	Sedation and withdrawal syndrome

Benzodiazepines

Drug	Dosing	Mechanism	Clinical target	Duration	Adverse effects
Diazepam	Treatment: 1–10 mg intravenous bolus	Central benzodiazepine receptors on GABA complexes in brain and spinal cord	Agitation, hypertension, tachycardia, and posturing	Intermediate	Sedation; use intravenous boluses with caution in patients without secure artificial airway
Lorazepam	Treatment: 1–4 mg intravenous bolus	Central benzodiazepine receptors on GABA complexes in brain and spinal cord	Agitation, hypertension, tachycardia, and posturing	Intermediate	Sedation; use intravenous boluses with caution in patients without secure artificial airway
Midazolam	Treatment: 1–2 mg intravenous bolus	Central benzodiazepine receptors on GABA complexes in brain and spinal cord	Agitation, hypertension, tachycardia, and posturing	Intermediate	Sedation; use intravenous boluses with caution in patients without secure artificial airway

(*continued*)

Table 13.2 Continued

	Prevention or treatment: dose and route	Site of action	Clinical features targeted	Evidence of efficacy	Cautionary notes
Clonazepam	Prevention: 0.5–8.0 mg/d, orally in divided doses	Central benzodiazepine receptors on GABA complexes in brain and spinal cord	Agitation, hypertension, tachycardia, and posturing	Intermediate	Sedation; use intravenous boluses with caution in patients without secure artificial airway
Sarcolemmal Ca²⁺ release blockers					
Dantrolene 46	Treatment: 0.5–2 mg/kg intravenous q6–12h; titrate to a maximum of 10 mg/kg/d	Ryanodine receptors in cell membranes of striated muscle fibre cells	Posturing and muscular spasms	Intermediate	Hepatotoxicity and respiratory depression

These data are provided as a record of published reports of drugs used to treat patients with PSH and not as recommendations for treatment. Drug doses and clinical impressions of efficacy are based on past publications of clinical trials, case series, and case reports[40–55] and are largely covered in four reviews on the subject.[1,46,56,57] Single case reports and other studies that did not add substantive information were excluded, but drug classes and specific agents that have been commonly used to treat patients with PSH are covered in this table. Combinations of drugs are commonly used in clinical practice (e.g., combining interventions for both prevention and treatment of paroxysms and using drugs in different therapeutic classes with different mechanisms). These drugs and drug combinations are based on local custom, rather than objective evidence.

Respiratory failure is common after TBI.[19] A study by Zygun et al. reported pulmonary complications in 80% of patients with severe TBI.[25] In the acute phase, neurogenic pulmonary edema and acute lung injury are common. Neurogenic pulmonary edema (NPO) can occur in the setting of TBI. The proposed the mechanism of NPO is thought to be the catecholamine surge after TBI, which increases the vascular tone of the pulmonary system and leads to hydrostatic edema. Additionally, there is most likely endothelial injury due to increased intravascular pressure and systemic inflammatory response.[19]

Treatment of acute lung injury is complicated in TBI because measures often used in treatment of acute lung injury are contraindicated in TBI. Increases in intracranial pressure can occur with prone ventilation, permissive hypercapnia, and increasing positive pressure ventilation and are therefore contraindicated.[19] The use of diuretics can exacerbate organ dysfunction in TBI because the catecholamine surge following TBI results in redistribution of blood from the systemic circulation into the pulmonary circulation, thereby reducing perfusion to organs. Therefore caution must be used when treating patients with TBI and acute lung injury.

In the chronic phase encountered in the rehabilitation setting, infection and venous thromboembolism (VTE) are more common. As patients with TBI may have difficulty protecting their airway, infection due to aspiration can arise. Ventilator associated pneumonia (VAP) can also occur in chronically ventilator-dependent patients with severe TBI. Last, VTE from immobility in severe TBI can lead to pulmonary embolism, a potentially deadly complication. Prevention strategies for both infection and VTE include mobilization, good oral hygiene, and mechanical and pharmacologic VTE prophylaxis.

Gastrointestinal

Commonly found GI complications after TBI include stress ulcers which can lead to GI bleeding and malnutrition.[26,27] In this section we discuss the pathophysiology, diagnostic methods, and therapy related to stress ulcers, along with an overview of malnutrition.

Stress Ulcers

Stress ulcers, along with GI bleeding, can commonly arise in the critically ill patient. Patients who have suffered from TBI and traumatic spinal cord injury (SCI) are among those at increased risk.[27]

Pathophysiology The pathophysiology behind these unfortunate outcomes is related to two main processes: impaired mucosal protection and increased secretion of the GI tract.[28,29] Critically ill patients produce increased levels of refluxed bile salts or uremic toxins compared to non–critically ill patient,[30] and this process can disrupt the mucosal lining of the stomach, which is normally protected by glycoproteins.[29] Another component is related particularly to the critically ill patient who has suffered a head injury in that increased levels of acid are produced secondary to overstimulation of parietal cells from gastrin.

Diagnosis Clues to diagnosis of stress ulcers are typically centered on physical exam findings related to bleeding from the GI tract such as coffee-ground emesis, emesis of frank blood, and melena. For patients who have nasogastric tubes, there may be evidence of blood while suctioning. Lab monitoring may also reveal a drop in hemoglobin level. Endoscopy is the imaging study of choice to reveal findings of ulcers.[29,31]

Prophylaxis and Pharmacotherapy Forms of prophylaxis include early enteral feeding and pharmacotherapy such as H_2- blockers, proton-pump inhibitors, and sucralfate.[27] When choosing pharmacotherapy, agents such as H_2 antihistamines (H_2A), sucralfate, and proton pump inhibitors (PPIs) have been shown to reduce the occurrence of GI bleeds.[32] Caution must be used when administering H_2A because an association has been noted with encephalopathy when these agents interact with anticonvulsant classes of medications; there is also an increased risk of developing hospital-acquired pneumonias, so avoiding H_2A is generally recommended, particularly in the patient with neurocritical illness.[32] PPIs should also be used with caution due to their increased propensity for the development of *Clostridium difficile* diarrhea.[33]

Malnutrition

Patients who suffer from severe TBI can develop complications within the GI tract leading to malnutrition, ultimately increasing their risk of mortality. Early enteral feeding is recommended in all patients with TBI.

Pathophysiology Many patients with TBI have elevated intracranial pressure and are treated with opiates for pain control. These entities can lead to sequelae such as delayed gastric emptying and alteration of normal gastric functions due to hypermetabolic, hypercatabolic, and hyperglycemic states contributing to a hyperdynamic response and breakdown of proteins.[32,34]

Prophylaxis and Pharmacotherapy Early enteral nutrition has been found to not only stimulate GI function but to prevent bacterial translocation from the GI tract, along with maintaining the composition of the mucosal structure and its function.[32,35,36] A study performed by Chiang et al. highlights that introduction of early enteral nutrition (within 48 hours of initial injury) to patients were severe TBI with a Glasgow Coma Score (GCS) of between 6 and 8 had improved survival, GCS recovery, and better outcomes.[36] Many times, patients with severe TBI can experience intolerance to feeds. In these cases, pharmacotherapy with prokinetic agents such as metoclopramide and erythromycin can be used. Gastric intolerance can also be avoided with postpyloric feeding. This method has also been shown to achieve higher caloric and nitrogen intake.[32]

Urologic Disorders

Urinary incontinence and urinary retention are common sequelae of TBI. In a study performed by Chau et al., it was found that in a group of 84 patients who had sustained TBI within 6 weeks, 62% had urinary incontinence and 9% had urinary retention. Of those patients affected with either form of bladder dysfunction, greater than half required external collecting systems or indwelling urinary catheters; overall, patients with urinary incontinence were found to have poorer functional outcomes.[37] In addition to urinary retention and incontinence, asymptomatic urodynamic abnormalities can occur in patients post TBI when there is a motor deficit.[38]

Early recognition of the patient presenting with urinary dysfunction is important. Identifying patients with urinary retention and urinary incontinence is first investigated with a thorough history and physical examination. Urine studies in the form of urinalysis and urine culture should be performed to identify infection that may be contributing to bladder dysfunction. A bladder scan can be used to measure the amount of retention within the bladder. In the acute setting, bladder decompression can be achieved with either urethral or suprapubic catheterization.[39] In patients with urinary incontinence, treatment is based on the type of incontinence presented (see the later section on urinary system disorders in the patient with SCI).

Endocrine System Disorders

Endocrine dysfunction is a common complication following TBI and can occur in both the acute phase and the chronic phase of TBI. The pathophysiology is thought to be multifactorial, including direct injury to the pituitary gland. In the acute phase of TBI abnormalities of the adrenal and thyroid glands are common, whereas growth hormone and gonadotropin dysfunction are more common in the latter phase.[19] In 2017, the British Neurotrauma Group published guidance for screening for pituitary dysfunction; the guidance for testing during the acute phase is represented in Figure 13.1.[40]

The chronic or late phase is considered to be 3–6 months, and the guidelines are represented in Figure 13.2.[40]

Dermatologic Disorders

Please see the section "Dermatologic Disorders" in the following section on SCI and also see Chapter 11 on management of pressure ulcers.

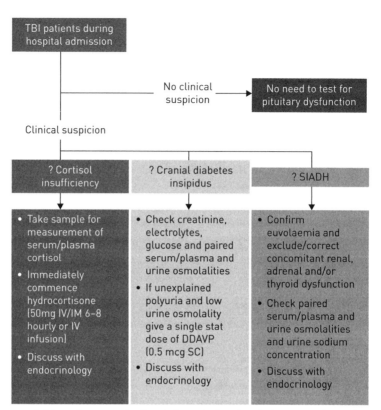

FIGURE 13.1 Guidance for screening for pituitary dysfunction during acute phase of traumatic brain injury.

THE PATIENT WITH SPINAL CORD INJURY
Neurologic System Disorders

According to the World Health Organization, the term "spinal cord injury" refers to damage to the spinal cord resulting from any trauma or from disease or degeneration. Examples include diseases such as cancer, transverse myelitis, and infarcts of the cord. "There is no reliable estimate of global prevalence, but estimated annual global incidence is 40 to 80 cases per million population. Up to 90% of these cases are due to traumatic causes, though the proportion of non-traumatic SCI appears to be growing."[41] According to US estimates, there are ap-proximately 40 new cases per million population, or just over 12,000 cases per year of SCI.[42]

Symptoms and sequelae of SCI depend on the severity of injury and its lo-cation on the spinal cord. "Symptoms may include partial or complete loss of sensory function or motor control of arms, legs and/or body. The most severe SCI affects the systems that regulate bowel or bladder control, breathing, heart rate and blood pressure. Most people with spinal cord injury experience chronic pain."[41]

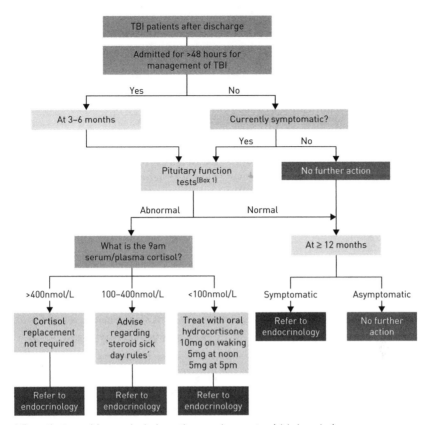

* For patients receiving regular hydrocortisone replacement or 'sick day rules' cover, parenteral hydrocortisone will be required in the event of vomiting/diarrhoea when oral absorption is uncertain

FIGURE 13.2 Guidance for screening for pituitary dysfunction during the chronic or late phase of traumatic brain injury.

Key Epidemiologic Spinal Cord Facts

- Every year, around the world, between 250 000 and 500 000 people suffer a SCI.
- Most SCIs are due to preventable causes such as road traffic crashes, falls, or violence.
- People with a SCI are two to five times more likely to die prematurely than people without a SCI, with worse survival rates in low- and middle-income countries.
- SCI is associated with lower rates of school enrollment and economic participation, and it carries substantial individual and societal costs.[41]

This section introduces topics that are very specific to SCI, although there is a great deal of overlap between the management of TBI and SCI. SCI on its own is a devastating disease, unfortunately there is also a significant incidence of co-occurring TBI in those with SCI, with estimates from 24% to 74%, and many of the medical complications are therefore also co-occurring.[42–44]

Musculoskeletal System Disorders

As seen in TBI, spasticity is a common complication after SCI and is seen in 70% of patients.[45] Guidelines for therapy are similar to those discussed for spasticity after TBI, including alternating heat and cold packs as well as antispasmodic medications such as baclofen, tizanidine, botulinum toxin, gabapentin, and pregabalin. Additional pharmacotherapy agents mentioned include dantrolene and benzodiazepines.[45] Early recognition of this complication is imperative in the acute setting, along with continual management after discharge. A study performed by Haisma et al. showed that after discharge to inpatient rehabilitation facilities, although pain levels improved, spasticity had worsened.[46]

In addition to spasticity, patients who suffer from SCI often have prolonged periods of immobilization which increase the risk of developing muscle contractures. These patients should be frequently repositioned while in bed and while sitting. These interventions not only aid in preventing muscle contractures, but also avoid the development of skin breakdown, which can ultimately lead to pressure ulceration. Range of motion exercises and splinting are additional methods that are attempted to stretch the soft tissues. These methods have not been formally studied, but they are likely to be effective in the therapy of contractures.[47,48]

Another complication related to the musculoskeletal system is pain. Patients who suffer from SCI are at risk for developing various types of pain, including nociceptive pain, musculoskeletal pain, and neuropathic pain. Treatment of this potential sequelae is guided by the type of pain the patient is experiencing.[45]

Last, when approaching the musculoskeletal complications of SCI and developing a treatment plan, a focus on treating and preventing other potential systemwide complications such as infection should be considered.[45]

Cardiovascular System Disorders

The chronic phase of SCI has many significant cardiovascular complications that may be encountered in the rehabilitation setting. These include:

- Orthostatic hypotension
- Impaired cardiovascular reflexes
- Autonomic dysreflexia (lesions above T6)
- Impaired transmission of cardiac pain (lesions above T4) resulting in impaired perception of chest pain
- Loss of reflex changes in the heart (lesions T1–T4)
- Atrophy of the heart with tetraplegia: loss of muscle mass in left ventricle
- Pseudo-myocardial infarction: rise in troponin with or without ECG changes without demonstrable cardiovascular cause[49]

Hypotension is common and has been reported to be as high as 21%.[50] It is treated in the same fashion as in TBI (see the "Cardiovascular System Disorders" section in TBI).

Autonomic dysreflexia (AD) is seen in lesions above T6 and occurs in the first 2–4 months after injury[51]; it is triggered by sensory stimulus below the level of the injury. The symptoms are the result of uncontrolled response of the sympathetic nervous system,[52] and in 85% of the cases the cause is a full and distended bladder.[53] The symptoms are an intense, pulsing headache, blurred vision, anxiety, agitation, shortness of breath, facial flushing, paradoxical sweating above the level of the injury, cold clammy skin, "goose pimples," and nausea.[53] AD can be life-threatening due to the associated hypertension that can result. Early recognition of AD and mitigation of the triggering stimuli are the cornerstones of its treatment, which is outlined in Figure 13.3.

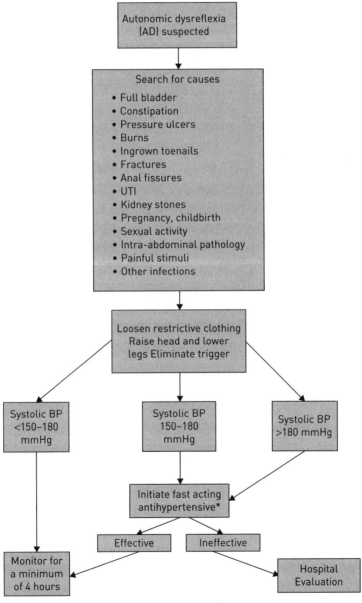

FIGURE 13.3 Treatment algorithm for autonomic dysreflexia.
From Sezer et al.[45]; MISSING REF[52]; Krassioukove et al.,[121]; Furlan et al.[122]

There is no consensus for specific antihypertensive drugs. Medications proposed include captopril, terazosin, prazosin, phenoxybenzamine, prostaglandin E2, and sildenafil.[45] In rehabilitation and SCI medicine the favorites are nifedipine, prazosin, and nitrates.[54]

Atrophy of the left ventricle can be diagnosed via ECG and should be suspected in patients with symptoms of congestive heart failure.

Respiratory System Disorders

Pulmonary complications are the leading cause of death in SCI patients and account for 37% of deaths in the first year after SCI.[55,56] Pulmonary compromise is related to level of injury (LOI) with more rostral injuries presenting with more severe respiratory dysfunction. The diaphragm (C3–C5, phrenic nerve) is the muscle primary responsible for breathing.[57] In addition to diaphragmatic weakness, weakness of other muscles of inspiration lead to a restrictive pattern of lung disease.[58] This is complicated by unopposed parasympathetic dominance in the tetraplegic patient resulting in increased cholinergic tone.[59] This increased cholinergic tone leads to increased mucous production and bronchospastic hypersensitivity, superimposing on an obstructive lung disease.[59,60]

It is a common misconception that the paraplegic patient does not have pulmonary complications. Most paraplegic (as well as tetraplegic) patients have abdominal wall weakness leading to increased abdominal wall compliance and a suboptimal length–tension ratio of the diaphragm, especially in the seated position due to the effects of gravity.[61] These factors predispose the patient to decreased tidal volume (TV), decreased ability to clear secretions, increased fatigue, atelectasis, infection, and further deconditioning.[61,62] These factors make pulmonary management extremely important after all SCI.

Acute Management of Respiratory Failure

After acute SCI respiratory failure requiring mechanical ventilation (MV) is present in up to 74% of those with tetraplegia and 95% of those with LOI of C5 or higher.[63] The preferred ventilator mode in the rehabilitation setting is assist-control (AC). For SCI individuals, a TV of more than 20 cc/kg of ideal body weight (IBW) is typically targeted,[63,64] which is significantly higher than the 6–8 cc/kg of IBW recommended in able-bodied individuals.[65] Using higher TV in the SCI population has been shown to decrease atelectasis, pneumonia, and total duration of ventilator-dependent days without increasing the risk of acute respiratory distress syndrome (ARDS).[63,64]

When weaning from the ventilator, progressive ventilator-free breathing (PVFB) is considered standard of care. During a PVFB weaning trial, a patient may start with as few as 2 minutes three times per day with as-needed supplemental oxygen or positive pressure support. As the patient improves, the duration of PVFB trials is increased until the patient is able to participate in 48 hours of ventilator-free breathing. It is important to think of PVFB as diaphragmatic and accessory muscle exercises that are best accompanied by periods of rest between sessions, which is why AC is the preferred ventilator mode in the rehabilitation setting.[63]

Chronic Management of Respiratory Failure

While most individuals are able to be weaned from MV, between 400 and 500 individuals with SCI each year are unable to do so.[66] Individuals with complete injuries between C1 and C3 will develop chronic respiratory failure with ongoing ventilatory requirements. Individuals with a partially intact phrenic nerve, typically seen in complete injuries at or between C3 and C4 or incomplete injuries at between C3 and C5, may be unable to completely wean from MV.[67]

In any of these patients some continuum of continuous MV, intermittent (usually nocturnal) MV, diaphragmatic pacing (DP), electrical phrenic nerve pacing (EPP), or noninvasive positive pressure ventilation (NIV) may be considered. It is important to understand that an intact phrenic nerve is required for EPP and DP, and thus complete injuries between C3 and C5 are often not appropriate while incomplete injuries or injuries above C3 often are. Preoperative electromyelography (EMG) and nerve conduction studies (NCS) of the diaphragm and phrenic nerve are required prior to insertion of either device.[66,68,69] EPP was first described in 1783 by Hufeland and first successfully completed in 1968 by Glenn and Judson.[70] EPP requires surgery to place an electrode around a viable bilateral phrenic nerves. A radio transmitter then can externally change the frequency at which the phrenic nerve fires.

DP has gained in popularity as laparoscopic surgery has made implantation of this device easier and less invasive than EPP.[69] In DP, electrodes are implanted near the highest concentration of motor units on the diaphragm. An external pacing device can be worn or stored on a wheelchair. Both DP and EPP have the advantage of aiding in diaphragm hypertrophy. They are also more physiologic forms of respiration, are less obtrusive to the patient, decrease tubes that can be accidentally dislodged, allow patients to transfer more easily, decrease wheelchair weight, improve speech and olfaction, and decrease rates of respiratory infections.[66,68,69] EPP and DP have the disadvantages of increased risk of surgery-related infection and device failure. It is also important to realize that EPP and DP do not aid expiratory muscles. NIV, which can be in the form of a mouthpiece, mask, or nocturnal lip seal device, is useful for those who do not have intact phrenic nerves as these devices also decrease the rate of respiratory infections.[71] Despite being more bulky, NIV devices still provide freedom to the individual, can be concealed on a wheelchair, and do not carry the risk of surgery-related infections.[71]

Nonmedical Treatment to Aid Respiratory Support

To help manage secretions, physical modalities are often used.

- *Abdominal binder*: These can help increase TV by displacing the diaphragm through compression of abdominal contents.
- *Postural percussion and drainage*: A trained individual performs chest percussion with a cupped hand to specific areas of the chest and back while the patient is turned and placed in positions to allow gravity to facilitate mucous drainage.

- *Chest vest/vibrating bed*: This is the same concept as used in postural percussion, except a vest and/or bed vibrates the patient's chest. This can also be done in conjunction with deep suction.
- *Manual assist "quad cough"*: The patient lies supine while a trained individual pushes in on the patient's abdomen as they are exhaling. This forces the diaphragm rostrally and aids in mucous expulsion.
- *Mechanical insufflation-exsufflation (Coughylator)*: This device provides positive pressure to the airway followed by immediate repetitive bouts of negative pressure. This change in pressure aids in dislodging and expulsion of mucous.
- *Bronchoscopy*: Reserved for severe cases of mucous plugging not helped with methods mentioned above.

Medical Treatment to Aid Respiratory Support

In the acute phase, SCI patients may require multiple bronchodilators and mucolytic agents in addition to the physical measures noted earlier. In the chronic phase, most tetraplegic patients are able to get by with just bronchodilators as needed. In general, anticholinergic medications for secretion management are not tolerated very well and have significant side effects,[72,73] however, botulinum toxin can be an effect antisecretion agent for individuals with sialorrhea.[74] Other agents used in the treatment of pulmonary disorders are listed here.

- Bronchodilators:
  - Albuterol 2.5 mg nebulized every 4–6 hours scheduled or as needed
  - Ipatropium 0.5 mg nebulized every 4–6 hours scheduled or as needed
- Mucolytic agents:
  - Hypertonic saline (2.1% to 7%) 2–4 mL nebulized every 12 hours or as needed
  - Guaifenesin 600–1,200 mg every 12 hours
  - N-Acetylcysteine (less common) 10% solution nebulized every 6–8 hours or as needed
  - Dornase alfa (expensive) 2.5 mg nebulized one to two times daily or as needed
- Antisialorrhea agents:
  - Botulinum toxin
  - Scopolamine
  - Hyoscyamine (less common)
  - Hyoscine (less common)
- Supplemental O_2

Gastrointestinal Disorders

After SCI there are several alterations in function of the GI system. Some aspects are minimally altered in the long run, while others are functionally changed for a lifetime. Some, such as dysphagia and poor gastric motility after an SCI, may improve with time. However, the resultant neurogenic bowel may have significant, physiologic, psychosocial, and emotional implications in the immediate and long term for individuals with SCI.[75]

In tetraplegia there are often permanent changes in gastric motility that may not abate after the initial trauma and neurogenic shock; this is not experienced by those with paraplegia. In tetraplegics there is dissociation of antral and duodenal motility, and gastric pacemaker potentials no longer originate in the antrum in most of these patients.[76,77] In the past, cisapride and tegaserod were often used, but now a trial metoclopramide may be initiated.

Neurogenic bowel occurs in most (68%) with chronic SCI and is ranked as the second largest impact on their life secondary to loss of mobility, causing significant distress in 54% of individuals.[78] The small and large bowel are innervated by the parasympathetic nervous system. The vagus nerve is responsible for peristalsis from the esophagus to the splenic flexure.[79,80] The descending colon receives its parasympathetic innervation from the pelvic nerve (S2–S4), and the external anal sphincter is innervated by the somatic pudendal (S2–S4) nerve.[80] After initial SCI, all reflexes are suppressed due to spinal shock.

Upper Motor Neuron Bowel

An injury above the conus medullaris will result in an upper motor neuron (UMN) bowel where the external sphincter is spastic.[81] Following spinal shock, the bulbocavernosus reflex is the first or second reflex to return and signifies the presence of a spastic external anal sphincter and thus a UMN bowel.[81,82] A UMN bowel is best managed by prophylactic medications with a daily bowel regimen which includes both medications and physical measures.[76] The goal of UMN bowel management is to produce a daily, consistent, and predictable bowel movement. Most frequently individuals with UMN bowel are started on a "3-2-1" protocol, with oral docusate sodium 100 mg three times a day (stool softener), two sennoside 8.6 mg tablets orally at noon (stimulant), and one Dulcolax 10 mg rectal suppository at bedtime (rectal stimulant). For optimal results this regimen should be started in the acute care setting. To aid bowel evacuation, timing a bowel movement after eating may elicit the gastrocolonic reflex while stimulation of the recto-colonic reflex with digital stimulation of the rectal wall is also recommended.[76,83] During digital stimulation a gloved and lubricated finger is inserted into the rectum; the finger is slowly rotated around the rectum until relaxation of the bowel wall is felt or stool passes.[76] This typically happens within 60 seconds. Digital stimulation can be repeated every 10 minutes until there are two bouts with no defecation, signaling emptying of bowel.[76] In addition to digital stimulation, digital evacuation of the rectal vault is sometimes helpful if firm stool is present.[76,83] It is also advantageous to get the patient on a commode chair during the bowel regimen to allow gravity to assist.

Lower Motor Neuron Bowel

An SCI below the conus medullaris will produce an areflexic or lower motor neuron (LMN) bowel. LMN bowel is characterized by a flaccid external sphincter and levator ani muscles that cause the lumen of the rectum to open.[83] The LMN bowel relies on slow stool propulsion with segmental colon peristalsis by the myenteric plexus alone.[76] LMN bowel is intrinsically more difficult to manage due to fecal incontinence with increasing abdominal pressure. The goal for an LMN bowel is to create a bulkier stool, often with the help of psyllium, Citrucel, or other bulk-forming agents. Digital evacuation is also often necessary.[84]

Urologic Disorders
Bladder Dysfunction

There are many alterations to bladder function that occur after SCI. Immediately following the injury it is common for the bladder to become flaccid during a period known as *spinal shock*, which lasts approximately 3 weeks.[85] During this time there is usually no reflexive bladder contraction. Bladder contractions begin to fully return at around 6–8 weeks.[42,86] It is recommended that during this time period an indwelling Foley catheter is placed until the patient is stabilized medically with low daily urine output of approximately 2 L.[86] Given the right clinical context, intermittent catheterization (IC) can be used as an alternative. As spinal shock resolves, it is common for patients to develop a neurogenic bladder. There are multiple types of neurogenic bladder dysfunction that occur after SCI; for the purposes of acute care, we will focus on UMN neurogenic bladder and LMN neurogenic bladder due to the higher risk of upper tract injury in these presentations.

For patients with SCI involving UMN lesions (above the sacral micturition center at S2, S3, S4) it is not uncommon to develop detrusor-sphincter dyssynergia (DSD) secondary to disruption of the descending inhibiting neuronal pathways from the pontine micturition center. In this condition there is uncoordinated detrusor and sphincter activity. The detrusor muscle involuntarily contracts against a closed sphincter, in turn increasing intravesicular pressure. With high pressures there is risk for vesicoureteral reflux, hydronephrosis, pyelonephritis, and, if severe enough, postobstructive renal failure.[87] Goal volumes are less than 500 cc, which usually equates to catheterization every 4–6 hours.[80] Larger volumes create the risk for bladder dilation and vesicoureteral reflux. To prevent reflexive voiding between IC, anticholinergic medications can be used. Some of the most popular agents are oxybutynin (Ditropan), tolterodine (Detrol), and miragebron (Myrbetriq) which all have anticholinergic effects. When these medications fail, there is large evidence for cystoscopically guided injections of botulinum toxin into the detrusor. This is the only therapy approved by the US Food and Drug Administration (FDA) for neurogenic overactive bladder refractory to oral medications.[88] Other medications are used to target the reflexive sphincter component of DSD, such as alpha blockers such as terazosin (Hytrin), tamsulosin (Flomax), and doxazosin (Cardura). Transperineal injections of Botox have also been investigated in small trials and demonstrated improved detrusor capacity and lower pressures during voiding.[89]

Patients with SCI involving the sacral segments and lower can present with uninhibited neurogenic bladder. This happens when the injury damages pathways from the sacral micturition center, resulting in a flaccid bladder. The bladder loses its inherent ability to reflexively contract and can become overdistended, causing dangerous vesicoureteral reflux. Treatment involves IC for patients who are unsuccessful with pelvic floor strengthening or Valsalva and Credé maneuvers. Medications such as urecholine (Bethanechol) can be used to stimulate parasympathetically mediated bladder contraction, but there is poor evidence supporting its use.[90]

There are clinical situations in which continuing an indwelling Foley catheter after acute care is preferred over IC. Specifically, patients who are tetraplegic and can't safely self-catheterize or in patients with repeated bouts of autonomic dysreflexia are two examples. Male patients with C6–C7 SCI may be able to urethral self-catheterize without assistance as can female patients who have had a Mitrofanoff procedure.[42] The clinical context must be carefully considered because indwelling catheters create a higher risk of urinary tract infections, bladder stone formation, prostate and epididymis infections, urethral erosion, and hypospadias.[91] Suprapubic catheters may be considered when anatomic abnormalities make IC difficult, in the presence of recurrent catheter obstructions or an increased risk of skin breakdown or wounds, or with patient preference secondary to body image or sexual function. They should be changed every 4 weeks (1–2 weeks if extensive calcification or obstruction is a recurrent problem).[80]

Endocrine Disorders

The brain and the spinal cord, when they incur injury, are affected by a cascade of events that "alter the normal homeostatic function of the neuro-endocrine system. These systems regulate cellular nutrition, energy consumption, oxygenation, and waste removal, which in turn control tissue growth and repair. Subsequently, these changes impact normal organ system functions that lead to various hematological, metabolic, and endocrine complications."[92] In this section, we will address some of the most common endocrine derangements during the acute phase of SCI.

Metabolism in the Acute Phase

Studies have demonstrated that persons with SCI remained in negative nitrogen balance for at least 8 weeks despite 120% caloric overfeeding and dietary protein supplementation of 2 g/kg/d; this contrasts with other types of trauma patients who were able to achieve positive nitrogen balance within 3 weeks. It is important to maintain higher nutritional vigilance for a longer period in patients with a traumatic SCI.[93,94]

Neuroendocrine

During the acute phase of SCI it is not uncommon for patients to suffer from the syndrome of inappropriate antidiuretic hormone (SIADH) secondary to trauma to the brain and pituitary function, as also occurs in TBI.[42–44]

SCI appears to have a profound impact on the hypothalamic-pituitary-gonadal axis, with a marked reduction in anabolic potential and a large effect on bone metabolism. Testosterone and estrogen levels are acutely lowered post injury and rarely return to normal levels in complete and high-level spinal cord injuries.[95]

Hypercalcemia and Bone Loss

Up to 23% of patients with acute SCI will suffer from hypercalcemia. Immediately after SCI there is rapid bone loss and excretion of free calcium into the bloodstream. Calcium levels increase within 10 days after SCI and peak between 1 and 6 months. Due to their high-density bone mass, young adult males are affected more than other populations.[42,96] The typical symptoms of hypercalcemia are vomiting, confusion, polydipsia, and polyuria. These symptoms can be difficult to recognize given the acuity of SCI and its concomitant management difficulties and can be mistaken for other issues.

Treatment consists of intravenous hydration with normal saline, early mobilization, and possibly furosemide to prevent volume overload and reabsorption of calcium by the kidney. Thiazides should not be used because they are calcium sparing.[96] After the acute management, a single dose of pamidronate will effectively resolve the problem for several weeks and has the added benefit of decreasing the simultaneously occurring rapid bone loss.[97]

Heterotopic Ossification

Heterotopic ossification (HO) is the formation of extraosseous lamellar bone in soft tissue surrounding peripheral joints below the level of injury. The incidence of HO in SCI is between 16% and 53%. Clinically significant HO develops in about 20% of patients with a SCI.

HO presents during the acute course of SCI, sometimes as early as a few weeks post injury. It will usually present as gradual loss of range of movement, with swelling and possibly erythema. It is also not uncommon to be accompanied by low-grade fever. The differential diagnosis in SCI with these symptoms is cellulitis, deep venous thrombosis (DVT), benign effusion, fracture, and hematoma.[98]

HO is most commonly found in the hips and knees in SCI, and sometimes at the shoulder and elbow,[98] sites that are more common in brain injury.

The four clinical stages of HO:

Stage 1 : Swelling, ↑ serum alkaline phosphatase, normal x-ray
Stage 2 : Swelling, ↑ serum alkaline phosphatase, positive x-ray
Stage 3 : No swelling, ↑ serum alkaline phosphatase, positive x-ray
Stage 4 : No swelling, normal serum alkaline phosphatase, positive x-ray

Based on data from Nicholas JJ. Ectopic bone formation in patients with SCI. *Arch Phys Med Rehabil.* Aug 1973;54(8):354–359.

Dermatologic Disorders
Pressure Injury

The insensate individual, such as those with SCI, is at increased risk for skin breakdown. For years, "pressure ulcer" was the term used to describe skin breakdown due to ischemia and necrosis, but, in 2016, to better characterize the type and extent of damage to the tissues, the term "pressure ulcer" was replaced with "pressure injury" (PI).[99] Unfortunately, PIs occur in approximately 25% of individuals with SCI between their acute care hospitalization and rehabilitation stay,[100] and a recent Canadian study showed an average increase in hospital cost of $18,758.[101] In the acute setting shortly after initial injury, PIs are most commonly seen on the sacrum (39%), calcaneus (13%), ischium (8%), occiput (6%), and scapula (5%).[100] Complications of PI include osteomyelitis, vascular fistulas, infection, and sepsis.[102]

Mechanism and Grading A PI occurs when perpendicular or shear forces are transmitted over a bony prominence.[99] The average venous capillary pressure is 6 mm Hg and the arteriolar limb capillary pressure is 32 mm Hg.[103] Tissue ischemia and necrosis will generally occur if tissue pressure becomes greater than 60 mm Hg for prolonged periods of time,[104] but it is important to note that greater pressures over shorter periods of time are equally injurious.[105] The staging of pressure injuries was first described in 1975[106] and has been modified numerous times over the years, most recently in 2016,[99] but it has always been based on four different stages (see Chapter 11). It is important to recognize that a PI can progress through these different stages. However, when it starts to heal it does not regress through the stages. This means that a stage IV PI will always be classified as a stage IV PI even if granulation tissue covers muscle, tendon, and bone in the future.

Prevention A proper risk assessment is vital for prevention of PIs. Smoking[107] and poor nutrition[108] are two modifiable risk factors for PI prevention. In the acute care setting the patient should be turned and repositioned every 2 hours if lying and for 2 minutes at a time every 20–30 minutes when sitting.[109] The lateral decubitus position should be avoided due to increased risk for greater trochanter PI,[110] and special care should be taken when reclining in bed or tilting in a space chair to ensure that sacral shearing does not occur. Patient education is probably the most important prevention tool.[110]

Pressure redistribution mattresses such as air-fluidized beds or alternating air mattresses are cost-effective and decrease healing time when compared to standard mattresses.[111–113]

Treatment Stage I and II PIs are managed nonoperatively. Stage III PIs may require surgical interventions, and stage IV PIs almost always require surgery. After acute SCI the patient is in a hypercatabolic and hypermetabolic state, the details of which are still relatively unknown.[114,115] Therefore providing adequate nutrition is an important part of the treatment of PI.

In general, the wound bed should be clean and free of necrotic tissue. This can be achieved by mechanical methods, enzymatic debridement, or surgical debridement. Wet-to-dry dressing changes for mechanical debridement and maintaining proper moisture is essential. Cleansing solutions can be used, and isotonic saline is the most common. The goal of local wound care is to provide appropriate hydration and decrease the wound's bioburden.[102] Sometimes antimicrobial cleansing solutions are used, including acetic acid and sodium hypochlorite (Dakin's), with the goal of decreasing bioburden and preserving fibroblasts for healing.[102] The use, indications for, and length of treatment with topical agents are debated.

Enzymatic and surgical debridement aid in the removal of necrotic tissue, eschar, and slough. Enzymatic debridement agents (collagenase, streptokinase, dornase) degrade collagen and liquify necrotic debris without damaging granulation tissue.[116] Alternatively, sharp debridement is achieved by removal of eschar and devitalized tissue. Both enzymatic and sharp debridement are helpful in creating a wound bed to promote granulation tissue.[102]

There are many wound care modalities used to stimulate growth of granulation tissue including ultrasound, hyperbaric oxygen, infrared, ultraviolet, and low-energy laser irradiation, but all lack robust data. Electrical stimulation of the wound bed is the only modality shown to increase circulation and granulation while decreasing bacterial counts.[117,118]

For nonhealing PIs, surgical reconstruction can be considered. Musculocutaneous and fasciocutaneous flaps involving the gluteus muscles are most common, although there are high rates of complications and failure.[119,120]

REFERENCES

1. Pervez M, Kitagawa RS, Chang TR. Definition of traumatic brain injury, neurosurgery, trauma orthopedics, neuroimaging, psychology, and psychiatry in mild traumatic brain injury. *Neuroimaging Clin N Am.* 2018;28(1):1–13.

2. *Association of Sleep with Neurobehavioral Impairments During Inpatient Rehabilitation After Traumatic Brain Injury.* IOS Press. 2018.

3. Kempf J, Werth E, Kaiser PR, Bassetti CL, Baumann CR. Sleep–wake disturbances 3 years after traumatic brain injury. 2010.

4. Zunzunegui C, Gao B, Cam E, Hodor A, Bassetti CL. Sleep disturbance impairs stroke recovery in the rat. *Sleep.* 2011;34(9):1261–1269.

5. Gao B, Cam E, Jaeger H, Zunzunegui C, Sarnthein J, Bassetti CL. Sleep disruption aggravates focal cerebral ischemia in the rat. *Sleep.* 2010;33(7):879–887.

6. Sleep, sleep disorders, and mild traumatic brain injury. What we know and what we need to know: Findings from a national working group. SpringerLink. 2018.

7. Barshikar S, Bell KR. Sleep disturbance after TBI. *Curr Neurol Neurosci Rep.* 2017;17(11):87.

8. Young T, Peppard P. Sleep-disordered breathing and cardiovascular disease: Epidemiologic evidence for a relationship. *Sleep.* 2000;23 Suppl 4:S122–S126.

9. Shahar E, Whitney CW, Redline S, et al. Sleep-disordered breathing and cardiovascular disease: Cross-sectional results of the Sleep Heart Health Study. *Am J Respir Crit Care Med.* 2001;163(1):19–25.

10. Chung F, Yegneswaran B, Liao P, et al. STOP questionnaire: A tool to screen patients for obstructive sleep apnea. *Anesthesiology.* 2008;108(5):812–821.

11. Trauer JM, Qian MY, Doyle JS, Rajaratnam SM, Cunnington D. Cognitive behavioral therapy for chronic insomnia: A systematic review and meta-analysis. *Ann Intern Med.* 2015;163(3):191–204.

12. Ouellet MC, Morin CM. Efficacy of cognitive-behavioral therapy for insomnia associated with traumatic brain injury: A single-case experimental design. *Arch Phys Med Rehabil.* 2007;88(12):1581–1592.

13. Zollman FS, Larson EB, Wasek-Throm LK, Cyborski CM, Bode RK. Acupuncture for treatment of insomnia in patients with traumatic brain injury: A pilot intervention study. *J Head Trauma Rehabil.* 2012;27(2):135–142.

14. Bajaj S, Vanuk JR, Smith R, Dailey NS, Killgore WDS. Blue-light therapy following mild traumatic brain injury: Effects on white matter water diffusion in the brain. *Front Neurol.* 2017;8:616.

15. Wright HR, Lack LC, Kennaway DJ. Differential effects of light wavelength in phase advancing the melatonin rhythm. *J Pineal Res.* 2004;36(2):140–144.

16. Gordon WA, Zafonte R, Cicerone K, et al. Traumatic brain injury rehabilitation: State of the science. *Am J Phys Med Rehabil.* 2006;85(4):343–382.

17. Pérez-Arredondo A, Cázares-Ramírez E, Carrillo-Mora P, et al. Baclofen in the therapeutic of sequela of traumatic brain injury: Spasticity. *Clin Neuropharmacol.* 2016;39:311–319.

18. Brown S, Hawker G, Beaton D, Colantonio A. Long-term musculoskeletal complaints after traumatic brain injury. *Brain Inj.* 2011;25(5):453–461.

19. Gaddam SS, Buell T, Robertson CS. Systemic manifestations of traumatic brain injury. *Handb Clin Neurol.* 2015;127:205–218.

20. Penfield W. Diencephalic autonomic epilepsy. *Arch Neurol Psychiatry.* 2019;22(2):358–374.

21. Baguley IJ, Perkes IE, Fernandez-Ortega JF, Rabinstein AA, Dolce G, Hendricks HT. Paroxysmal sympathetic hyperactivity after acquired brain injury: Consensus on conceptual definition, nomenclature, and diagnostic criteria. *J Neurotrauma.* 2014;31(17):1515–1520.

22. Baguley IJ, Nicholls JL, Felmingham KL, Crooks J, Gurka JA, Wade LD. Dysautonomia after traumatic brain injury: A forgotten syndrome? *J Neurol Neurosurg Psychiatry.* 1999;67(1):39–43.

23. Meyfroidt G, Baguley IJ, Menon DK. Paroxysmal sympathetic hyperactivity: The storm after acute brain injury. *Lancet Neurol.* 2017;16(9):721–729.

24. Thomas A, Greenwald BD. Paroxysmal sympathetic hyperactivity and clinical considerations for patients with acquired brain injuries: A narrative review. *Am J Phys Med Rehabil.* 2019;98(1):65–72.

25. Berthiaume L, Zygun D. Non-neurologic organ dysfunction in acute brain injury. *Crit Care Clin.* 2006;22(4):753–766; abstract x.

26. Bansal V, Costantini T, Kroll L, et al. Traumatic brain injury and intestinal dysfunction: Uncovering the neuro-enteric axis. *J Neurotrauma.* 2009;26(8):1353–1359.

27. Haddad SH, Arabi YM. Critical care management of severe traumatic brain injury in adults. *Scand J Trauma Resusc Emerg Med.* 2012;20(1):12.

28. Bowen JC, Houston T, Division of Surgery, et al. Increased gastrin release following penetrating central nervous system injury. *Surgery.* 1974;75(5):720–724.

29. Gerald L Weinhouse, MD. https://www.uptodate.com/contents/stress-ulcer-prophylaxis-in-the-intensive-care-unit?search=stress%20ulcer%20prophylaxis&source=search_

result&selectedTitle=1~150&usage_type=default&display_rank=1#H4. 2019. Last updated 01, 2019.

30. Schindlbeck NE, Lippert M, Heinrich C, Muller-Lissner SA. Intragastric bile acid concentrations in critically ill, artificially ventilated patients. *Am J Gastroenterol.* 1989;84(6):624–628.

31. Moody FG, Cheung LY. Stress ulcers: Their pathogenesis, diagnosis, and treatment. *Surg Clin North Am.* 1976;56(6):1469–1478.

32. Schirmer CM, Kornbluth J, Heilman CB, Bhardwaj A. Gastrointestinal prophylaxis in neurocritical care. *Neurocrit Care.* 2012;16(1):184–193.

33. Howell MD, Novack V, Grgurich P, et al. Iatrogenic gastric acid suppression and the risk of nosocomial Clostridium difficile infection. *Arch Intern Med.* 2010;170(9):784–790.

34. Pepe JL, Barba CA. The metabolic response to acute traumatic brain injury and implications for nutritional support. *J Head Trauma Rehabil.* 1999;14(5):462–474.

35. Sevim A, Hülya U, Haydar U, Esin Y, Ümit Ç, Kemalettin A, Engin Y, Suat K. Effects of early versus delayed nutrition on intestinal mucosal apoptosis and atrophy after traumatic brain injury. SpringerLink. 2019. https://link.springer.com/article/10.1007/s00595-005-3034-3. Accessed September, 2005.

36. Chiang YH, Chao DP, Chu SF, et al. Early enteral nutrition and clinical outcomes of severe traumatic brain injury patients in acute stage: A multi-center cohort study. *J Neurotrauma.* 2012;29(1):75–80.

37. Chua K, Chuo A, Kong KH. Urinary incontinence after traumatic brain injury: Incidence, outcomes and correlates. *Brain Inj.* 2003;17(6):469–478.

38. Moiyadi AV, Devi BI, Nair KP. Urinary disturbances following traumatic brain injury: Clinical and urodynamic evaluation. *NeuroRehabilitation.* 2007;22(2):93–98.

39. UpToDate. Acute urinary retention. 2019. https://www.uptodate.com/contents/acute-urinary-retention. Last updated 01, 2019.

40. Tan CL, Alavi SA, Baldeweg SE, et al. The screening and management of pituitary dysfunction following traumatic brain injury in adults: British Neurotrauma Group guidance. *J Neurol Neurosurg Psychiatry.* 2017;88:971–981.

41. World Health Organization. Spinal cord injury. November 19, 2013. https://www.who.int/news-room/fact-sheets/detail/spinal-cord-injury. Accessed January 25, 2019.

42. Kirshblum S, Campagnolo DI. *Spinal Cord Medicine.* 2nd ed. Philadelphia: Wolters Kluwer; 2011.

43. Macciocchi S, Seel RT, Thompson N, Byams R, Bowman B. Spinal cord injury and co-occurring traumatic brain injury: Assessment and incidence. *Arch Phys Med Rehabil.* 2008;89(7):1350–1357.

44. Tolonen A, Turkka J, Salonen O, Ahoniemi E, Alaranta H. Traumatic brain injury is under-diagnosed in patients with spinal cord injury. *J Rehabil Med.* 2007;39(8):622–626.

45. Sezer N, Akkuş S, Uğurlu FG. Chronic complications of spinal cord injury. *World J Orthop.* 2015;6(1):24–33.

46. Haisma JA, van der Woude LH, Stam HJ, et al. Complications following spinal cord injury: Occurrence and risk factors in a longitudinal study during and after inpatient rehabilitation. *J Rehabil Med.* 2007;39(5):393–398.

47. UpToDate. Chronic complications of spinal cord injury and disease. 2019. https://www.uptodate.com/contents/chronic-complications-of-spinal-cord-injury-and-disease. Last updated 12, 2018.

48. Harvey LA, Herbert RD. Muscle stretching for treatment and prevention of contracture in people with spinal cord injury. *Spinal Cord.* 2002;40(1):1–9.

49. Phillips WT, Kiratli BJ, Sarkarati M, et al. Effect of spinal cord injury on the heart and cardiovascular fitness. *Curr Probl Cardiol.* 1998;23(11):641–716.

50. Sisto SA, Lorenz DJ, Hutchinson K, Wenzel L, Harkema SJ, Krassioukov A. Cardiovascular status of individuals with incomplete spinal cord injury from 7 NeuroRecovery Network rehabilitation centers. *Arch Phys Med Rehabil.* 2012;93(9):1578–1587.

51. Karlsson AK. Autonomic dysfunction in spinal cord injury: Clinical presentation of symptoms and signs. *Prog Brain Res.* 2006;152:1–8.

52. Cardiovascular complications of spinal cord injury. 2019. https://tidsskriftet.no/en/ 2012/05/cardiovascular-complications-spinal-cord-injury

53. Shergill IS, Arya M, Hamid R, Khastgir J, Patel HR, Shah PJ. The importance of autonomic dysreflexia to the urologist. *BJU Int.* 2004;93(7):923–926.

54. Medicine CfSC. Acute management of autonomic dysreflexia: Individuals with spinal cord injury presenting to health-care facilities. *J Spinal Cord Med.* 2002;25 Suppl 1:S67–S88.

55. DeVivo MJ, Krause JS, Lammertse DP. Recent trends in mortality and causes of death among persons with spinal cord injury. *Arch Phys Med Rehabil.* 1999;80(11):1411–1419.

56. NSCISC. Home page. 2019. https://www.nscisc.uab.edu/. Accessed.

57. Schilero GJ, Bauman WA, Radulovic M. Traumatic spinal cord injury: Pulmonary physiologic principles and management. *Clin Chest Med.* 2018;39(2):411–425.

58. Hemingway A, Bors E, Hobby RP. An investigation of the pulmonary function of paraplegics. *J Clin Invest.* 1958;37(5):773–782.

59. Schilero GJ, Hobson JC, Singh K, Spungen AM, Bauman WA, Radulovic M. Bronchodilator effects of ipratropium bromide and albuterol sulfate among subjects with tetraplegia. *J Spinal Cord Med.* 2018;41(1):42–47.

60. Dicpinigaitis PV, Spungen AM, Bauman WA, Absgarten A, Almenoff PL. Bronchial hyperresponsiveness after cervical spinal cord injury. *Chest.* 1994;105(4):1073–1076.

61. Goldman JM, Rose LS, Williams SJ, Silver JR, Denison DM. Effect of abdominal binders on breathing in tetraplegic patients. *Thorax.* 1986;41(12):940–945.

62. Julia PE, Sa'ari MY, Hasnan N. Benefit of triple-strap abdominal binder on voluntary cough in patients with spinal cord injury. *Spinal Cord.* 2011;49(11):1138–1142.

63. Early acute management in adults with spinal cord injury: A clinical practice guideline for health-care professionals. *J Spinal Cord Med.* 2008;31(4):403–479.

64. Peterson WP, Barbalata L, Brooks CA, Gerhart KA, Mellick DC, Whiteneck GG. The effect of tidal volumes on the time to wean persons with high tetraplegia from ventilators. *Spinal Cord.* 1999;37(4):284–288.

65. Brower RG, Matthay MA, Morris A, Schoenfeld D, Thompson BT, Wheeler A. Ventilation with lower tidal volumes as compared with traditional tidal volumes for acute lung injury and the acute respiratory distress syndrome. *N Engl J Med.* 2000;342(18):1301–1308.

66. DiMarco AF. Diaphragm pacing. *Clin Chest Med.* 2018;39(2):459–471.

67. Como JJ, Sutton ER, McCunn M, et al. Characterizing the need for mechanical ventilation following cervical spinal cord injury with neurologic deficit. *J Trauma.* 2005;59(4):912–916; discussion 916.

68. Dalal K, DiMarco AF. Diaphragmatic pacing in spinal cord injury. *Phys Med Rehabil Clin N Am.* 2014;25(3):619–629, viii.

69. Gater DR, Jr., Dolbow D, Tsui B, Gorgey AS. Functional electrical stimulation therapies after spinal cord injury. *NeuroRehabilitation.* 2011;28(3):231–248.

70. Judson JP, Glenn WW. Radio-frequency electrophrenic respiration. Long-term application to a patient with primary hypoventilation. *JAMA.* 1968;203(12):1033–1037.

71. Bach JR. Noninvasive respiratory management of high level spinal cord injury. I*J Spinal Cord Med.* 2012;35:72–80.

72. Banfi P, Ticozzi N, Lax A, Guidugli GA, Nicolini A, Silani V. A review of options for treating sialorrhea in amyotrophic lateral sclerosis. *Respir Care.* 2015;60(3):446–454.

73. Jongerius PH, van Tiel P, van Limbeek J, Gabreels FJ, Rotteveel JJ. A systematic review for evidence of efficacy of anticholinergic drugs to treat drooling. *Arch Dis Child.* 2003;88(10):911–914.

74. Ondo WG, Hunter C, Moore W. A double-blind placebo-controlled trial of botulinum toxin B for sialorrhea in Parkinson's disease. *Neurology.* 2004;62(1):37–40.

75. Bauman WA, Korsten MA, Radulovic M, Schilero GJ, Wecht JM, Spungen AM. 31st g. Heiner Sell lectureship: Secondary medical consequences of spinal cord injury. *Top Spinal Cord Inj Rehabil.* 2012;18(4):354–378.

76. Stiens SA, Bergman SB, Goetz LL. Neurogenic bowel dysfunction after spinal cord injury: Clinical evaluation and rehabilitative management. *Arch Phys Med Rehabil.* 1997;78(3 Suppl):S86–S102.

77. Rajendran SK, Reiser JR, Bauman W, Zhang RL, Gordon SK, Korsten MA. Gastrointestinal transit after spinal cord injury: Effect of cisapride. *Am J Gastroenterol.* 1992;87(11):1614–1617.

78. Glickman S, Kamm MA. Bowel dysfunction in spinal-cord-injury patients. *Lancet.* 1996;347(9016):1651–1653.

79. Barr J, Fraser GL, Puntillo K, et al. Clinical practice guidelines for the management of pain, agitation, and delirium in adult patients in the intensive care unit. *Crit Care Med.* 2013;41(1):263–306.

80. *Braddom's Physical Medicine and Rehabilitation,* 5th ed. Elsevier; 2019.

81. Previnaire JG. The importance of the bulbocavernosus reflex. *Spinal Cord Ser Cases.* 2018;4:2.

82. Ditunno JF, Little JW, Tessler A, Burns AS. Spinal shock revisited: A four-phase model. *Spinal Cord.* 2004;42(7):383–395.

83. Krassioukov A, Eng JJ, Claxton G, Sakakibara BM, Shum S. Neurogenic bowel management after spinal cord injury: A systematic review of the evidence. *Spinal Cord.* 2010;48(10):718–733.

84. Yim SY, Yoon SH, Lee IY, Rah EW, Moon HW. A comparison of bowel care patterns in patients with spinal cord injury: Upper motor neuron bowel vs lower motor neuron bowel. *Spinal Cord.* 2001;39(4):204–207.

85. *The Physiological Basis of Rehabilitation Medicine,* 2nd ed. Elsevier; 2019.

86. Burns AS, Rivas DA, Ditunno JF. The management of neurogenic bladder and sexual dysfunction after spinal cord injury. *Spine (Phila Pa 1976).* 2001;26(24 Suppl):S129–S136.

87. Bladder management for adults with spinal cord injury: A clinical practice guideline for health-care providers. *J Spinal Cord Med.* 2006;29(5):527–573.

88. Cooley LF, Kielb S. A review of botulinum toxin A for the treatment of neurogenic bladder. *Pm r.* 2018.

89. Gallien P, Robineau S, Verin M, Le Bot MP, Nicolas B, Brissot R. Treatment of detrusor sphincter dyssynergia by transperineal injection of botulinum toxin. *Arch Phys Med Rehabil.* 1998;79(6):715–717.

90. Finkbeiner AE. Is bethanechol chloride clinically effective in promoting bladder emptying? A literature review. *J Urol.* 1985;134(3):443–449.

91. Weld KJ, Dmochowski RR. Effect of bladder management on urological complications in spinal cord injured patients. *J Urol.* 2000;163(3):768–772.

92. Stephen R. Lebduska M, Bhargav Mudda, MD. Hematological, metabolic and endocrine complications. PM&R Knowledge NOW Web site. September 20, 2014. https://now.aapmr.org/hematological-metabolic-and-endocrine-complications/#references. Accessed January 20, 2019.

93. Rodriguez DJ, Clevenger FW, Osler TM, Demarest GB, Fry DE. Obligatory negative nitrogen balance following spinal cord injury. *JPEN J Parenter Enteral Nutr.* 1991;15(3):319–322.

94. Rodriguez DJ, Benzel EC, Clevenger FW. The metabolic response to spinal cord injury. *Spinal Cord.* 1997;35(9):599–604.

95. Maïmoun L, Lumbroso S, Paris F, et al. The role of androgens or growth factors in the bone resorption process in recent spinal cord injured patients: A cross-sectional study. *Spinal Cord.* 2006;44(12):791–797.

96. Maynard FM. Immobilization hypercalcemia following spinal cord injury. *Arch Phys Med Rehabil.* 1986;67(1):41–44.

97. Maïmoun L ea. The role of androgens or growth factors in the bone resorption process in recent spinal cord injured patients: A cross-sectional study. PubMed—NCBI. 2019.

98. Kedlaya D. Heterotopic ossification in spinal cord injury. Medscape. 2018. https://emedicine.medscape.com/article/322003-overview. Accessed January 25, 2019.

99. Edsberg LE, Black JM, Goldberg M, McNichol L, Moore L, Sieggreen M. Revised National Pressure Ulcer Advisory Panel pressure injury staging system: Revised pressure injury staging system. *J Wound Ostomy Continence Nurs.* 2016;43(6):585–597.

100. Chen D, Apple DF, Jr., Hudson LM, Bode R. Medical complications during acute rehabilitation following spinal cord injury: Current experience of the Model Systems. *Arch Phys Med Rehabil.* 1999;80(11):1397–1401.

101. White BAB, Dea N, Street JT, et al. The economic burden of urinary tract infection and pressure ulceration in acute traumatic spinal cord injury admissions: Evidence for comparative economics and decision analytics from a matched case-control study. *J Neurotrauma.* 2017;34(20):2892–2900.

102. Kruger EA, Pires M, Ngann Y, Sterling M, Rubayi S. Comprehensive management of pressure ulcers in spinal cord injury: Current concepts and future trends. *J Spinal Cord Med.* 2013;36(6):572–585.

103. Landis E. Microinjection studies of capillary blood pressure in human skin. *Heart.* 1930;15:209.

104. *Physical Medicine and Rehabilitation Board Review,* 2nd ed.. American Journal of Physical Medicine & Rehabilitation; 2019.

105. Kosiak M, Kubicek WG, Olson M, Danz JN, Kottke FJ. Evaluation of pressure as a factor in the production of ischial ulcers. *Arch Phys Med Rehabil.* 1958;39(10):623–629.

106. Shea JD. Pressure sores: Classification and management. *Clin Orthop Relat Res.* 1975(112):89–100.

107. Lane CA, Selleck C, Chen Y, Tang Y. The impact of smoking and smoking cessation on wound healing in spinal cord-injured patients with pressure injuries: A retrospective comparison cohort study. *J Wound Ostomy Continence Nurs.* 2016;43(5):483–487.

108. Posthauer ME, Banks M, Dorner B, Schols JM. The role of nutrition for pressure ulcer management: National pressure ulcer advisory panel, European pressure ulcer advisory panel, and pan Pacific pressure injury alliance white paper. *Adv Skin Wound Care.* 2015;28(4):175–188; quiz 189–190.

109. Reddy M, Gill SS, Rochon PA. Preventing pressure ulcers: A systematic review. *JAMA.* 2006;296(8):974–984.

110. Groah SL, Schladen M, Pineda CG, Hsieh CH. Prevention of pressure ulcers among people with spinal cord injury: A systematic review. *Pm r.* 2015;7(6):613–636.

111. McInnes E, Jammali-Blasi A, Bell-Syer SE, Dumville JC, Middleton V, Cullum N. Support surfaces for pressure ulcer prevention. *Cochrane Database Syst Rev.* 2015(9):cd001735.

112. Allman RM, Walker JM, Hart MK, Laprade CA, Noel LB, Smith CR. Air-fluidized beds or conventional therapy for pressure sores. A randomized trial. *Ann Intern Med.* 1987;107(5):641–648.

113. Ferrell BA, Keeler E, Siu AL, Ahn SH, Osterweil D. Cost-effectiveness of low-air-loss beds for treatment of pressure ulcers. *J Gerontol A Biol Sci Med Sci.* 1995;50(3):M141–M146.

114. Thibault-Halman G, Casha S, Singer S, Christie S. Acute management of nutritional demands after spinal cord injury. *J Neurotrauma.* 2011;28(8):1497–1507.

115. Planas Vila M. Nutritional and metabolic aspects of neurological diseases. *Nutr Hosp.* 2014;29(Suppl 2):3–12.

116. Smith F, Dryburgh N, Donaldson J, Mitchell M. Debridement for surgical wounds. *Cochrane Database Syst Rev.* 2011(5):cd006214.

117. Baker LL, Rubayi S, Villar F, Demuth SK. Effect of electrical stimulation waveform on healing of ulcers in human beings with spinal cord injury. *Wound Repair Regen.* 1996;4(1):21–28.

118. Liu L, Moody J, Gall A. A quantitative, pooled analysis and systematic review of controlled trials on the impact of electrical stimulation settings and placement on pressure ulcer healing rates in persons with spinal cord injuries. *Ostomy Wound Manage.* 2016;62(7):16–34.

119. Lefevre C, Bellier-Waast F, Lejeune F, et al. Ten years of myocutaneous flaps for pressure ulcers in patients with spinal lesions: Analysis of complications in the framework of a specialised medical-surgical pathway. *J Plast Reconstr Aesthet Surg.* 2018;71(11):1652–1663.

120. Levine SM, Sinno S, Levine JP, Saadeh PB. An evidence-based approach to the surgical management of pressure ulcers. *Ann Plast Surg.* 2012;69(4):482–484.

121. Krassioukov A, Warburton DE, Teasell R, Eng JJ. A systematic review of the management of autonomic dysreflexia following spinal cord injury. *Arch Phys Med Rehabil.* 2009;90(4):682–695.

122. Furlan JC, Fehlings MG. Cardiovascular complications after acute spinal cord injury: Pathophysiology, diagnosis, and management. *Neurosurg Focus.* 2008;25(5):E13.

14 Palliative Care in the Neurosurgical Patient

Michael Liquori, Kathleen Mechler, John Liantonio, and Adam Pennarola

INTRODUCTION TO PALLIATIVE CARE

Palliative care is defined by the Center for the Advancement of Palliative Care (CAPC) as specialized medical care for people living with serious illness. "It focuses on providing relief from the symptoms and stress of a serious illness, and its goal is to improve quality of life for both the patient and the family."[1] Similarly, the American Academy of Hospice and Palliative Medicine (AAHPM), the national governing body of the specialty, describes palliative care as focusing on improving a patient's quality of life by managing pain and other distressing symptoms of a serious illness.[2] As described in further depth here, palliative care is often provided to patients in conjunction with disease-modifying therapy and should be differentiated from hospice. In this chapter, we describe key roles for palliative care including understanding the difference between palliative care and hospice care and when and how to identify appropriate patients for palliative care referral. Please see Box 14.1 for an outline of situations in which referral to palliative care is appropriate. We also describe some of the expertise that palliative care provides including communicating often difficult information and providing symptom management of pain and nonpain symptoms like nausea, constipation, or delirium. Finally, while it is important to identify appropriate patients for palliative care referral, it is equally important to understand when patients would be appropriate for hospice referral.

PALLIATIVE CARE VERSUS HOSPICE CARE

The terminology used to describe care provided for patients who are seriously ill or at the end of life can be confusing for both patients and providers. Terms including "palliative care" and "hospice care" are used to describe services provided for such patients; however, even these basic and foundational concepts are defined differently throughout the literature.[3-5] Further complicating this language are the many shared and overlapping elements between these terms, inconsistent usage of each of them by practitioners and patients, and a certain stigma surrounding descriptions of care provided for patients who are nearing death.[3,6,7] Despite this, there are components to each term that remain consistent throughout the literature

> **Box 14.1** When to Refer to Palliative Care
>
> Pain management, typically for patients with serious and life-limiting illness.
> Symptom management, including:
>
> - Anorexia
> - Nausea and vomiting
> - Constipation and diarrhea
> - Cough and dyspnea
> - Anxiety and depression
> - Confusion and delirium
>
> Communicating and coordinating care with patients' families where there may be distress or discord.
> Palliative care can also be useful in helping to establish underlying goals of care.
> Patients and families with psychosocial distress.

and therefore can provide a common framework for defining care provided to the seriously ill.[3] In comparing and contrasting the terms "palliative care" and "hospice care," it is possible to better grasp the essential elements of each care model. A working understanding of these two terms is crucial for any practitioner caring for patients nearing the end of life.

Both palliative and hospice care have a primary focus on symptom management and seek to preserve and prioritize quality of life for patients.[3–5] Care in both models is interdisciplinary, relying heavily on nurses, physicians, social workers/care coordinators, and chaplains to support patients and their families as they face their own (or their loved one's) mortality.[5,8] Each approach also assists patients and families with decision-making at multiple levels of the illness process.[5]

Palliative care is generally provided earlier in the course of disease than hospice care and may take place in conjunction with curative medical treatment of a potentially terminal condition.[3,5,9] Such care is provided by interdisciplinary teams and seeks to address the physical, emotional, and spiritual needs of patients and families. Multiple agencies, professional societies, and organizations provide definitions for palliative care, including the World Health Organization (WHO), which provides the following definition: "Palliative care is an approach that improves the quality of life of patients and their families facing the problem associated with life-threatening illness, through the prevention and relief of suffering by means of early identification and impeccable assessment and treatment of pain and other problems, physical, psychosocial and spiritual."[10] The WHO definition highlights features that are characteristic of palliative care: emphasizing quality of life, relief of suffering, early identification, and holistic management of a patient's clinical condition. Additionally, while palliative care is not exclusively an academic or institutional discipline, such care is more frequently provided either directly within or in close conjunction with a hospital system.

As described, hospice care is also focused on preserving and prioritizing quality of life for seriously ill patients. In contrast to patients who receive palliative care, patients who receive hospice care typically have advanced, terminal disease and are relatively closer to the end of life.[3,4,11] Most patients who receive hospice care have made the decision to forgo curative treatment of their underlying terminal condition.[5] Absent this decision, a patient's eligibility to receive hospice care will likely be effected. An additional differentiating factor between palliative care and hospice care is that the services provided by the latter are more heavily influenced by policies set by insurance providers. In the United States specifically, Medicare is the socialized primary insurance provider for most patients who are eligible to receive hospice care; in 2014, greater than 85% of US hospice services were paid for through Medicare.[12] The two basic eligibility requirements for patients to qualify for hospice care under Medicare are a prognosis of 6 months or less as verified by two physicians, and an agreement to receive care directed at symptom management and quality of life as opposed to cure of a terminal condition.[13] Furthermore, while institution-based inpatient hospice units are relatively common, the vast majority of hospice care is delivered outside of the hospital, in the community, with 94% or hospice services provided at the "routine home care" level in 2014.[3,4,11,12] Outpatient hospice services are also characterized by the presence of community-based volunteers who assist with provision of care.[12]

To summarize, both palliative care and hospice care are provided to patients who are seriously ill and emphasize quality of life for patients and families. Each approach is multidisciplinary and requires a team of providers in order to function effectively. Palliative care is more hospital-based, is often utilized relatively earlier in the disease course, may be delivered in conjunction with curative medical therapies, and has no strict eligibility restrictions. Hospice care is more community- and home-based, is usually reserved for patients close to the end of life, and has eligibility criteria that patients must meet in order to qualify for services. The correct usage of terminology itself is important so that patients and fellow providers can best understand the strengths and limitations of each model.

COMMUNICATION

The neurosurgery hospitalist plays an important role in the primary care management of both acutely and chronically ill neurosurgical patients. While the neurosurgeon has an important operative role, the neurosurgery hospitalist is often tasked with daily symptoms management, chronic disease management with coordination of consulting teams, disclosure of imaging and biopsy results, discussions of goals of care, and complex discharge planning. Effective communication skills are essential to the completion of these tasks, which may include the communication of bad or serious news and the sharing of life-altering information defined as information that poses "a threat to a person's mental or physical well-being or upsets an established life" or is "perceive(d) as causing a significant change in the health or quality of life of the patient and family."[14,15] It can also be news carrying great uncertainty, such as the unknown potential for neurologic recovery and future quality of life as is common for patients with neurological cancers, traumatic brain injury, spinal cord injury, large strokes, or neurosurgical complications.[16,17]

Communication skills were once thought to be an innate part of bedside manner for the good clinician; however, as our patients' conditions and available interventions become more complex, these conversations for shared decision-making can also become complex. Once considered harmful to deliver serious news directly to a patient, it is now accepted that a patient wants to know,[18] has a right to all information about their health, and that after receiving information patients do not experience more anxiety or depression.[19] Neurological literature reflects that patients and families have better experiences with clinicians who have comprehensive communication skills such as balancing hope and advanced illness or who adhere to protocols such as SPIKES.[19-23] However, a stress reaction is often felt on the part of the clinician prior to initiating a difficult conversation,[23-25] and repeating this cycle of distress without considering how to improve upon communication can lead to burnout. Studies have demonstrated that communication skills can be learned through practice, simulation,[26-28] and through online experiences or reading,[29] and we will outline the SPIKES protocol with reference to the neurosurgical patient.

The SPIKES tool was developed by Baile et al.[30] and published in 2000 in response to a 1998 survey of oncologists that showed that fewer than 10% had received formal training in communication, and only 32% had observation and feedback on communication of bad news. Although developed for oncology SPIKES is applicable to the neurosurgical patient population, with the major difference being that these patients are more likely to be incapacitated earlier in the disease and clinicians are often working with proxies/agents and surrogates for the communication of bad news and for complex decisions. It is important to the care of the incapacitated patient to determine if the patient has a health care proxy or power of attorney for health care naming a decision-maker (called "proxy" or "agent"). In the absence of this document a "surrogate" decision-maker would be used for decision-making. Each state determines its own statute for the order of surrogacy; resources for learning your state's regulations can be found through hospital administration or at the American Bar Association website (www.americanbar.org).

Communication and Discussing Bad or Serious News

Following a stepwise plan helps ensure that a discussion of serious news can reliably accomplish four goals: determine the patient's and family's knowledge and expectations, provide information to the level the patient desires, provide support to patient and family emotions, and develop a plan through shared decision-making with the patient and family.[30]

Step 1: S—Setting Up

Preparation for the discussion includes internal and practical considerations. To prepare the physical setting, it is important to consider who will be involved: Is the patient able to be involved, so that the meeting should take place in his or her room?

Or is the patient in an altered state of consciousness and another space is needed? A private room is preferable, but if not available ensure privacy by using dividing curtains and speaking as quietly as possible. Many patients will want an important family member or friend present; if not it is reasonable to recommend that they ask someone to be present in person or by phone for the purpose of helping to absorb all the details likely to be discussed. Create uninterrupted time as much as possible by silencing devices or consider asking a colleague to cover your phone or pager. In a survey of amyotrophic lateral sclerosis (ALS) patients and families recalling their diagnosis conversations, better conversation performance was associated with more time spent on the encounter.[21] In addition to opening your time, opening your body language also creates the rapport needed for serious conversations. Sit down at the patient's level and at a distance close enough to allow you to maintain good eye contact and to be able reach for their arm or hand to give comfort if the patient is comfortable with this. Neurologic patients often experience depersonalization due changes in memory or mental status due to their illness: be aware of this and try to involve them as much as possible.[16,22]

Consider, additionally, giving time to internal reflection prior to initiating serious discussions. Ask yourself: Which consultants may need to be there? If not present, am I current on their plan and have I anticipated patient and family questions? Mental rehearsal is especially practical for preparation.

Step 2: P—Assessing the Patient's Perception

Before discussing any new medical findings, it is most useful to have the patient or family summarize their understanding of the current medical condition or hospital course. This "before you tell, ask" method along with follow-up open-ended questioning is useful to assess understanding and view their impression of the gravity and implications of the condition. For example, "What have you been told about your medical condition so far?" or "Can someone please quickly summarize this hospitalization to date so I can give the next update?" This patient or family-based summary allows you to correct any details and provides an opportunity to assess the patient and family for use of coping strategies such as denial or unrealistic expectations. If they struggle to do this step independently, you may have to start the summary: speak in small segments, checking for nodding or "oh yeah," perhaps even empowering them to take over and complete the summary.

Step 3: I—Obtaining the Patient's Invitation

Studies show that most patients want realistic information about their illness and prognosis and that they are not harmed by this knowledge.[18] However some patients do not want to know this information, either to aid in coping or as a cultural norm. You can determine their desire by asking, "How would you like me to discuss the test results?" or "Do you want to know all information about your condition or are there certain things you don't want to know and prefer discussed with a loved one? If so, who should the doctors speak with?" The patient has a right not to know certain information; however, when that undesired information is needed for appropriate decision-making and care planning it is necessary that the patient chooses someone who is participating in decisions to receive this information.

Step 4: K—Giving Knowledge and Information

After obtaining the patient's invitation to give information, if the information is of a serious nature it is helpful to patients and families to use a warning statement alerting that serious news is coming. Examples include "Unfortunately, I have some bad news to tell you," or "I'm sorry to have to tell you that. . . ." These statements allow patients and families to have a moment to prepare for the news, be alerted to pay attention, and may facilitate information processing.[30] Proceed with disclosing the medical facts in small amounts using common language and avoiding medical jargon. Consider using phrases like "bruising of the brain" instead of "contusions," using "a stroke from bleeding/a blood clot in the brain" instead of "hemorrhagic/ischemic stroke," using "the cancer is growing and pushing against the healthy parts of brain causing damage" instead of "the tumor is enlarged causing midline shift," and using "the scan shows severe brain damage" instead of describing the radiographic terms from the report. Avoid using excess bluntness or dismissive statements such as "there is nothing more we can do for you" as this is divisive and not true for all therapeutic goals—perhaps there is nothing we can medically do to reverse their spinal cord damage or to stop them from dying from their large stroke, but we can always treat their symptoms and provide medical supportive care with dignity. Offer to give prognostic information if they desire and you are able; instead of specific numbers, use ranges such as hours to days, days to weeks, weeks to months, etc. Check frequently for understanding, offer to repeat information or answer follow-up questions, and, although difficult, consider allowing for silence because it leaves space for emotional processing.

Step 5: E—Addressing the Patient's Emotions with Empathetic Responses

When patients and families receive serious or bad news they may undergo a range of emotions from silence or disbelief, to crying, to anger and denial. It is important for the clinician to observe, identify, and respond so that he or she can validate these emotions. Emotions need to be addressed before any additional information can be shared or before treatment plans can be discussed. Effective strategies include using empathetic statements such as "I know this is not the information you wanted to hear" or "I can see how upsetting this is to you." If the patient's or family's expressions of understanding are vague or emotions are not clear, you can follow-up with exploratory questions such as "Please explain what you mean by that?" or "Could you please tell me what is worrying you most now?" before your empathetic response. The patient and family can feel most supported when you try to understand on an individual basis what they are experiencing rather than making assumptions. Again, this is where sitting in close proximity directly facing the patient with a relaxed body language is meaningful. This can be the most challenging step for many clinicians due to discomfort with unpredictable emotional reactions, but mental rehearsal and practice with responses is helpful.

Step 6: S—Strategy and Summary

When the patient and family are emotionally ready to move to planning, having a strategy is important to reduce anxiety because it provides them with less uncertainty and more control over next steps. If not ready, however, the next best step is to establish a time to continue the conversation at a later date. With the permission to discuss a treatment plan, the clinician will be prepared to make a patient-centered plan by building on the rapport and information gathered in steps 2–5. Again asking for a summary of the updates presented in Step 4 and their implications allows for final errors and omissions to be corrected.

Shared decision-making is now the standard of practice in the United States and is accepted in the neurological community.[31–33] Shared decision-making is defined as a collaborative process involving both the clinician and the patient or surrogate working together to combine the goals and desires of the patient and family with the expertise of the clinician, using evidence-based medicine to make the best healthcare decisions for the individual patient.[31] Start by asking open-ended questions such as "Knowing this new information, what are your thoughts or concerns about what's next/after the hospital?" or "Have you considered how you would want to be treated in a condition like we discussed?" or "To help with care planning, can you please share thoughts about how this impacts your goals for the future or changes what's important to you?" These questions may need to be more directed, but patients and families may take this opening to express their preferences enough to guide strategy. The role of the physician in discussing treatment options is to educate patients about all reasonable treatment options, including palliative and symptom-focused treatment, and to present options not as equal but as more or less in line with elicited goals. Another useful strategy is to explain each treatment option with "big picture" end points and timelines in mind by summarizing what could be possible with each treatment option in a "best case/worst case/most likely outcome" fashion.[18,34,35] This differentiation between "best" and "most likely" outcomes can help to give hope but avoid false or unrealistic hope.[35,36] Consider asking the patient and family if a medical recommendation, based on your medical experience in combination with their preferences shared with you, would be helpful.[23,37] When information and decisions are shared, patients and families feel listened to and clinicians can experience less feelings of failure if the decided-on treatments are ultimately not successful. If patients and families ask for private time to discuss options, set up a distinct follow-up plan because patient care is optimal when there is a defined patient-centered care plan.

Advance Directives

Advance directives are documents made in advance of incapacitating illness that outline patient desires for medical care and decisions. Examples include *health care proxy* or *power of attorney for health care* documents and *living wills*. The clinician's responsibility in regards to these documents is to examine the patient and conclude if they are in a condition that the document requires if it is to be placed in effect. For the health care proxy to be in effect the clinician must determine that the patient does not have the capacity to make medical decisions required and that the proxy is needed. If capacity is regained, such as after hypernatremia is reversed, then the document is no longer in effect and the patient makes his or her own decisions. For the living will, typical language requires the clinician to determine if the patient is either "comatose or persistently vegetative" or "terminal within 6 months regardless of treatments rendered *and* incapacitated"; at that point, the care directives for treatments that the patient does or does not want go into effect.[38] If there is uncertainty about the patient's condition or the patient does not meet these criteria, then the living will is not in effect; neither is it in effect if the patient has a terminal condition but *retains* decision-making capacity.

SYMPTOMS

The role of palliation in the neurosurgical patient varies based on illness stage. Patients with new symptoms and a long prognosis require workup of and conservative management for their condition; however, in the setting of known chronic or progressive neurologic or neurosurgical illnesses the palliative management of severe symptoms becomes an important role for the neurosurgical hospitalist. The following treatment recommendations are for these palliative patients.

Pain
Pain Assessment

Pain is a ubiquitous symptom in surgical populations, and the neurosurgical patient is no exception. Postoperative pain was discussed in Chapter 12. Here, we focus instead on the approach to pain management in an end-of-life population. Perhaps not surprisingly, pain is very common in this population. It is estimated that one-fifth of patients who die in the hospital experience pain during their last admission[39] while approximately 60% of community-dwelling adults experience pain in their final year of life.[40] These patients with advanced illness and life-limiting disease often have their pain go underrecognized and undertreated.[41,42] Reasons for this are likely multifactorial, relating to clinician, patient, and system issues. A common patient issue at the end-of-life that may lead to unrecognized and undertreated pain is the loss of the ability to effectively communicate.[43] In order to decrease the chances of not recognizing pain, especially in those who are noncommunicative, it is important to have a systematic approach to the assessment of pain.

The initial step in pain assessment is to obtain a detailed characterization of the pain. A simple method for doing this is to utilize the "OPQRST" structure for evaluating medical complaints. Specific questions should be directed to the location, onset, palliating and provoking factors, quality, related symptoms, response to prior treatments, severity, and timing. A key goal of this assessment is to determine the etiology of the pain and to categorize the pain if possible. One such categorization is along nociceptive and neuropathic lines. *Nociceptive pain*, which is derived from pain receptors, may be visceral or somatic.[44] *Visceral pain* is often poorly localized and described as deep, aching, or colicky. *Somatic pain* is often more localized and described as constant, aching, or gnawing. *Neuropathic pain* is due to damage to peripheral nerves, the spinal cord, or the central nervous system. Neuropathic pain is frequently described as burning, shooting, or electric. Each of these components thus far is entirely subjective. A crucial step in the assessment is to utilize an objective measure of severity. There are many ways of doing this but common methods are to use a numerical pain scale or the visual analog scale (VAS).

While pain is often thought of solely in the sense of the physical discomfort it may cause, it is important to keep the concept of "total pain" in mind. Thus, a thorough pain assessment requires the clinician to recognize that pain is a "complex of physical, emotional, social, and spiritual elements"[45] and to direct questions at the impact that patients' physical pain may have on their ability to function, physical activity, mood, and relationships. Similarly, it is necessary to ask about the patient's goals in relation to pain control. Some patients prefer to endure slightly more pain in order to be alert and to have time with loved ones. For other patients, though, their goal is to experience no pain at all, and they are willing to sacrifice time with loved ones in order to achieve that goal. Knowledge of this piece of information can be crucial in choosing appropriate treatments and their respective titrations.

Pain Assessment of the Noncommunicative Patient

The assessment of pain when a patient is unable to communicate is challenging. In these scenarios it is recommended to follow a hierarchy approach to information gathering and to assimilate multiple sources of information.[43] An attempt should be made at allowing the patient to self-report pain. This can be accomplished by using yes/no questions and allowing the patient use other vocalizations or gestures if needed. If the patient is unable to self-report any information, proxy reporting of pain from a family member or caregiver who knows the patient well should be sought. The next step is to search for potential causes of pain such as trauma, wounds, history of pain, or positioning.[43] Next is to observe patient behaviors and utilize behavioral pain assessment tools. There are a variety of tools available, but few have been validated in multiple populations. For palliative care and end-of-life populations, tools that have some evidence to support their use are the Multidimensional Objective Pain Assessment Tool (MOPAT),[43,46] Pain Assessment in Advanced Dementia Tool (PAINAD),[43] and the Checklist of Nonverbal Pain Indicators (CNPI).[46] If questions still remain about the presence of pain, it is sometimes practical to assume that pain is present and to attempt an empiric trial of analgesia.[43]

Pain Management

There are many options for pain management, but pharmacotherapy is the mainstay for patients as they approach the end of life. There are three main categories of pharmacotherapy: opioids, nonopioid analgesics, and adjuvant analgesics. In today's climate of appropriate concern over the opioid prescribing epidemic it is essential to keep a patient's history of dependence or addiction, or the potential to develop such issues, in mind. However, as patients approach the end of life, the risk–benefit analysis changes and it is generally acceptable to provide patients with the appropriate treatment to ensure symptom control and a comfortable quality of life. While there are multiple pharmacotherapy options available for pain, any patient with pain of moderate or greater severity should be given a trial of opioid therapy, and, in fact, most patients with severe pain will require the use of opioids. In this section, we only discuss the opioid analgesics. For a discussion of nonopioid and adjuvant analgesics, please refer to Chapter 12. In general, the preferred treatment approach in this patient population is to begin with immediate-release opioids, especially in opioid-naïve patients. As the clinician begins to understand the patient's requirements to achieve adequate pain control, a long-acting opioid should be added on a scheduled basis while still continuing the "as-needed" immediate-release opioid with the goal of using two to three (or fewer) doses of the immediate-release agent in a 24-hour period.

There is currently no consensus regarding a preferred agent, and choice of therapy should be individualized to each patient. The most common opioids in the United States include morphine, oxycodone, hydrocodone, hydromorphone, oxymorphone, and fentanyl. Due to cost, availability, and analgesic potency, morphine is the most commonly prescribed opioid.[47] Morphine is available in a variety of formulations, including sustained- and immediate-release, tablets, solutions, elixirs, and injectable solutions. In cases of known, or expected, renal insufficiency one needs to thoughtful with the use of morphine. As renal function deteriorates, morphine metabolites can accumulate and lead to neurotoxicity.[48] In cases of renal insufficiency, hydromorphone and fentanyl are preferred. Hydromorphone, similar to morphine, is available in multiple formulations including oral tablets, oral solutions, and injectable solutions. Importantly, there is no long-acting formulation available in the United States. Fentanyl, which is approximately 80 times more potent than morphine,[49] is available as transdermal patches and intravenous formulations. Use of fentanyl, especially in its transdermal formulation, is limited by the inability to rapidly titrate dose and increased fentanyl release with fevers.[49] In cases of stable, chronic pain, though, transdermal fentanyl is a viable option. Whenever possible, the oral route is preferred as it provides a slower onset of action and a longer duration of action.[49] As patients approach end of life and enter the active dying phase, it is quite common to develop dysphagia. In these times, options include switching from tablets to concentrated oral solutions, providing

Table 14.1 Equianalgesic doses of common opioids

Opioid	Oral Dose (mg)	Parenteral dose (mg)
Morphine	30	10
Hydrocodone	30	–
Oxycodone	20	–
Hydromorphone	7.5	1.5
Oxymorphone	10	1
Fentanyl	–	0.1

medications per rectum, or using intravenous or subcutaneous formulation. To safely initiate, titrate, change formulations and/or convert between opioids, understanding equianalgesic dosing is paramount. There is some variability in the data underlying opioid equivalency, and so it is important that you remain consistent in the equivalencies that you use. See Table 14.1 for a common equianalgesic dosing table that we use. Notably, this table includes a fentanyl conversion ratio but only for the intravenous formulation. When converting to or from fentanyl transdermal patches, a common short cut, sometimes referred to as "Levy's Rule," is to use a ratio of *2 mg* of morphine *per day* as equivalent to *1 µg per hour* of transdermal fentanyl.[50] As an example, for a person requiring 50 mg of oral morphine per day, switching to a 25 µg/h fentanyl patch would be safe and likely effective. Given some of the inherent complications with fentanyl conversions, asking palliative care for assistance is encouraged.

Anorexia

Anorexia, a poor or decreased appetite, is a common symptom in neurologic illnesses and in all illnesses at end of life. This anorexia is typically bothersome to the family and not to the patient, and the best management is family education regarding this predictable and painless symptom. Nonpharmacologic treatments include multiple small frequent meals, eating only when sitting upright and most awake, and bringing favorite foods from home.[51] Treatment with appetite stimulants can be burdensome, and only poor evidence exists for their use. On a case-by-case basis, if a trial of appetite stimulation is decided, consider treatments that may have a secondary beneficial effect. Dexamethasone is a commonly used treatment after neurosurgery for cerebral edema or inflammatory pain and can cause increased appetite and feelings of well-being.[52] Mirtazapine can be used when poor mood or sleep are also present; in a small study of dementia patients use was associated with weight gain and well-tolerated.[53] Dronabinol is also indicated for treatment of chemo-induced nausea and vomiting and has been shown to maintain weight when patients lost weight on placebo treatments.[54] Megestrol use outside of cancer is not supported by evidence and has only a limited role in palliation due to its side-effect profile.[55] Anorexia associated with stroke or brain injury can improve with time, rehabilitation, and nonpharmacologic interventions; however, if nutrition is impeding recovery and it is within patient goals, then supplementation with artificial nutrition via gastrostomy tube must be considered.[56]

Nausea and Vomiting

Nausea, the painless sensation that you are about to vomit, is an unfortunately common symptom in neurosurgical illnesses and is more treatment-resistant than the vomiting itself.[57] Causes include conditions and chemicals that affect the chemoreceptor trigger zone (CTZ), the autonomic nervous system, the cerebral cortex, or the gastric system: chemotherapy, medications (for seizure, Parkinson's disease, antibiotics, pain), increased intracranial pressure (ICP), cerebritis, anxiety, and constipation. It is important to consider the cause when making management choices. History is often sufficient to reach the diagnosis; however, if there is concern for a GI etiology, it is reasonable to consider abdominal imaging. For medication- or chemo-induced nausea and vomiting impacting the CTZ, consider ondansetron, dronabinol, low-dose haloperidol or olanzapine, prochlorperazine, or promethazine. For anticipatory or anxiety-related symptoms, use low-dose benzodiazepine, especially before emetogenic events.[51,57] Dexamethasone is the treatment of choice for increased ICP and cerebritis.[58–61] For GI causes, treat constipation and give excellent mouth care; consider metoclopramide use 30 minutes before meals. Chronic nausea, like chronic pain, requires multimodal treatment with antidepressants and support.[51] Use intravenous or rectal formulations of medications until patient can tolerate oral medications.

Constipation and Diarrhea

Constipation, or small hard feces passed infrequently and with difficulty, is a common symptom in neurosurgical patients and is associated with higher pain medication use and a trend toward longer postoperative hospitalization.[62] Causes include immobility, low enteral intake, cauda equina syndrome, and medication or opioid use, and it is observed with regularity in about half of patients with advanced Parkinson's disease and in stroke patients in rehabilitation centers.[63–66] Diarrhea, frequent loose stools, is less common and can be due to infection or chemotherapy. Treatment for both should include privacy with access to a commode and a balanced diet if possible. Avoid bulk agents in neurology patients because these agents require the intake of a large amount of water, and docusate is rarely sufficient monotherapy. For the goal of a soft bowel movement every 1–2 days, start with a gentle stimulant laxative such as 1–2 tabs of senna 1–4 times daily or bisacodyl 1–3 oral tabs daily. If no results, add daily lactulose, sorbitol, or milk of magnesia.[51,61] If constipation is opioid-induced and not improved by these agents, consider methylnaltrexone dosed every other day or naloxegol every morning. If no bowel movement occurs for several days, perform a digital rectal exam to rule out fecal impaction, which would need to be removed manually, and to assess if a suppository or an enema would be effective to treat. If a malignant bowel obstruction is suspected and nonoperative management is appropriate, consult palliative medicine. For diarrhea, treat with antibiotics if infectious; otherwise give rehydration and consider loperamide.

Cough and Dyspnea

Respiratory symptoms in neurosurgical patients in the absence of pulmonary, cardiac, or infectious diseases are often due to respiratory muscle neuropathy or brainstem dysfunction. A cough is generally considered protective and not suppressed; treat with guaifenesin and humidified air. In respiratory muscle dysfunction due to ALS or other traumatic or progressive myopathies or neuropathies, noninvasive ventilation can improve symptoms of dyspnea; with time, this may progress to a need for invasive ventilation if this decision is in line with patient and family goals.[67-69] Brainstem respiratory dysfunction is often treated with invasive ventilatory support in temporary or permanent fashion. If, however, the patient is at end of life or continued invasive support is not in line with patient goals, a palliative extubation may be warranted along with aggressive treatment for dyspnea. Mild dyspnea can be treated with supplemental oxygen or air movement across the face with a fan. The standard of treatment for more severe dyspnea is oral, sublingual, or intravenous opioids.[51] A conservative starting dose is 5 mg oral or 2 mg intravenous morphine every 3–4 hours as needed, titrated for comfort and normal respiratory rate. Anxiolytics can be used but only if anxiety is suspected or paradoxical breathing motions are noted and distressing; otherwise, for pure tachypnea opioids are recommended. For the management of secretions causing deep rattling noises without associated tachypnea consider turning the patient, changing the angle of the bed head, or educating family about their expected nature to decrease distress. If associated with tachypnea or if distressing to family, treat with scopolamine patch, intravenous glycopyrrolate 0.2–0.4 mg every 6 hours as needed, or atropine ophthalmic drops 2 drops sublingual every 6 hours as needed. Deep suctioning is not recommended due to discomfort.

Anxiety and Depression

Clinically diagnosed or subclinical mood disorders such as anxiety and depression occur in the neurosurgical patient population, but these are neither expected nor normal and treatment is indicated. Special populations in which mood symptoms are present at higher rates than in the general public are those with traumatic brain and spinal cord injuries, stroke, epilepsy, Parkinson's disease and other dementias, chronic back pain, and cancer.[70-79] Anxiety related to cancer and planned spine surgery has been found to be clustered most symptomatically near time of diagnosis or surgery, with a natural course of improvement with time and information, although treatment could be indicated with short-term low-dose benzodiazepines if symptoms are severe. In patients with pain before planned spinal surgery consider preoperative treatment with duloxetine or nortriptyline to improve mood and pain outcomes.[70,71,76,78] In the elderly, avoid benzodiazepines for anxiety and consider hydroxyzine or BuSpar; for depression, consider mirtazapine if sleep and appetite complaints are present, or try newer tricyclic antidepressants.[61] Selective serotonin or serotonin and norepinephrine reuptake inhibitors (SSRI or SNRIs) are overall well tolerated for depression but need a commitment to use for 4 weeks before stopping for treatment failure. Atypical antipsychotics can be considered if the patient has failed other treatments or presents with psychotic features. For a patient at end of life with severe depression in need of rapid relief, consider the use of a psychostimulant such as methylphenidate at 8 AM and noon.[51] Always refer for mental health aftercare if the concerning symptoms may be ongoing or impact functioning.

Confusion and Delirium

New-onset confusion and delirium in the typical patient require workup and conservative management for patient safety. Evidence is against the use of antipsychotics.[80] However, in the patient at the end of life and with a focus on comfort, their use can be indicated. Haloperidol is a useful medication; it is available in oral pill and liquid formulations and also can be administered rectally or by intravenous or subcutaneous injection (avoid intramuscular injections unless the situation is an emergency). Consider atypical antipsychotics such as quetiapine (Seroquel) if the patient can swallow or has Parkinson's disease.[61] As with all patients, management begins with keeping a consistent and calm environment, maintaining day–night cycles, providing welcome family and familiar objects, keeping fluid intake and nutrition normal, and avoiding monitors and restraints.[51]

HOSPICE
Hospice Definition and Background

Hospice is both a philosophy and a model of care which is focused on providing optimal quality of life to patients and their families at the end of life through care which is consistent with the patient's values. The modern conception of hospice care is credited to Dame Cicely Saunders after she started St. Christopher's Hospice in 1967 to provide care for patients with advanced cancer. Since that time, her model of hospice has spread throughout the world. In the United States, the first hospice was started in 1974, at the New Haven Connecticut Hospice.[81] This hospice was slightly different from those in Britain in that most care was provided in the patient's home as opposed to a hospital/institutional setting. To this day, this is the most common form of hospice in the United States.[81]

Hospice Model of Care

Hospice provides medical care and supportive services to a patient with a life-limiting illness and to their family with the focus being on quality of life and not life prolongation. The goal of hospice is to alleviate suffering in the dying patient, which arises from Cicely Saunders concept of "total pain"—the combination of physical, psychological, spiritual, and social imbalance that leads to symptoms and impairments.[82] To achieve this goal, an interdisciplinary team comprised of physicians (the hospice physician and the primary physician), nurses, social workers, chaplains, home health aides, volunteers, and bereavement counselors work closely together to address each component of suffering.[83,84]

In addition to the services aimed at providing relief of symptoms, the Medicare Hospice Benefit, which covers approximately 80% of all hospice patients in the United States,[85,86] also entitles patients to a variety of other services. Among these services are durable medical equipment (such as a hospital bed, commode, oxygen, etc.), all medications for the palliation of the terminal illness, 24-hour accessibility to a provider (usually a hospice nurse) to assess and manage any changes, nursing care, home health aides, and bereavement care to the family after the patient's death.[86] It is important to note, however, that continuous nursing or home health aide care is *not* covered. Typically, nurses visit the patient one to three times per week depending on illness severity, and home health aides visit for a couple hours per day up to 4 times per week. When a patient is receiving home hospice, the bulk of patient care responsibility falls to the family. As such, the Medicare Hospice Benefit also provides for 5 days of respite care in a facility within each benefit period to help alleviate caregiver burden.[81]

In the United States, hospice care is most frequently delivered in the patient's place of residence. Generally, this means their private home, but also includes assisted-living facilities and nursing homes. Other locations include a residential hospice facility and inpatient hospice units.

Candidates for Hospice and Eligibility

There are two main criteria for hospice eligibility according to the Medicare Hospice Benefit (and most private insurers by proxy, as they generally base their coverage on the Medicare benefit): (1) a life expectancy of 6 months or less if the disease follows its expected course, as certified by two physicians, and (2) the patient agrees to forego Medicare reimbursement for curative medical treatments related to the terminal illness.[85] It is important to note that patients may continue to receive care for diseases unrelated to the terminal illness (commonly, dialysis for end-stage renal disease, provided it is not caused by the terminal illness) under their regular Medicare coverage. Information on disease-specific requirements, which is beyond the scope of this review, can be found on the Centers for Medicare & Medicaid Services website (www.cms.gov). One barrier to hospice referral is difficulty with certifying that a patient has 6 months or less to live, especially with non–cancer related diagnoses. There is ongoing research in this domain, however, and a useful website for clinicians is http://eprognosis.ucsf.edu/calculators, which helps prognosticate a patient's estimated survival based on a variety of comorbidities. Some clinicians may also hesitate to refer to hospice if a patient does not wish to have a do-not-resuscitate order. While a do-not-resuscitate order is in line with the hospice philosophy, it is not a requirement for enrollment and should not delay referral.

Benefits of Hospice Care

There is some evidence that utilization of hospice leads to decreased healthcare costs in some[87,88] but not all settings.[89] More important than potential cost savings, though, is the impact on patients and their families. Hospice care is associated with improved quality of life for the patient, and quality of life scores increase with increasing time on hospice.[90,91] Family members of those who die on hospice tend to be more satisfied with the care that the patient received and are less likely to experience posttraumatic stress disorder.[92,93] From a survival standpoint, a few studies have shown a survival advantage for those enrolled in hospice versus those who were not enrolled, among a variety of illnesses.[94,95] Interestingly, hospice care may also have a survival benefit for spouses as it has been associated with a lower rate of mortality following the death of a spouse, especially among women.[96]

REFERENCES

1. Center for the Advancement of Palliative Care (CAPC). Palliative Care Definition. What is palliative care? https://www.capc.org/about/palliative-care/. Accessed September 1, 2018.

2. AAHPM and the Specialty of Hospice and Palliative Medicine. http://aahpm.org/about/about. Accessed April 1, 2019.

3. Hui D, De La Cruz M, Mori M, et al. Concepts and definitions for "supportive care," "best supportive care," "palliative care," and "hospice care" in the published literature, dictionaries, and textbooks. *Support Care Cancer.* 2013;21(3):659–685. doi: 10.1007/s00520-012-1564-y.

4. Davis MP, Gutgsell T, Gamier P. What is the difference between palliative care and hospice care? *Cleve Clin J Med.* 2015;82(9):569–571. doi: 10.3949/ccjm.82a.14145.

5. Bonebrake D, Culver C, Call K, Ward-Smith P. Clinically differentiating palliative care and hospice. *Clin J Oncol Nurs.* 2010;14(3):273–275. doi: 10.1188/10.CJON.273-275.

6. Hanks G. Palliative care: Careless use of language undermines our identity. *Palliat Med.* 2008;22(2):109–110. doi: 10.1177/0269216308089301.

7. Doyle D. Editorial. *Palliat Med.* 2003;17(1):9–10. doi: 10.1191/0269216303pm651ed.

8. Finlay IG, Jones RVH. Definitions in palliative care. *BMJ.* 1995;311(7007):754. doi: 10.1136/bmj.311.7007.754a.

9. Billings JA. What is palliative care? *J Palliat Med.* 1998;1(1):73–81. doi: 10.1089/jpm.1998.1.73.

10. World Health Organization. WHO definition of palliative care. 2012. http://www.who.int/cancer/palliative/definition/en/. Accessed August 17, 2018.

11. Batchelor NH. Palliative or hospice care? Understanding the similarities and differences. *Rehabil Nurs.* 2010;35(2):60–64. doi: 10.1002/j.2048-7940.2010.tb00032.x.

12. National Hospice and Palliative Care Organization, Hospice Action Network. *The Medicare Hospice Benefit*; 2015. https://www.nhpco.org/sites/default/files/public/communications/Outreach/The_Medicare_Hospice_Benefit.pdf. Accessed August 8, 2017.

13. Medicare.gov. Hospice & respite care. https://www.medicare.gov/coverage/hospice-and-respite-care.html. Accessed August 17, 2018.

14. Ptacek JT, Eberhardt TL. Breaking bad news. *JAMA*. 1996;276(6):496. doi: 10.1001/jama.1996.03540060072041.

15. Wolfe AD, Frierdich SA, Wish J, Kilgore-Carlin J, Plotkin JA, Hoover-Regan M. Sharing life-altering information: Development of pediatric hospital guidelines and team training. *J Palliat Med*. 2014;17(9):1011–1018. doi: 10.1089/jpm.2013.0620.

16. Lou S, Carstensen K, Jørgensen CR, Nielsen CP. Stroke patients' and informal carers' experiences with life after stroke: An overview of qualitative systematic reviews. *Disabil Rehabil*. 2017;39(3):301–313. doi: 10.3109/09638288.2016.1140836.

17. Turner-Stokes L, Sykes N, Silber E, Khatri A, Sutton L, Young E. From diagnosis to death: Exploring the interface between neurology, rehabilitation and palliative care in managing people with long-term neurological conditions. *Clin Med (Northfield Il)*. 2007;7(2):129–136. doi: 10.7861/clinmedicine.7-2-129.

18. Pfeifer MP, Sidorov JE, Smith AC, et al. The discussion of end-of-life medical care by primary care patients and physicians. *J Gen Intern Med*. 1994;9(2):82–88. doi: 10.1007/BF02600206.

19. Schofield PE, Butow PN, Thompson JF, Tattersall MHN, Beeney LJ, Dunn SM. Psychological responses of patients receiving a diagnosis of cancer. *Ann Oncol*. 2003;14(1):48–56. doi: 10.1093/annonc/mdg010.

20. Schutz REC, Coats HL, Engelberg RA, Curtis JR, Creutzfeldt CJ. Is there hope? Is she there? How families and clinicians experience severe acute brain injury. *J Palliat Med*. 2017;20(2):170–176. doi: 10.1089/jpm.2016.0286.

21. Mccluskey L, Casarett D, Siderowf A. Breaking the news: A survey of ALS patients and their caregivers. *Amyotroph Lateral Scler Other Mot Neuron Disord*. 2004;5(3):131–135. doi: 10.1080/14660820410020772.

22. Boersma I, Miyasaki J, Kutner J, Kluger B. Palliative care and neurology: Time for a paradigm shift. *Neurology*. 2014;83(6):561–567. doi: 10.1212/WNL.0000000000000674.

23. Back AL, Curtis JR. Communicating bad news. *West J Med*. 2002;176(3):177–180.

24. Shaw J, Brown R, Heinrich P, Dunn S. Doctors' experience of stress during simulated bad news consultations. *Patient Educ Couns*. 2013;93(2):203–208. doi: 10.1016/j.pec.2013.06.009.

25. Studer RK, Danuser B, Gomez P. Physicians' psychophysiological stress reaction in medical communication of bad news: A critical literature review. *Int J Psychophysiol*. 2017;120:14–22. doi: 10.1016/j.ijpsycho.2017.06.006.

26. Alelwani SM, Ahmed YA. Medical training for communication of bad news: A literature review. *J Educ Health Promot*. 2014;3:51. doi: 10.4103/2277-9531.134737.

27. Goelz T, Wuensch A, Stubenrauch S, et al. Specific training program improves oncologists' palliative care communication skills in a randomized controlled trial. *J Clin Oncol*. 2011;29(25):3402–3407. doi: 10.1200/JCO.2010.31.6372.

28. Lamba S, Tyrie LS, Bryczkowski S, Nagurka R. Teaching surgery residents the skills to communicate difficult news to patient and family members: A literature review. *J Palliat Med*. 2016;19(1):101–107. doi: 10.1089/jpm.2015.0292.

29. Daetwyler CJ, Cohen DG, Gracely E, Novack DH. eLearning to enhance physician patient communication: A pilot test of "doc.com" and "WebEncounter" in teaching bad news delivery. *Med Teach*. 2010;32(9):e381–e390. doi: 10.3109/0142159X.2010.495759.

30. Baile WF, Buckman R, Lenzi R, Glober G, Beale EA, Kudelka AP. SPIKES—A six-step protocol for delivering bad news: Application to the patient with cancer. *Oncologist*. 2000;5(4):302–311. doi: 10.1634/theoncologist.5-4-302.

31. Khan MW, Muehlschlegel S. Shared decision making in neurocritical care. *Neurol Clin.* 2017;35(4):825–834. doi: 10.1016/j.ncl.2017.06.014.

32. Armstrong MJ, Shulman LM, Vandigo J, Mullins CD. Patient engagement and shared decision-making: What do they look like in neurology practice? *Neurol Clin Pract.* 2016;6(2):190–197. doi: 10.1212/CPJ.0000000000000240.

33. Armstrong MJ. Shared decision-making in stroke: An evolving approach to improved patient care. *Stroke Vasc Neurol.* 2017;2(2):84–87. doi: 10.1136/svn-2017-000081.

34. Kruser JM, Nabozny MJ, Steffens NM, et al. "Best case/worst case": Qualitative evaluation of a novel communication tool for difficult in-the-moment surgical decisions. *J Am Geriatr Soc.* 2015;63(9):1805–1811. doi: 10.1111/jgs.13615.

35. Belagaje SR. Stroke rehabilitation. *Contin Lifelong Learn Neurol.* 2017;23(1):238–253. doi: 10.1212/CON.0000000000000423.

36. Sreekrishnan A, Leasure AC, Shi F-D, et al. Functional improvement among intracerebral hemorrhage (ICH) survivors up to 12 months post-injury. *Neurocrit Care.* 2017;27(3):326–333. doi: 10.1007/s12028-017-0425-4.

37. Rose M, Parks S, Swartz K, Wagner B. Communication with patients with cancer. In: Rose MG, Devita Jr VT, Lawrence TS, Rosenberg SA, eds. *Oncology in Primary Care.* Philadelphia, PA: Lippincott Williams & Wilkins; 2013:197–201.

38. American Academy of Family Physicians. Sample Advance Directive Form. *Am Fam Physician.* 1999;59(3):617–620.

39. Von Gunten CF. Interventions to manage symptoms at the end of life. *J Palliat Med.* 2005;8(Suppl 1):s88–s94. doi: 10.1089/jpm.2005.8.s-88.

40. Singer AE, Meeker D, Teno JM, Lynn J, Lunney JR, Lorenz KA. Symptom trends in the last year of life from 1998 to 2010: A cohort study. *Ann Intern Med.* 2015;162(3):175. doi: 10.7326/M13-1609.

41. The SUPPORT Principle Investigators. A controlled trial to improve care for seriously ill hospitalized patients. The study to understand prognoses and preferences for outcomes and risks of treatments (SUPPORT). The SUPPORT Principal Investigators. *JAMA.* 1995;274(20):1591–1598. doi: 10.1001/jama.274.20.1591.

42. Teno JM, Freedman VA, Kasper JD, Gozalo P, Mor V. Is care for the dying improving in the United States? *J Palliat Med.* 2015;18(8):662–666. doi: 10.1089/jpm.2015.0039.

43. Herr K, Coyne PJ, McCaffery M, Manworren R, Merkel S. Pain assessment in the patient unable to self-report: Position statement with clinical practice recommendations. *Pain Manag Nurs.* 2011;12(4):230–250. doi: 10.1016/j.pmn.2011.10.002.

44. Hanson MM, Swartz K, Worster BK. Palliative and end-of-life care for the elderly. In: Busby-Whitehead J, Arenson C, Durso S, Swagerty D, Mosqueda L, Fiatarone Singh M, eds. *Reichel's Care of the Elderly: Clinical Aspects of Aging.* 7th ed. New York: Cambridge University Press; 2016:671–684. doi: 10.1017/9781107294967.049.

45. Saunders C. A personal therapeutic journey. *BMJ.* 1996;313(7072):1599–1601. doi: 10.1136/bmj.313.7072.1599.

46. McGuire DB, Kaiser KS, Haisfield-Wolfe ME, Iyamu F. Pain assessment in noncommunicative adult palliative care patients. *Nurs Clin North Am.* 2016;51(3):397–431. doi: 10.1016/j.cnur.2016.05.009.

47. Lopez G, Reddy S. Pain assessment and management. In: Yennurajalingam S, Bruera E, eds. *Oxford American Handbook of Hospice and Palliative Medicine.* New York: Oxford University Press; 2011:31–71.

48. Mercadante S, Arcuri E. Opioids and renal function. *J Pain.* 2004;5(1):2–19. doi: 10.1016/j.jpain.2003.09.007.

49. Fallon MT, Cherny NI. Opioid therapy: Optimizing analgesic outcomes. In: Cherny NI, Fallon MT, Kaasa S, Portenoy RK, Currow DC, eds. *Oxford Textbook of Palliative Medicine*. 5th ed. New York: Oxford University Press; 2015:525–559.

50. McPherson M. Transdermal and parenteral fentanyl dosage calculations and conversions. In: McPherson M, ed. *Demystifying Opioid Conversion Calculations: A Guide For Effective Dosing*. 1st ed. Bethesda, MD: American Society of Health-System Pharmacists; 2010:83–106.

51. Frederich ME. Nonpain symptom management. *Prim Care*. 2001;28(2):299–316. doi: 10.1016/S0095-4543(05)70023-3.

52. Miller S, McNutt L, McCann M-A, McCorry N. Use of corticosteroids for anorexia in palliative medicine: A systematic review. *J Palliat Med*. 2014;17(4):482–485. doi: 10.1089/jpm.2013.0324.

53. Segers K, Surquin M. Can mirtazapine counteract the weight loss associated with Alzheimer disease? A retrospective open-label study. *Alzheimer Dis Assoc Disord*. 2014;28(3):291–293. doi: 10.1097/WAD.0b013e3182614f52.

54. Beal JE, Olson R, Laubenstein L, et al. Dronabinol as a treatment for anorexia associated with weight loss in patients with AIDS. *J Pain Symptom Manage*. 1995;10(2):89–97. doi: 10.1016/0885-3924(94)00117-4.

55. Taylor JK, Pendleton N. Progesterone therapy for the treatment of non-cancer cachexia: A systematic review. *BMJ Support Palliat Care*. 2016;6(3):276–286. doi: 10.1136/bmjspcare-2015-001041.

56. Paquereau J, Allart E, Romon M, Rousseaux M. The long-term nutritional status in stroke patients and its predictive factors. *J Stroke Cerebrovasc Dis*. 2014;23(6):1628–1633. doi: 10.1016/j.jstrokecerebrovasdis.2014.01.007.

57. Singh P, Yoon SS, Kuo B. Nausea: A review of pathophysiology and therapeutics. *Therap Adv Gastroenterol*. 2016;9(1):98–112. doi: 10.1177/1756283X15618131.

58. Van Samkar A, Poulsen MNF, Bienfait HP, Van Leeuwen RB. Acute cerebellitis in adults: A case report and review of the literature. *BMC Res Notes*. 2017;10(1):610. doi: 10.1186/s13104-017-2935-8.

59. Williams JR, Venchiarutti RL, Smee R. A prospective patient-focused evaluation of the tolerance and acceptability of a stereotactic radiosurgery procedure. *J Clin Neurosci*. 2017;40:91–96. doi: 10.1016/j.jocn.2017.02.027.

60. Lonjaret L, Guyonnet M, Berard E, et al. Postoperative complications after craniotomy for brain tumor surgery. *Anaesth Crit Care Pain Med*. 2017;36(4):213–218. doi: 10.1016/j.accpm.2016.06.012.

61. Rakel RE, Trinh TH. Care of the dying patient. In: Rakel RE, Rakel D, eds. *Textbook of Family Medicine*. 9th ed.; Philadelphia, PA: Elsevier Saunders 2015:54–72.

62. Stienen MN, Smoll NR, Hildebrandt G, Schaller K, Tessitore E, Gautschi OP. Constipation after thoraco-lumbar fusion surgery. *Clin Neurol Neurosurg*. 2014;126:137–142. doi: 10.1016/j.clineuro.2014.08.036.

63. Engler TMN de M, Aguiar MH de A, Furtado ÍAB, et al. Factors associated with intestinal constipation in chronic patients with stroke sequelae undergoing rehabilitation. *Gastroenterol Nurs*. 2016;39(6):432–442. doi: 10.1097/SGA.0000000000000163.

64. Leclair-Visonneau L, Magy L, Volteau C, et al. Heterogeneous pattern of autonomic dysfunction in Parkinson's disease. *J Neurol*. 2018;265(4):933–941. doi: 10.1007/s00415-018-8789-8.

65. Rodríguez-Violante M, de Saráchaga AJ, Cervantes-Arriaga A, et al. Self-perceived pre-motor symptoms load in patients with Parkinson's disease: A retrospective study. *J Parkinsons Dis*. 2016;6(1):183–190. doi: 10.3233/JPD-150705.

66. Gan J, Wan Y, Shi J, Zhou M, Lou Z, Liu Z. A survey of subjective constipation in Parkinson's disease patients in Shanghai and literature review. *BMC Neurol.* 2018;18(1):29. doi: 10.1186/s12883-018-1034-3.

67. Borasio GD, Miller RG. Clinical characteristics and management of ALS. *Semin Neurol.* 2001;21(02):155–166. doi: 10.1055/s-2001-15268.

68. Tiirola A, Korhonen T, Surakka T, Lehto JT. End-of-life care of patients with amyotrophic lateral sclerosis and other nonmalignant diseases. *Am J Hosp Palliat Med.* 2017;34(2):154–159. doi: 10.1177/1049909115610078.

69. Georges M, Morélot-Panzini C, Similowski T, Gonzalez-Bermejo J. Noninvasive ventilation reduces energy expenditure in amyotrophic lateral sclerosis. *BMC Pulm Med.* 2014;14(1):17. doi: 10.1186/1471-2466-14-17.

70. Piil K, Jakobsen J, Christensen KB, et al. Needs and preferences among patients with high-grade glioma and their caregivers: A longitudinal mixed methods study. *Eur J Cancer Care (Engl).* 2018;27(2):e12806. doi: 10.1111/ecc.12806.

71. Dunn LK, Durieux ME, Fernández LG, et al. Influence of catastrophizing, anxiety, and depression on in-hospital opioid consumption, pain, and quality of recovery after adult spine surgery. *J Neurosurg Spine.* 2018;28(1):119–126. doi: 10.3171/2017.5.SPINE1734.

72. Lim S-W, Shiue Y-L, Ho C-H, et al. Anxiety and depression in patients with traumatic spinal cord injury: A nationwide population-based cohort study. Hu W, ed. *PLoS One.* 2017;12(1):e0169623. doi: 10.1371/journal.pone.0169623.

73. Mameniškienė R, Guk J, Jatužis D. Family and sexual life in people with epilepsy. *Epilepsy Behav.* 2017;66:39–44. doi: 10.1016/j.yebeh.2016.10.012.

74. Rana AQ, Qureshi ARM, Kachhvi HB, Rana MA, Chou KL. Increased likelihood of anxiety and poor sleep quality in Parkinson's disease patients with pain. *J Neurol Sci.* 2016;369:212–215. doi: 10.1016/j.jns.2016.07.064.

75. Brandel MG, Hirshman BR, McCutcheon BA, et al. The association between psychiatric comorbidities and outcomes for inpatients with traumatic brain injury. *J Neurotrauma.* 2017;34(5):1005–1016. doi: 10.1089/neu.2016.4504.

76. Adogwa O, Elsamadicy AA, Cheng J, Bagley C. Pretreatment of anxiety before cervical spine surgery improves clinical outcomes: A prospective, single-institution experience. *World Neurosurg.* 2016;88:625–630. doi: 10.1016/j.wneu.2015.11.014.

77. Kayhan F, Albayrak Gezer İ, Kayhan A, Kitiş S, Gölen M. Mood and anxiety disorders in patients with chronic low back and neck pain caused by disc herniation. *Int J Psychiatry Clin Pract.* 2016;20(1):19–23. doi: 10.3109/13651501.2015.1100314.

78. Piil K, Jakobsen J, Christensen KB, Juhler M, Jarden M. Health-related quality of life in patients with high-grade gliomas: A quantitative longitudinal study. *J Neurooncol.* 2015;124(2):185–195. doi: 10.1007/s11060-015-1821-2.

79. Hyer L, Scott C, Mullen CM, McKenzie LC, Robinson Jr JS. Randomized double-blind placebo trial of duloxetine in perioperative spine patients. *J Opioid Manag.* 2015;11(2):147–155. doi: 10.5055/jom.2015.0264.

80. Agar MR, Lawlor PG, Quinn S, et al. Efficacy of oral risperidone, haloperidol, or placebo for symptoms of delirium among patients in palliative care. *JAMA Intern Med.* 2017;177(1):34–42. doi: 10.1001/jamainternmed.2016.7491.

81. Twaddle ML, Kelley SA. Hospice. In: Berger AM, Shuster JL, Von Roenn JH, eds. *Principles and Practice of Palliative Care and Supportive Oncology.* 4th ed. Philadelphia, PA: Lippincott Williams & Wilkins; 2013:604–612.

82. Saunders C. Introduction: History and challenge. In: Saunders C, Sykes N, eds. *The Management of Terminal Malignant Disease*. 3rd ed. London: Hodder and Stoughton; 1993:1–14.

83. Buss MK, Rock LK, McCarthy EP. Understanding palliative care and hospice. *Mayo Clin Proc*. 2017;92(2):280–286. doi: 10.1016/j.mayocp.2016.11.007.

84. Kelley AS, Morrison RS. Palliative care for the seriously ill. *N Engl J Med*. 2015;373(8):747–755. doi: 10.1056/NEJMra1404684.

85. Aldridge Carlson MD, Twaddle ML. What are the eligibility criteria for hospice? In: Goldstein NE, Morrison RS, eds. *Evidence-Based Practice of Palliative Medicine*. Philadelphia: Elsevier Saunders; 2013:443–447.

86. Harrold JK, von Gunten CF. Hospice approach to palliative care. In: Yennurajalingam S, Bruera E, eds. *Oxford American Handbook of Hospice and Palliative Medicine and Supportive Care*. 2nd ed. New York: Oxford University Press; 2016:231–243.

87. Brumley R, Enguidanos S, Jamison P, et al. Increased satisfaction with care and lower costs: Results of a randomized trial of in-home palliative care. *J Am Geriatr Soc*. 2007;55(7):993–1000. doi: 10.1111/j.1532-5415.2007.01234.x.

88. Obermeyer Z, Makar M, Abujaber S, Dominici F, Block S, Cutler DM. Association between the medicare hospice benefit and health care utilization and costs for patients with poor-prognosis cancer. *JAMA*. 2014;312(18):1888–1896. doi: 10.1001/jama.2014.14950.

89. Gozalo P, Plotzke M, Mor V, Miller SC, Teno JM. Changes in Medicare costs with the growth of hospice care in nursing homes. *N Engl J Med*. 2015;372(19):1823–1831. doi: 10.1056/NEJMsa1408705.

90. Wallston K, Burger C, Smith R, Baugher R. Comparing the quality of death for hospice and non-hospice cancer patients. *Med Care*. 1988;26(2):177–182.

91. Wright AA, Zhang B, Ray A, et al. Associations between end-of-life discussions, patient mental health, medical care near death, and caregiver bereavement adjustment. *JAMA*. 2008;300(14):1665–1673. doi: 10.1001/jama.300.14.1665.

92. Teno JM, R CB, Casey V, et al. Family perspectives on end of life care at the last place of care. *JAMA*. 2004;291(1):88–93.

93. Wright AA, Keating NL, Balboni TA, Matulonis UA, Block SD, Prigerson HG. Place of death: Correlations with quality of life of patients with cancer and predictors of bereaved caregivers' mental health. *J Clin Oncol*. 2010;28(29):4457–4464. doi: 10.1200/JCO.2009.26.3863.

94. Connor SR, Pyenson B, Fitch K, Spence C, Iwasaki K. Comparing hospice and nonhospice patient survival among patients who die within a three-year window. *J Pain Symptom Manage*. 2007;33(3):238–246. doi: 10.1016/j.jpainsymman.2006.10.010.

95. Saito AM, Landrum MB, Neville BA, Ayanian JZ, Weeks JC, Earle CC. Hospice care and survival among elderly patients with lung cancer. *J Palliat Med*. 2011;14(8):929–939. doi: 10.1089/jpm.2010.0522.

96. Christakis NA, Iwashyna TJ. The health impact of health care on families: A matched cohort study of hospice use by decedents and mortality outcomes in surviving, widowed spouses. *Soc Sci Med*. 2003;57(3):465–475. doi: 10.1016/S0277-9536(02)00370-2.

Index

Page numbers followed by *t*, *f*, or *b* denote tables, figures, or boxes respectively.

For the benefit of digital users, indexed terms that span two pages (e.g., 52–53) may, on occasion, appear on only one of those pages.